PET Imaging of Lymphoma

Guest Editors

REBECCA L. ELSTROM, MD
STEPHEN J. SCHUSTER, MD

PET CLINICS

www.pet.theclinics.com

Consulting Editor
ABASS ALAVI, MD, PhD (Hon), DSc (Hon)

January 2012 • Volume 7 • Number 1

SAUNDERS an imprint of ELSEVIER, Inc.

W.B. SAUNDERS COMPANY
A Division of Elsevier Inc.

1600 John F. Kennedy Boulevard • Suite 1800 • Philadelphia, Pennsylvania 19103-2899

http://www.theclinics.com

PET CLINICS Volume 7, Number 1
January 2012 ISSN 1556-8598, ISBN-13: 978-1-4557-3915-8

Editor: Sarah Barth
Developmental Editor: Donald Mumford

PET Clinics (ISSN 1556-8598) is published quarterly by Elsevier Inc., 360 Park Avenue South, New York, NY 10010-1710. Months of issue are January, April, July, and October. Periodicals postage paid at New York, NY, and additional mailing offices. Subscription prices per year are $215.00 (US individuals), $297.00 (US institutions), $110.00 (US students), $244.00 (Canadian individuals), $332.00 (Canadian institutions), $124.00 (Canadian students), $260.00 (foreign individuals), $332.00 (foreign institutions), and $134.00 (foreign students). To receive student and resident rate, orders must be accompanied by name of affiliated institution, date of term, and the signature of program/residency coordinator on institution letterhead. Orders will be billed at individual rate until proof of status is received. Foreign air speed delivery is included in all Clinics subscription prices. All prices are subject to change without notice. POSTMASTER: Send address changes to PET Clinics, Elsevier Health Sciences Division, Subscription Customer Service, 3251 Riverport Lane, Maryland Heights, MO 63043. **Customer Service: 1-800-654-2452 (U.S. and Canada); 314-447-8871 (outside U.S. and Canada). Fax: 314-447-8029. E-mail: journalscustomerservice-usa@elsevier.com (for print support); journalsonlinesupport-usa@elsevier.com (for online support).**

Reprints. For copies of 100 or more of articles in this publication, please contact the Commercial Reprints Department, Elsevier Inc., 360 Park Avenue South, New York, NY 10010-1710. Tel.: 212-633-3812; Fax: 212-462-1935; E-mail: reprints@elsevier.com.

Printed and bound by CPI Group (UK) Ltd, Croydon, CR0 4YY

Transferred to Digital Print 2012

Contributors

CONSULTING EDITOR

ABASS ALAVI, MD, PhD (Hon), DSc (Hon)
Professor of Radiology, Division of Nuclear
Medicine, University of Pennsylvania School
of Medicine, Philadelphia, Pennsylvania

GUEST EDITORS

REBECCA L. ELSTROM, MD
Assistant Professor, Division of Hematology/
Oncology, Department of Internal Medicine,
Weill Medical College, Cornell University,
New York, New York

STEPHEN J. SCHUSTER, MD
Robert and Margarita Louis-Dreyfus Associate
Professor in Chronic Lymphocytic Leukemia
and Lymphoma Clinical Care and Research
Attending Physician, Department of Medicine,
Division of Hematology-Oncology, Hospital of
the University of Pennsylvania; Director,
Lymphoma Program, Abramson Cancer
Center of the University of Pennsylvania
Director, Lymphoma Translational Research,
Abramson Cancer Center of the University of
Pennsylvania School of Medicine, Philadelphia,
Pennsylvania

AUTHORS

SCOTT R. AKERS, MD, PhD
Department of Radiology, Philadelphia VA
Medical Center, Philadelphia, Pennsylvania

ABASS ALAVI, MD, PhD (Hon), DSc (Hon)
Professor of Radiology, Division of Nuclear
Medicine, University of Pennsylvania School
of Medicine, Philadelphia, Pennsylvania

FERNANDO ARIAS-MENDOZA, MD, PhD
Senior Research Associate, Department of
Radiology and Hatch Imaging Center,
Columbia University College of Physicians
and Surgeons, New York, New York

SANDIP BASU, MBBS (Hons), DRM, DNB
Radiation Medicine Center (Bhabha Atomic
Research Center), Tata Memorial Center
Annexe, Mumbai, Maharashtra, India; Division
of Nuclear Medicine, Department of Radiology,
Hospital of the University of Pennsylvania,
Philadelphia, Pennsylvania

JULIANO JULIO CERCI, MD, PhD
Quanta – Diagnóstico e Terapia, Curitiba; Heart
Institute (InCor), University of São Paulo
Medical School, São Paulo, Brazil

GANG CHENG, MD, PhD
Department of Radiology, Philadelphia VA
Medical Center, Philadelphia, Pennsylvania

SO HYUN CHUNG, PhD
Postdoctoral Researcher, Department
of Physics and Astronomy, University
of Pennsylvania, Philadelphia, Pennsylvania

E. JAMES DELIKATNY, PhD
Research Associate Professor, Laboratory of
Molecular Imaging, Department of Radiology,
The University of Pennsylvania School of
Medicine, Philadelphia, Pennsylvania

STEFANO FANTI, MD, PhD
Policlinico S. Orsola, University of Bologna,
Bologna, Italy

GEOFFREY GEIGER, MD
Department of Radiation Oncology, Perelman
Center for Advanced Medicine, Philadelphia,
Pennsylvania

ELI GLATSTEIN, MD
Professor and Vice Chairman, Department
of Radiation Oncology, Perelman Center for
Advanced Medicine, Philadelphia,
Pennsylvania

JERRY D. GLICKSON, PhD
Professor of Radiology and Director
of Molecular Imaging, Laboratory of Molecular
Imaging, Department of Radiology,
University of Pennsylvania, Philadelphia,
Pennsylvania

ANDRE GOY, MD, MS
John Theurer Cancer Center at Hackensack
University Medical Center, Hackensack,
New Jersey

LALE KOSTAKOGLU, MD, MPH
Professor of Radiology, Director, PET/CT
Oncology and Research, Division of Nuclear
Medicine, Department of Radiology,
Mount Sinai School of Medicine, New York,
New York

THOMAS C. KWEE, MD, PhD
Department of Radiology, University Medical
Center Utrecht, Utrecht, The Netherlands

SEUNG-CHEOL LEE
Laboratory of Molecular Imaging, Department
of Radiology, The University of Pennsylvania
School of Medicine, Philadelphia, Pennsylvania

MICHAL MARZEC, MD, PhD
Associate Fellow, Department of Pathology
and Laboratory Medicine, The University of
Pennsylvania School of Medicine, Philadelphia,
Pennsylvania

ANTHONY R. MATO, MD, MSCE
John Theurer Cancer Center at Hackensack
University Medical Center, Hackensack,
New Jersey

JOSÉ C. MENEGHETTI, MD, PhD
Heart Institute (InCor), University of São Paulo
Medical School, São Paulo, Brazil

SUNITA D. NASTA, MD
Assistant Professor of Clinical Medicine;
Attending Physician, Hematology-Oncology,
Department of Medicine, Hospital of The
University of Pennsylvania School of Medicine,
Philadelphia, Pennsylvania

RUTGER A.J. NIEVELSTEIN, MD, PhD
Department of Radiology, University Medical
Center Utrecht, Utrecht, The Netherlands

OWEN A. O'CONNOR, MD, PhD
Associate Professor of Medicine, Department
of Hematology/Oncology, Columbia University
Medical Center, New York, New York

RODOLFO PERINI, MD
Clinical Instructor, Division of Nuclear Medicine
and Molecular Imaging, Department of
Radiology; Division of Hematology and
Oncology, Department of Medicine, University
of Pennsylvania, Philadelphia, Pennsylvania

JOHN P. PLASTARAS, MD, PhD
Assistant Professor, Director of Clinical
Research, Department of Radiation Oncology,
Perelman Center for Advanced Medicine,
University of Pennsylvania, Philadelphia,
Pennsylvania

HARISH POPTANI, PhD
Research Associate Professor, Laboratory
of Molecular Imaging, Department of
Radiology, The University of Pennsylvania
School of Medicine, Philadelphia, Pennsylvania

STEPHEN J. SCHUSTER, MD
Robert and Margarita Louis-Dreyfus Associate
Professor in Chronic Lymphocytic Leukemia
and Lymphoma Clinical Care and Research
Attending Physician, Department of Medicine,
Division of Hematology-Oncology, Hospital of
the University of Pennsylvania; Director,
Lymphoma Program, Abramson Cancer
Center of the University of Pennsylvania
Director, Lymphoma Translational Research,
Abramson Cancer Center of the University of
Pennsylvania School of Medicine, Philadelphia,
Pennsylvania

MITCHELL R. SMITH, MD, PhD
Director, Lymphoma Service, Fox Chase
Cancer Center, Philadelphia, Pennsylvania

JAKUB SVOBODA, MD
Division of Hematology-Oncology, Department
of Medicine, The University of Pennsylvania
School of Medicine, Philadelphia,
Pennsylvania

DREW A. TORIGIAN, MD, MA
Department of Radiology, Hospital of the
University of Pennsylvania, Philadelphia,
Pennsylvania

MARIUSZ WASIK, MD
Associate Professor; Director of Experimental
Hematology and Associate Director of
Hematology Laboratory, Department of
Pathology and Laboratory Medicine, The
University of Pennsylvania School of Medicine,
Philadelphia, Pennsylvania

LUCIA ZANONI, MD
Policlinico S. Orsola, University of Bologna,
Bologna, Italy

HONGMING ZHUANG, MD, PhD
Department of Radiology, Children's Hospital
of Philadelphia, Philadelphia, Pennsylvania

Contents

Preface xiii

Rebecca L. Elstrom and Stephen J. Schuster

Role of Structural Imaging in Lymphoma 1

Thomas C. Kwee, Rutger A.J. Nievelstein, and Drew A. Torigian

The lymphomas, Hodgkin lymphoma and non-Hodgkin lymphoma, are among the most common types of cancer in the United States. Imaging plays an important role in the evaluation of patients with lymphoma, because it aids in treatment planning and in the determination of prognosis. Structural imaging entails the assessment of morphologic features of normal tissues and organs of the body and of malignant lesions within these structures, and plays a major role in the noninvasive assessment of lymphoma. This article reviews cross-sectional structural imaging modalities with an emphasis on computed tomography and magnetic resonance imaging, with some mention of ultrasonography.

FDG-PET in Lymphoma: Nuclear Medicine Perspective 21

Juliano Julio Cerci, Lucia Zanoni, José C. Meneghetti, and Stefano Fanti

Positron emission tomography (PET) is a sectional molecular imaging procedure that allows evaluation of the metabolism at a molecular and cellular level. For a PET scan, the patient is injected with a radiotracer, such as ^{18}F-fluorodeoxyglucose (FDG). FDG PET–computed tomography has become an established modality for metabolic staging and plays an important role in the major steps of evaluation and treatment of most lymphoma subtypes, with significant impact in the initial staging, posttherapy evaluation, and suspect of relapse of disease. However, whenever the information of PET results is translated to changing treatment, especially in cases of further treatment, biopsy confirmation should always be made when possible.

**The Evolving Role of Medical Imaging in Lymphoma Management:
The Clinician's Perspective** 35

Jakub Svoboda and Stephen J. Schuster

Hodgkin and non-Hodgkin lymphomas are a heterogeneous group of hematologic neoplasms which arise from malignant lymphocytes. Imaging plays an important role in management of lymphoma patients during diagnosis, staging, and response assessment. Functional imaging may also provide prognostic information and improve the ability to detect extranodal disease. This article provides an overview of the evolving role of various imaging techniques in lymphoma from the clinician's perspective. It serves as an introduction to the other articles in this issue that focus on specific areas of lymphoma imaging.

**Review of Clinical Applications of Fluorodeoxyglucose-PET/Computed Tomography
in Pediatric Patients with Lymphoma** 47

Gang Cheng, Scott R. Akers, Hongming Zhuang, and Abass Alavi

[^{18}F]fluorodeoxyglucose (FDG) positron emission tomography (PET)/computed tomography (CT) imaging is routinely used in the initial diagnosis and response assessment during and immediately after therapy, as well as in the follow-up surveillance. FDG PET/CT outperforms diagnostic CT and other conventional imaging modalities in the evaluation of pediatric patients with lymphoma, with higher sensitivity and specificity, leading to more accurate staging/restaging and modifications of therapeutic strategies. Resolution of FDG-avid lesions in the early post-therapy phase often indicates good response to treatment and better prognosis. FDG PET/CT also outperforms bone marrow biopsy in detecting bone marrow infiltration of lymphoma.

Role of Positron Emission Tomography with Fludeoxyglucose F 18 in Personalization
of Therapy in Patients with Lymphoma   57
Anthony R. Mato and Andre Goy

The widespread availability of functional imaging in clinical practice has revolutionized the care (staging, response assessment, surveillance) of patients with lymphoma. Using positron emission tomography/computed tomography (PET/CT) with fludeoxyglucose F 18 (FDG), the potential exists for prognostic risk stratification and therapeutic adjustment. This review focuses on personalization of therapy using these 2 modalities in 2 lymphoma subtypes: diffuse large B-cell lymphoma and Hodgkin lymphoma.

The Use of PET in Radiation Therapy for Lymphoma   67
John P. Plastaras, Geoffrey Geiger, Rodolfo Perini, and Eli Glatstein

Positron emission tomography (PET) with 18-fluorodeoxyglucose (FDG) and computed tomography (CT) has essentially replaced CT alone for staging of lymphomas. FDG-PET has been incorporated into the revised response criteria, but response adapted strategies are still being evaluated. The role of FDG-PET/CT in radiation treatment planning is still being developed. It is unclear how to use FDG-PET/CT to determine whether to give consolidative radiation, where to radiate, and what dose. Ongoing efforts are underway to use early interim FDG-PET/CT to limit therapy in good prognosis patients. A multidisciplinary team is important in the management of patients with lymphoma, leading to individualized treatment plans and better outcomes.

Evolving Importance of Diffusion-Weighted Magnetic Resonance Imaging in Lymphoma   73
Thomas C. Kwee, Sandip Basu, Drew A. Torigian, Rutger A.J. Nievelstein, and Abass Alavi

Diffusion-weighted magnetic resonance imaging (DWI) is a rapidly evolving functional imaging modality that can now be used for the evaluation of lymphomatous lesions throughout the body. This article describes the basics of (whole-body) DWI, and reviews and discusses the evolving importance of whole-body DWI for the staging and therapy response assessment of lymphoma.

Novel PET Radiotracers for Potential Use in Management of Lymphoma   83
Lale Kostakoglu

This article discusses possible roles for emerging novel positron emission tomography (PET) radiotracers for diagnosis and follow-up of lymphomas. Novel imaging probes are being developed to fulfill the need of a more specific radiopharmaceutical to target subcomponents of tumor microenvironment to individualize management approaches. Noninvasive molecular imaging probes are being developed to revolutionize characterization of tumor biology and response to therapy in more specific ways for the host, tumor microenvironment, and therapeutic regimens. The new clinical PET probes seem promising in fostering clinical gains that would lead to better survival outcomes, although further studies are warranted to prove a role in the management of lymphomas.

Prediction and Early Detection of Response by NMR Spectroscopy and Imaging   119

Seung-Cheol Lee, Fernando Arias-Mendoza, Harish Poptani, E. James Delikatny, Mariusz Wasik, Michal Marzec, Stephen J. Schuster, Sunita D. Nasta, Jakub Svoboda, Owen A. O'Connor, Mitchell R. Smith, and Jerry D. Glickson

Pretreatment ^{31}P magnetic resonance (MRS) when applied to a cadre of 41 non-Hodgkin's lymphoma (NHL) regardless of disease type or stage and regardless of therapeutic regimen, was able to predict about two thirds of the patients that exhibited a complete response (CR; sensitivity 0.92, specificity 0.79). However, when the study was restricted to 27 NHL patients with the most common form of NHL, diffuse large B-cell lymphoma, all of whom were treated with RCHOP (rituximab plus CHOP chemotherapy) or "RCHOP-like" therapy, was able to predict CR and non-CR with a sensitivity of 1.0 and specificity of 0.90 by Fisher analysis). Patients predicted not to exhibit a CR could be directed to more vigorous therapeutic regimens followed by bone marrow transplantation or to experimental new therapeutic agents. This article highlights a general strategy for non-invasively monitoring response to inhibitors of specific signal transduction pathways by monitoring the corresponding metabolic pathway that is modified by signal transduction inhibition.

Diffuse Optical Technology: A Portable and Simple Method for Noninvasive Tissue Pathophysiology   127

So Hyun Chung

Noninvasive diffuse optical technologies are introduced for the future application for lymphoma diagnosis/treatment monitoring. Diffuse optical technologies measure tumor physiology in deep tissues in vivo, and demonstrate efficacy for tumor detection and chemotherapy response monitoring. Light has been used to see tumors in thick human tissues for several decades. Based on the idea that the interaction between the light and tumor provides its pathology related information, biomedical optics technology has advanced to be more quantitative and more accurate so that it can be used for tumor diagnosis and treatment monitoring.

Index   133

PET Clinics

FORTHCOMING ISSUES

April 2012

PET Imaging of Infection and Inflammation
Hongming Zhuang, MD, PhD, and
Abass Alavi, MD, *Guest Editors*

July 2012

Clinical Utility of NaF in Benign and Malignant Disorders
Mohsen Beheshti, MD, FASNC, FEBNM,
Guest Editor

RECENT ISSUES

October 2011

Cardiac PET Imaging
Wengen Chen, MD, PhD, and
Amol M. Takalkar, MD, MS, *Guest Editors*

July 2011

PET Imaging of Thoracic Disease
Drew A. Torigian, MD, and Abass Alavi, MD,
Guest Editors

THE CLINICS ARE NOW AVAILABLE ONLINE!

Access your subscription at:
www.theclinics.com

GOAL STATEMENT

The goal of the *PET Clinics* is to keep practicing radiologists and radiology residents up to date with current clinical practice in positron emission tomography by providing timely articles reviewing the state of the art in patient care.

ACCREDITATION

PET Clinics is planned and implemented in accordance with the Essential Areas and Policies of the Accreditation Council for Continuing Medical Education (ACCME) through the joint sponsorship of the University of Virginia School of Medicine and Elsevier. The University of Virginia School of Medicine is accredited by the ACCME to provide continuing medical education for physicians.

The University of Virginia School of Medicine designates this enduring material activity for a maximum of 15 *AMA PRA Category 1 Credit*(s)™ *for each issue*, 60 credits per year. Physicians should only claim credit commensurate with the extent of their participation in the activity.

The American Medical Association has determined that physicians not licensed in the US who participate in this CME enduring material activity are eligible for a maximum of 15 *AMA PRA Category 1 Credit*(s)™ for each issue, 60 credits per year.

Credit can be earned by reading the text material, taking the CME examination online at http://www.theclinics.com/home/cme, and completing the evaluation. After taking the test, you will be required to review any and all incorrect answers. Following completion of the test and evaluation, your credit will be awarded and you may print your certificate.

FACULTY DISCLOSURE/CONFLICT OF INTEREST

The University of Virginia School of Medicine, as an ACCME accredited provider, endorses and strives to comply with the Accreditation Council for Continuing Medical Education (ACCME) Standards of Commercial Support, Commonwealth of Virginia statutes, University of Virginia policies and procedures, and associated federal and private regulations and guidelines on the need for disclosure and monitoring of proprietary and financial interests that may affect the scientific integrity and balance of content delivered in continuing medical education activities under our auspices.

The University of Virginia School of Medicine requires that all CME activities accredited through this institution be developed independently and be scientifically rigorous, balanced and objective in the presentation/discussion of its content, theories and practices.

All authors/editors participating in an accredited CME activity are expected to disclose to the readers relevant financial relationships with commercial entities occurring within the past 12 months (such as grants or research support, employee, consultant, stock holder, member of speakers bureau, etc.). The University of Virginia School of Medicine will employ appropriate mechanisms to resolve potential conflicts of interest to maintain the standards of fair and balanced education to the reader. Questions about specific strategies can be directed to the Office of Continuing Medical Education, University of Virginia School of Medicine, Charlottesville, Virginia.

The faculty and staff of the University of Virginia Office of Continuing Medical Education have no financial affiliations to disclose.

The authors/editors listed below have identified no professional or financial affiliations for themselves or their spouse/ partner:

Scott R. Akers, MD, PhD; Abass Alavi, MD, PhD (Hon), DSc (Hon) (Consulting Editor); Fernando Arias-Mendoza, MD, PhD; Sarah Barth, (Acquisitions Editor); Sandip Basu, MBBS (Hons), DRM, DNB; Juliano Julio Cerci, MD, PhD; Gang Cheng, MD, PhD; So Hyun Chung, PhD; E. James Delikatny, PhD; Rebecca Elstrom, MD (Guest Editor); Stefano Fanti, MD, PhD; Geoffrey Geiger, MD; Eli Glatstein, MD; Jerry D. Glickson, PhD; Andre Goy, MD, MS; Lale Kostakoglu, MD, MPH; Thomas C. Kwee, MD, PhD; Seung-Cheol Lee, PhD; Michal Marzec, MD; José C. Meneghetti, MD, PhD; Sunita D. Nasta, MD; Rutger A.J. Nievelstein, MD, PhD; Rodolfo Perini, MD; John P. Plastaras, MD, PhD; Patrice Rehm, MD (Test Editor); Jakub Svoboda, MD; Mariusz Wasik, MD; Lucia Zanoni, MD; and Hongming Zhuang, MD, PhD.

The authors/editors listed below identified the following professional or financial affiliations for themselves or their spouse/partner:

Anthony R. Mato, MD, MSCE is a consultant for Celgene, Genentech, and Millenium.

Owen A. O'Connor, MD, PhD is an industry funded research/investigator, and is a consultant and on the Advisory Board, for Seattle Genetic and Allos Pharmaceuticals; is an industry funded research/investigator and on the Advisory Board for Millennium; and is an industry funded research/investigator for Merck.

Harish Poptani, PhD is a consultant for the American College of Radiology Image Metrix.

Stephen J. Schuster, MD (Guest Editor) is an industry funded research/investigator for Celgene Corp., GlaxoSmithKline, and Gilead Sciences, Inc.

Mitchell R. Smith, MD, PhD is on the Speakers' Bureau for Cephalon/TEVA, Genentech, Allos, and Seattle Genetics, is an industry funded research/investigator for Seattle Genetics, and is on the Advisory Board for Cephalon/TEVA.

Drew A. Torigian, MD, MA is an industry funded research/investigator for Pfizer, Inc.

Disclosure of Discussion of Non-FDA Approved Uses for Pharmaceutical Products and/or Medical Devices

The University of Virginia School of Medicine, as an ACCME provider, requires that all faculty presenters identify and disclose any off-label uses for pharmaceutical and medical device products. The University of Virginia School of Medicine recommends that each physician fully review all the available data on new products or procedures prior to clinical use.

TO ENROLL

To enroll in the PET Clinics Continuing Medical Education program, call customer service at 1-800-654-2452 or visit us online at www.theclinics.com/home/cme. The CME program is available to subscribers for an additional fee of $196.00.

Preface
PET Imaging of Lymphoma

Structural imaging techniques have become essential to the management of patients with lymphomas. While these modalities, mostly CT scanning, have served as the standard approach for staging, response assessment, and follow-up, functional imaging with FDG-PET has emerged over the last decade as a complementary tool that can enhance detection and guide clinical care of patients with specific lymphomas. FDG-PET, particularly in combination with CT as the standard of care in most centers, has improved the ability to detect lymphomas at specific extranodal sites not visualized by CT (eg, bone marrow, liver) and in lymph nodes that appear normal by size criteria. However, other potential applications of FDG-PET, such as interim response assessment (evaluation early in a specific treatment course intended to determine the ultimate outcome with respect to a complete course of that treatment) and surveillance following achievement of a complete remission, are somewhat controversial at this time. In addition, many new imaging modalities, both structural and molecular, with potential utility in the care of patients with lymphoma, are under investigation.

In this issue of *PET Clinics*, these topics are addressed in great detail by a variety of renowned investigators from diverse specialties and viewpoints. The current standards of structural imaging, including not only CT scanning but also ultrasound and advanced MRI technology, are reviewed in the article by Kwee and colleagues. The current role of FDG-PET in standard care of patients with lymphomas is addressed from both the radiologist's and the clinician's perspectives in articles by Cerci and colleagues and by Svoboda and Schuster. Cheng and colleagues specifically address pediatric patients and Mato and Goy review the potential to personalize therapy based on FDG-PET imaging. Plastaras and colleagues discuss the role of FDG-PET imaging specifically for optimization of radiation therapy.

In addition to these more well-established and commonly used imaging techniques, new imaging modalities that may improve assessment of disease state in a variety of settings are under investigation. Kwee and colleagues review the evolving role of diffusion MRI in the imaging of lymphoma. Kostakoglu provides a comprehensive review of the state of novel PET tracers in oncology, such as compounds for imaging proliferation, apoptosis, and hypoxia, and examines how these agents could be useful in the care of patients with lymphoma. Lee and colleagues review their experience using NMR spectroscopy in evaluating the metabolic profile of lymphoma at baseline, which may be predictive of responsiveness to therapy, and changes in that profile in response to therapeutic agents. These changes may provide insight into the mechanisms by which specific targeted agents exert their effects on cells. Finally, Chung discusses the potential applications of diffuse optical spectroscopy in the assessment of tumor pathophysiology, tumor targeting by therapeutic agents, and response to treatment in a noninvasive, office-based setting.

These articles provide a comprehensive overview of the current state of structural and molecular imaging in lymphoma and provide exciting prospects for future developments in this discipline.

Rebecca L. Elstrom, MD
Division of Hematology/Oncology
Department of Internal Medicine
Weill Medical College
Cornell University
New York, NY 10065, USA

Stephen J. Schuster, MD
Division of Hematology/Oncology
Department of Medicine
The University of Pennsylvania School of Medicine
Philadelphia, PA 19104, USA

E-mail addresses:
ree2001@med.cornell.edu (R.L. Elstrom)
Stephen.Schuster@uphs.upenn.edu
(S.J. Schuster)

PET Clin 7 (2012) xiii
doi:10.1016/j.cpet.2012.01.001
1556-8598/12/$ – see front matter © 2012 Elsevier Inc. All rights reserved.

Role of Structural Imaging in Lymphoma

Thomas C. Kwee, MD, PhD[a],
Rutger A.J. Nievelstein, MD, PhD[a],
Drew A. Torigian, MD, MA[b],*

KEYWORDS

- Structural imaging • CT • MR imaging • Ultrasonography
- Lymphoma • Hodgkin • Non-Hodgkin

STAGING AND RESPONSE ASSESSMENT IN LYMPHOMA

The lymphomas, Hodgkin lymphoma (HL) and non-Hodgkin lymphoma (NHL), comprise approximately 5% to 6% of all malignancies, and are the fifth most frequently occurring type of cancer in the United States.[1] Annually, in the United States, approximately 8490 new cases of HL and 65,540 new cases of NHL are diagnosed, and an estimated number of 1320 patients with HL and 20,120 patients with NHL die because of their disease.[1] Once a lymphoma has been diagnosed histologically (frequently by means of excisional biopsy), extent of disease has to be assessed (ie, staging), because this allows appropriate treatment planning, aids in the determination of prognosis, and knowledge of all sites of involvement permits monitoring of the effects of therapy.[2,3] In HL, the extent of disease directly influences choice of the most appropriate therapy, whereas in NHL, therapy is influenced more by the pathologic subtype of tumor bulk of disease and symptoms. In both HL and NHL, assessment of disease bulk provides important prognostic information, as does the presence of extranodal disease. In NHL in particular, staging provides a baseline assessment against which future imaging studies can be compared.[4] Lymphomas are staged using the Ann Arbor staging system (**Table 1**).[2,3] However, pediatric NHLs are staged using the St Jude staging system described by Murphy, which takes into account the more frequent presence of extranodal disease (with frequent involvement of the gastrointestinal tract, solid abdominal viscera, and sites in the head and neck) in this condition (**Table 2**).[4–6] The revised International Working Group response criteria are used to assess therapeutic response (**Table 3**).[7,8]

GROWTH AND DISTRIBUTION PATTERNS OF HL AND NHL

Lymphomas tend to form conglomerate masses and show expansive growth, but generally respect organ boundaries and compartments (unlike other solid tumors and their metastases). An important difference between HL and NHL is that spread of disease in HL tends to be contiguous via the lymphatics from 1 nodal group to the next, whereas spread in NHL is hematogenous and, therefore, often discontiguous.[4,9]

Table 4 lists the differences in distribution patterns that may differentiate HL from NHL. In general, NHL tends to have a generalized distribution, whereas HL is often localized.[4,9] Primary lymphomas of the internal organs are rare, and most are NHLs. Secondary involvement is more common; it is characteristic of higher disease stages, which usually are generalized. The incidence of organ involvement is also increased in lymphomas associated with immunosuppression in patients after organ transplantation.[4,9]

[a] Department of Radiology, University Medical Center Utrecht, Heidelberglaan 100, 3584 CX Utrecht, The Netherlands
[b] Department of Radiology, Hospital of the University of Pennsylvania, 3400 Spruce Street, Philadelphia, PA 19102, USA
* Corresponding author.
E-mail address: Drew.Torigian@uphs.upenn.edu

PET Clin 7 (2012) 1–19
doi:10.1016/j.cpet.2011.11.002

Table 1
Ann Arbor staging classification of lymphoma

Stage	Involvement
I	Single lymphatic region (I) or 1 extralymphatic site (IE)
II	Two or more lymph node regions on same side of diaphragm (II) or 1 localized extralymphatic site plus 1 or more lymph node regions on same side of the diaphragm (IIE)
III	Lymph node regions on both sides of diaphragm (III), which may be accompanied by extralymphatic extension (IIIE), splenic involvement (IIIS), or both (IIIE,S)
IV	Diffuse involvement of 1 or more extralymphatic organs or sites

Suffix	Features
A	No B symptoms
B	Presence of at least one of the following: unexplained weight loss >10% of usual body weight in 6 months before diagnosis; unexplained fever >38°C; drenching night sweats
X	Bulky tumor is defined as either a single mass of tumor tissue exceeding 10 cm in largest diameter or a mediastinal mass with size greater than or equal to one-third of the maximum intrathoracic diameter measured on a standard posterior-anterior chest radiograph

Data from Armitage JO. Staging non-Hodgkin lymphoma. CA Cancer J Clin 2005;55(6):368–76; and Connors JM. State-of-the-art therapeutics: Hodgkin's lymphoma. J Clin Oncol 2005;23(26):6400–8.

ROLE OF CROSS-SECTIONAL STRUCTURAL IMAGING IN LYMPHOMA

Cross-sectional imaging plays a crucial role in staging and follow-up of lymphoma, because it provides a noninvasive means to evaluate lymphomatous lesions throughout the body. Imaging technologies used to assess patients with cancer, including lymphoma, may be grossly subdivided into structural and functional imaging categories. Structural imaging entails the assessment of morphologic features of normal tissues and organs of the body and of malignant lesions within these structures. Functional imaging comprises a multitude of quantitative imaging techniques that can be used to study tumor physiology, to probe tumor molecular processes, and to study tumor molecules and metabolites in vitro and in vivo.[10] Computed tomography (CT), magnetic resonance (MR) imaging, and ultrasonography (US) are the prototypical imaging technologies that are used to perform oncological structural imaging. These technologies can be used to assess the morphologic features of lesions and of changes in these features over time through use of serial imaging.[10]

Table 2
St Jude staging system described by Murphy for pediatric NHL

Stage	Involvement
I	Single tumor (extranodal) or single anatomic area (nodal) outside mediastinum or abdomen
II	Single tumor (extranodal) with regional nodal involvement OR Two or more nodal areas, same side of diaphragm OR Two single extranodal sites, same side of diaphragm OR Primary gastrointestinal tract tumor, completely resectable
III	Two single tumors (extranodal) on opposite sides of diaphragm OR Two or more nodal areas above and below diaphragm OR All primary intrathoracic tumors OR All extensive primary intra-abdominal disease, incompletely resectable OR All paraspinal or epidural tumors
IV	Any of the above with initial central nervous system or bone marrow involvement

Data from Murphy SB. Classification, staging and end results of treatment of childhood non-Hodgkin's lymphomas: dissimilarities from lymphomas in adults. Semin Oncol 1980;7(3):332–9; and Murphy SB, Fairclough DL, Hutchison RE, et al. Non-Hodgkin's lymphomas of childhood: an analysis of the histology, staging, and response to treatment of 338 cases at a single institution. J Clin Oncol 1989;7(2):186–93.

Table 3
Revised International Working Group response criteria for clinical trials in lymphoma

Response	Definition	Nodal Masses	Spleen, Liver	Bone Marrow
Complete remission (CR)	Disappearance of all evidence of disease	a. FDG avid or PET positive before therapy; mass of any size permitted if PET negative b. Variably FDG avid or PET negative; regression to normal size on CT	Not palpable, nodules disappeared	Infiltrate cleared on repeat biopsy; if indeterminate by morphology, immunohistochemistry should be negative
Partial remission (PR)	Regression of measurable disease and no new sites	≥50% decrease in sum of the product of the diameters (SPD) of up to 6 largest dominant masses; no increase in size of other nodes a. FDG avid or PET positive before therapy; 1 or more PET positive at previously involved site b. Variably FDG avid or PET negative; regression on CT	≥50% decrease in SPD of nodules (for single nodule in greatest transverse diameter); no increase in size of liver or spleen	Irrelevant if positive before therapy; cell type should be specified
Stable disease	Failure to attain CR/PR or progressive disease (PD)	a. FDG avid or PET positive before therapy; PET positive at prior sites of disease and no new sites on CT or PET b. Variably FDG avid or PET negative; no change in size of previous lesions on CT	–	–
Relapsed disease or PD	Any new lesion or increase by ≥50% of previously involved sites from nadir	Appearance of a new lesion(s) >1.5 cm in any axis, ≥50% increase in longest diameter of a previously identified node >1 cm in short axis or in SPD of more than 1 node Lesions PET positive if FDG avid lymphoma or PET positive before therapy	>50% increase from nadir in SPD of any previous lesions	New or recurrent involvement

Data from Cheson BD, Pfistner B, Juweid ME, et al. International Harmonization Project on Lymphoma. Revised response criteria for malignant lymphoma. J Clin Oncol 2007;25(5):579–86; and Seam P, Juweid ME, Cheson BD. The role of FDG-PET scans in patients with lymphoma. Blood 2007;110(10):3507–16.

Table 4
Differences between HL and NHL

Involvement	HL (%)	NHL (%)
Mediastinum	85	<50
Lung parenchyma	15	5
Para-aortic lymph nodes	25	50
Mesenteric lymph nodes	5	50
Liver	10	15
Diffuse liver involvement	+	+
Nodular liver involvement	–	+
Liver involvement with hepatomegaly	<30	60
Spleen	<40	>40
Gastrointestinal tract	–	+
Kidney	–	+
Adrenal gland	–	+

Abbreviations: –, less common; +, more common.

Data from Van der Molen AJ, Schaefer-Prokop C, Leppert A. Lymphatic system. In: Prokop M, Galanski M, editors. Spiral and multislice computed tomography of the body. New York: Georg Thieme Verlag; 2003. p. 755–7.

Accurate detection and delineation of disease also enable radiotherapy planning for localized lymphoma. Furthermore, structural imaging may identify relevant space-occupying consequences of cancer such as spinal cord compression, bone lesions at risk of fracture, and vascular, biliary, or ureteral obstruction (**Fig. 1**). Structural imaging is complementary to functional imaging. An example of a functional imaging method that currently plays a central role in the evaluation of lymphoma is positron emission tomography (PET) using the radiotracer [^{18}F]-2-fluoro-2-deoxy-D-glucose (FDG).[7,11] Correlative structural imaging is used to improve the anatomic localization, segmentation, and quantification of areas with abnormal

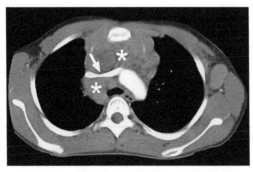

Fig. 1. Axial contrast-enhanced CT image in patient with HL shows large mediastinal mass (*asterisks*) compressing left brachiocephalic vein (*arrow*).

FDG uptake. The aim of this article is to review cross-sectional structural imaging modalities with an emphasis on CT and MR imaging, with some mention of US, because these are most often used in lymphoma.

CROSS-SECTIONAL STRUCTURAL IMAGING MODALITIES IN LYMPHOMA: GENERAL CONSIDERATIONS
CT

Before the CT era, patients with a diagnosis of lymphoma were subjected to a battery of radiologic studies that included chest radiography, intravenous pyelography, lymphangiography, skeletal surveys, and isotope scans. In addition, most patients with HD underwent staging laparotomy, with its attendant risks.[12] The introduction of CT in the early 1970s was a breakthrough, and its potential for evaluating lymphoma was soon recognized and investigated.[13] Since then, CT has gradually become the imaging modality of choice for staging lymphoma. CT technology has continuously been developed and refined; major milestones include the introduction of spiral CT in the early 1990s, the advent of multidetector row CT in 1998, and the more recent development of dual-source and dual-energy CT systems. Using state-of-the-art CT technology (ie, ≥16-detector row CT), a volumetric whole-body CT scan can be obtained within a few seconds, allowing for the detection of lymph nodes of 5 mm or less throughout the body. In combination with powered injectors for rapid bolus administration of intravenous contrast medium, focal extranodal lesions on the order of a few millimeters can be identified.[4,14] CT is currently the mainstay for the structural imaging evaluation of lymphoma, particularly in combination with FDG-PET using integrated PET/CT systems. An important disadvantage of CT is the use of ionizing radiation, which may be associated with induction of second cancers in later life.[15] This health risk caused by ionizing radiation is especially of concern in children, because they have a higher radiosensitivity than adults and have more years ahead in which cancerous changes might occur.[15] Another disadvantage of CT is the administration of iodinated contrast agents, which may cause adverse reactions, including contrast-induced nephrotoxicity and rarely occurring but life-threatening anaphylactic shock.[16]

HL and NHL have identical CT morphologies. Lymph node enlargement is the most common manifestation of lymphoma at CT. Any lymph node station in the body may be affected.[4,9] Regardless of location, affected lymph nodes have approximately the same CT attenuation as muscle tissue (**Fig. 2**).[4,9] Most lymphomas have a homogeneous appearance, but necrotic areas are occasionally seen, especially in large nodal masses (particularly in the anterior mediastinum). However, the presence of necrosis does not have any prognostic significance,[4,9,17] nor does it indicate a certain pathologic subtype. Necrosis may also occur after radiation therapy or chemotherapy. Calcification, although rare before therapy, can occur in large nodal masses. Although seen in the more aggressive subtypes, it too does not have any prognostic impact.[4,9,18] It has been suggested that in NHL, high-grade tumors tend to be more heterogeneous on precontrast and postcontrast scans than low-grade tumors of comparable size,[4,9,19] but the clinical implications of this are uncertain. Most lymph nodes affected by lymphomatous infiltration display only a slight degree of contrast enhancement. More intensely enhancing lymph nodes are occasionally found in certain types of NHL.[4,9]

One of the major limitations of CT scanning in lymphoma is that recognition of nodal involvement depends almost entirely on size criteria. The short-axis diameter is accepted as being the most helpful measurement because it is the most reproducible.[4,9] Lymph nodes with a short-axis diameter greater than or equal to 10 mm are generally considered as positive. Detection of disease in normal-sized nodes remains difficult, where clustering of multiple normal-sized but prominent lymph nodes in areas such as the anterior mediastinum (see **Fig. 2**) and the mesentery is suggestive of disease, particularly when they are rounded in shape. Conversely, CT cannot distinguish between enlargement caused by reactive hyperplasia and involvement with lymphoma. The use of intravenous contrast medium is not helpful, because moderate enhancement is typically seen.[4,9,20] Nevertheless, intravenous contrast facilitates nodal recognition in the neck and retroperitoneum of patients with a paucity of adipose tissue, and helps to differentiate nodal enlargement from large venous tributaries.[4,9] General criteria for extranodal involvement are areas of abnormal attenuation in the spleen, bone, bone marrow, or liver; presence of a nodule or infiltration in the lung; and presence of a soft tissue attenuation mass in other extranodal sites.[4,9]

MR Imaging

The concept that MR imaging might become the ultimate whole-body imaging tool was initially proposed by Damadian[21] and Lauterbur[22] more than 3 decades ago. The high spatial resolution and excellent soft tissue contrast make MR imaging an ideal tool for the detection of parenchymal and bone marrow lesions. Furthermore, MR imaging does not use ionizing radiation (which is particularly advantageous in children and pregnant women), and the safety profile of MR imaging contrast agents is favorable when compared with that of iodinated contrast agents for CT.[23] However, because of long scan times, limited availability, and extensive costs, MR imaging was previously used as a tool to image only limited anatomic areas of the body. Considerable improvements in MR imaging technology (including the development of high-performance magnetic field gradients, multichannel surface coils, parallel acquisition techniques, multisource radiofrequency transmission technology, and digital broadband technology) have resulted in the availability of sufficiently fast and diagnostic sequences for whole-body MR imaging. In addition, the availability of sliding table platforms and whole-body surface coil designs allows for sequential (or continuous) movement of the patient through the

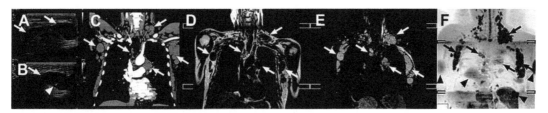

Fig. 2. B-mode US image of left axilla (*A*) in 48-year-old man with mantle cell lymphoma shows homogeneously hypoechoic enlarged lymphomatous lymph nodes. Color Doppler US image (*B*) shows striking hilar vascularity (*arrowhead*) in one of these lymphomatous lymph nodes (*arrow*). Coronal contrast-enhanced CT image (*C*) in same patient shows left cervical/supraclavicular, mediastinal, and bilateral axillary enlarged/clustered lymphomatous lymph nodes with homogeneous attenuation (*arrows*) similar to muscle. Coronal T1-weighted (*D*) and T2-weighted STIR MR images (*E*) and grayscale inverted DWI (*F*) show same lymphomatous lymph nodes (*arrows*), which appear homogeneously slightly hyperintense to muscle on T1-weighted MR imaging (*D*), hyperintense to muscle on T2-weighted STIR MR imaging (*E*), and hyperintense to spinal cord on DWI (*F*). Note poorly suppressed fat on DWI (*F, arrowheads*).

bore of the magnet without patient repositioning, which further decreases scan times. As a result, whole-body MR imaging has become a clinically feasible imaging modality for staging malignancies, including lymphoma (**Fig. 3**).[24–29] A state-of-the-art whole-body MR imaging examination (including T1-weighted, T2-weighted, or short inversion time inversion recovery [STIR], and diffusion-weighted imaging [DWI] sequences) can be performed in approximately 30 to 60 minutes. MR imaging systems operating at 1.5 T are widely available and can provide diagnostic image quality in most body regions within reasonable scan times. Nevertheless, because signal-to-noise ratio (SNR) increases linearly with field strength, there is interest to perform whole-body MR imaging at higher field strength (3.0 T). On the other hand, whole-body MR imaging at high field strength is challenging because of the higher risk of B0 and B1 inhomogeneities and susceptibility artifacts.[30] Whole-body MR imaging at 3.0 T has not yet proved to be superior to whole-body MR imaging at 1.5 T.[30,31] The use of a phased-array surface coil is preferred because it provides an increased SNR/spatial resolution compared with an integrated body coil. There is no standard whole-body MR imaging protocol for the evaluation of lymphoma; data regarding preferred sequences

and imaging planes are lacking. Nevertheless, commonly applied sequences for whole-body MR imaging tumor/lymphoma staging are T1-weighted (without and with intravenous contrast material), fat-suppressed T2-weighted, STIR, and DWI.[24–29] Because MR imaging is a versatile imaging tool that can be used to extract anatomic, physiologic, and molecular information from tumors, its role in the management of patients with lymphoma is expected to increase.

In general, lymphomas are relatively homogeneous on T1-weighted and T2-weighted images. In general, solid portions of lymphoma are isointense to slightly hyperintense relative to muscle on T1-weighted images and hyperintense relative to muscle on T2-weighted images (see **Fig. 2**). Low-grade, intermediate-grade, and high-grade NHLs have identical imaging characteristics. Lymphomas enhance variably after the administration of gadolinium-based contrast agents, although a lower degree of enhancement relative to organ enhancement is usually observed, and delayed enhancement may also occur because of presence of fibrosis.[32]

Although MR imaging provides excellent soft tissue contrast and has the potential to characterize lesions from signal characteristics, T1 and T2 relaxation times of benign and malignant lymph

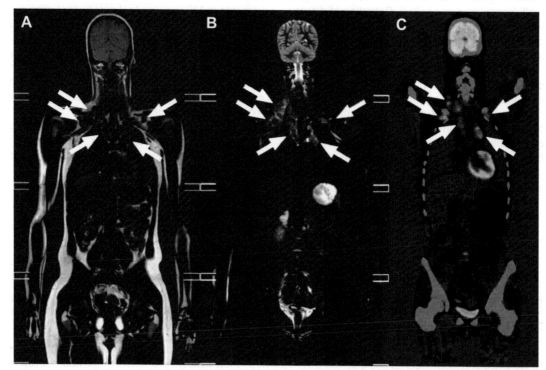

Fig. 3. Coronal T1-weighted (*A*) and T2-weighted STIR MR images (*B*) in 24-year-old woman with HL show right cervical, bilateral supraclavicular, and mediastinal lymph node involvement (*arrows*). Coronal low-dose FDG-PET/CT (*C*) shows same lesions (*arrows*).

nodes show considerable overlap,[33,34] as a result of which assessment of nodal involvement is still based on size criteria, by which lymph nodes with a short-axis diameter greater than or equal to 10 mm are generally considered positive (similar to CT). General criteria for extranodal involvement are any signal abnormalities or mass lesions involving soft tissues, bone marrow, parenchymal organs, and serosal cavities.

US

US is a radiation-free and inexpensive imaging modality that provides real-time high-resolution images, and has long been used to investigate lymphadenopathy.[35] Lymphomatous nodal masses are usually strikingly hypoechoic (see **Fig. 2**), and frequently have a septumlike hyperechoic border. They should not be confused with cysts, the latter of which typically have posterior acoustic enhancement.[36] Before therapy, lymphomatous lymph nodes are rarely hyperechoic (which is even less common than in nodal metastases from other solid tumors).[36] It has been reported that in low-grade lymphomas, the hyperechoic hilum of the lymph node can often still be differentiated from the hypoechoic periphery. In contrast, in high-grade lymphomas, the hilum of the lymph node can often not be recognized.[36,37] Color Doppler US can show increased hilar vascularity (see **Fig. 2**), although the presence of peripheral subcapsular vessels, which is typical of metastasis, is rare in lymphoma (with the possible exception in the uncommon subtypes of high-grade lymphomas).[36,38] However, some investigators[39] suggest that lymphomatous lymph nodes may have high perfusion both in the center and periphery. The differentiation between lymphoma and lymphadenitis from color Doppler patterns is frequently impossible.[38]

Despite the appearances of lymphoma described earlier, the short-axis diameter is still the main US criterion used to evaluate nodal disease in staging lymphoma. As in CT, the detection of lymphomatous involvement in normal-sized lymph nodes and the discrimination between enlargement caused by reactive hyperplasia and involvement by lymphoma is not possible based on size criteria alone. US may also be used to detect extranodal involvement, such as in the liver, spleen, gastrointestinal tract, kidneys, and adrenal glands, which, like lymphoma elsewhere, typically appears as 1 or more solid hypoechoic masses.

Although US is a useful method to evaluate superficial tissues (**Fig. 4**), it is less useful for the evaluation of deeper-lying tissues, and for tissues located behind bones or air-containing structures.

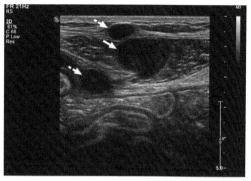

Fig. 4. B-mode US image of right abdominal wall in 38-year-old man with Burkitt lymphoma shows large rounded hypoechoic lymphomatous lesion in right rectus abdominis muscle (*continuous arrow*) and 2 more similar-appearing lymphomatous lesions in subcutis/anterior rectus sheath and peritoneum (*dashed arrows*).

Therefore, US is of limited use in the chest, deep retroperitoneum, and in the evaluation of most organs in obese patients. US is also a highly operator-dependent imaging modality.[36] As a result, the main role of US in routine clinical practice is to help ascertain the nature of palpable masses and to guide biopsy procedures, although its role in staging of lymphoma is limited.[4] Therefore, the following section mainly focuses on the usefulness of CT and MR imaging in several body regions.

USEFULNESS OF CT AND MR IMAGING (AND US) IN SEVERAL BODY REGIONS
Central and Peripheral Nervous System

Unlike primary central nervous system (CNS) lymphoma, which comprises approximately 5% of all primary brain tumors,[40] secondary involvement of the CNS in lymphoma is uncommon. NHL occasionally involves the CNS (occurring more often in high-grade cases, implicating a poor prognosis),[41] whereas CNS involvement in HL is rare.[42] Diagnosis is achieved by recognizing the clinical manifestations, followed by neuroradiologic studies and laboratory examination of the cerebrospinal fluid. Nevertheless, normal studies based on these methods do not exclude such a diagnosis. Although MR imaging and CT have equivalent sensitivities in detecting intracerebral lymphoma, MR imaging can show more subtle meningeal, subdural, and epidural disease within the cranium and spinal column because of its superior soft tissue contrast.[4] Furthermore, MR imaging provides superior assessment of the spinal cord, and also allows for the evaluation of neurolymphomatosis (ie, diffuse infiltration of peripheral nerves including cranial nerves by lymphoma, the least common metastatic presentation of CNS lymphoma) (**Fig. 5**).[43] US is also a useful method to evaluate (superficial) peripheral nerve involvement, and may be complementary to MR imaging.[44]

Extracranial Head and Neck

In HL, 70% to 80% of cases present as a painless enlarging cervical mass, most frequently in the lower neck or supraclavicular region, often associated with contiguous disease in the mediastinum. HL typically affects only lymph nodes, and an isolated extranodal or a combined nodal and extranodal presentation is uncommon. On the other hand, NHL accounts for 5% of head and neck cancer, and frequently presents as extranodal disease, with or without lymph node involvement. In this respect, the head and neck region is the second most common site of lymphoma after the gastrointestinal tract. Most extranodal NHL lesions are located in the Waldeyer ring, whereas other areas of involvement include the paranasal sinuses, orbits, salivary glands, thyroid, larynx, and the ear. Lymphoma of the paranasal sinuses, orbits, and temporal bones usually occur in an older age group. Fewer NHL patients have truly localized disease than those with HL, and 40% to 60% of those presenting with head and neck NHL also have systemic manifestations.[45] US can be used to assess for superficial cervical lymphadenopathy, parotid and submandibular gland involvement, and thyroid gland involvement, but is of less value in evaluating deeper-lying structures. MR imaging performs as well as or better than CT in the imaging of nodal disease in the neck and supraclavicular fossa.[4,46] Furthermore, MR imaging may be better than CT for the evaluation of extranodal disease in the extracranial head and neck region, and for the assessment of lymphoma extension in the intracranial cavity,

whereas CT is preferred for the evaluation of cortical bone (eg, the temporal bone).[46]

Chest

Intrathoracic disease occurs in about 70% to 85% of patients with HL and in 25% to 50% of patients with NHL. The frequency of intrathoracic disease also changes with age: children, especially those with HL, tend to have fewer thoracic manifestations than adults. Anterior mediastinal, paratracheal, and tracheobronchial lymph nodes are involved in almost all cases of HL with intrathoracic disease. All mediastinal lymph nodes are seen to be involved on imaging more frequently in patients with HL (3–4 times more commonly than in those with NHLs), with the exception of the paracardiac and posterior mediastinal groups. Furthermore, anterior mediastinal lymphadenopathy is found in about 90% of patients with HL showing intrathoracic localization of the disease. Involvement of hilar lymph nodes is the next most common site of disease in HL, occurring in up to 22% of patients with intrathoracic disease, usually in association with mediastinal lymphadenopathy. Isolated hilar lymph node involvement is rare in HL, because of the characteristic contiguous pattern of spread, but can occasionally be seen. In patients with NHL, the involvement of different nodal groups is more commonly observed, often without anterior mediastinal lymphadenopathy: enlarged subcarinal, posterior mediastinal, and paracardiac nodes can be found in up to 13%, 10%, and 7% of cases, respectively. Enlarged posterior mediastinal and paracardiac nodes are sometimes the only sites of intrathoracic manifestations of the disease in untreated patients with NHL.[47] Extranodal thoracic manifestations of lymphoma include the thymus (in up to 30% of patients presenting with HL), lung (in 10%–12% and 4% presenting with HL and NHL, respectively), pleura (in 26%–30% of cases at autopsy), pericardium (in 5%–8% of cases,

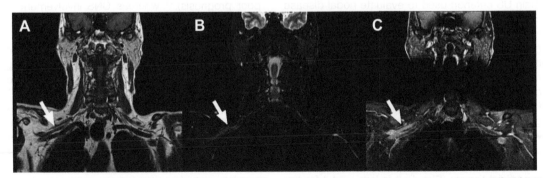

Fig. 5. Coronal T1-weighted (A), T2-weighted STIR (B), and fat-suppressed contrast-enhanced T1-weighted MR images (C) in 62-year-old man with HL, and motor deficits of right arm show thickening and contrast enhancement of right-sided brachial plexus (*arrows*), consistent with neurolymphomatosis.

particularly in patients presenting with a large mediastinal mass), and chest wall (in 2%–5% of cases, particularly in patients with bulky mediastinal disease).

CT is the most frequently used structural imaging modality for the evaluation of the chest. Its high scan speed minimizes the risk of motion artifacts, allowing for the detection of enlarged intrathoracic lymph nodes and pulmonary parenchymal involvement (which may appear as a mass or masslike consolidation, parenchymal nodules, peribronchial thickening, or alveolar and interstitial infiltrates) (**Fig. 6**).[47] Despite its higher susceptibility to motion artifacts and the risk of signal loss because of magnetic field inhomogeneities, MR imaging is also a feasible method for the evaluation of intrathoracic disease. MR imaging can readily detect enlarged lymph nodes in the chest (see **Fig. 6**), provided an appropriate respiratory motion compensation technique (ie, breath-hold or respiratory-gated acquisition) is used. Furthermore, although CT is still regarded as the method of choice for the evaluation of the lung, it has been shown that pulmonary MR imaging is feasible as part of a whole-body MR imaging protocol. Particularly, STIR imaging has been shown to yield high accuracy (sensitivity greater than 90%) compared with chest CT for pulmonary lesions 3 mm or larger in size.[48] An advantage of MR imaging is that it can readily depict pericardial, pleural, and chest wall involvement that may not be evident on CT.[47,49,50] It has also been reported that MR imaging outperforms CT in detecting subpectoral or interpectoral lymphadenopathy and anterior chest wall invasion.[47,51] MR imaging also proved to be particularly beneficial in outlining disease extending from posterior mediastinal nodes into the vertebral body or spinal canal.[47]

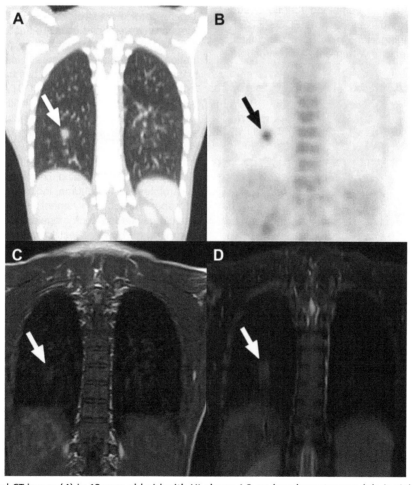

Fig. 6. Coronal CT image (*A*) in 13-year-old girl with HL shows 1.3-cm lymphomatous nodule in right lower lobe (*arrow*), which shows high FDG uptake on coronal PET image (*B, arrow*). T1-weighted (*C*) and T2-weighted STIR MR images (*D*) also show same lesion (*arrow*), although its visibility is poorer because of respiratory motion artifacts.

Abdomen and Pelvis

Retroperitoneal nodal disease is seen at presentation in up to 25% to 35% of patients with HL and up to 55% of patients with NHL. Sites commonly involved by NHL include the mesentery, porta hepatis, and splenic hilum. Furthermore, both HL and NHL can involve any nodal group in the pelvis. Involved lymph nodes in NHL tend to be markedly enlarged, forming conglomerate masses, whereas in HL nodal enlargement may be minimal, complicating recognition of the affected nodes.[4,52] Both CT and MR imaging are appropriate imaging modalities to detect abdominal lymphadenopathy, whereas the use of US for this purpose is mainly limited to the pediatric population.

The abdomen is the most common location of extranodal disease, which mostly occurs in NHL. Laparotomy data have shown that the spleen is involved in up to 30% to 40% of patients with HL and 10% to 40% of those with NHL (**Fig. 7**).[4,53,54] Unlike combined functional/structural imaging modalities such as FDG-PET/CT,[55] structural imaging alone may have difficulties in detecting splenic involvement. This situation is partly because involvement often takes the form of diffuse infiltration and nodules larger than 1 cm occur in only a few cases. In addition, the size of the spleen is not helpful because diffuse infiltration may be present in spleens of normal size, whereas mild to moderate reactive splenomegaly occurs in about 30% of patients in the absence of lymphoma deposits. On the other hand, marked splenomegaly almost always indicates infiltration.[4,42] Focal nodules larger than 1 cm can be detected equally well by CT, MR imaging, and US. Nodules tend to be hypoattenuating at CT, enhance less than normal splenic parenchyma, generally have intermediate T2-weighted signal intensity relative to spleen at MR imaging, and are hypoechoic at US. Coexistent splenic hilar lymphadenopathy detected by any imaging modality is suggestive of presence of splenic lymphoma.[4,42]

Hepatic involvement is seen at presentation in 8% of patients with HL and 25% of those with NHL at laparoscopy or laparotomy (**Figs. 8** and **9**).[56,57] Hepatic involvement is usually diffuse, with discrete nodular lesions seen in only 10% of cases. A combination of the 2 patterns occurs in less than 3% of patients. Nodular liver disease has the same characteristics as splenic disease at CT, MR imaging, and US, whereas diffuse hepatic infiltration is more difficult to detect with structural imaging.[4,42]

The gastrointestinal tract is the most common site of primary extranodal lymphoma, which is nearly always caused by NHL (**Fig. 10**).[4] There are strict criteria for the diagnosis of primary gastrointestinal lymphoma, including the absence of hepatosplenic involvement and nodal involvement confined to the drainage area of the affected segment of bowel. Gastric mucosa-associated

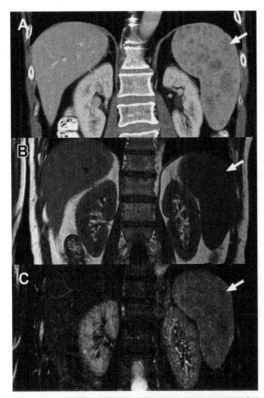

Fig. 7. Coronal contrast-enhanced CT image (*A*), T1-weighted MR image (*B*), and T2-weighted STIR MR image (*C*) in 45-year-old man with follicular lymphoma show hypoattenuating and hypointense lymphomatous nodules in spleen (*arrows*).

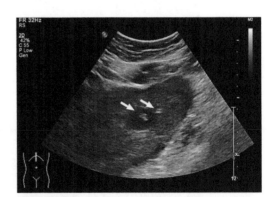

Fig. 8. B-mode US image of left hepatic lobe in sagittal plane in 51-year-old, human immunodeficiency virus-positive woman shows 2 lesions with hyperechoic centers and hypoechoic rims (*arrows*) (so-called target or bull's eye lesions), which were histologically proved to be Burkitt lymphoma.

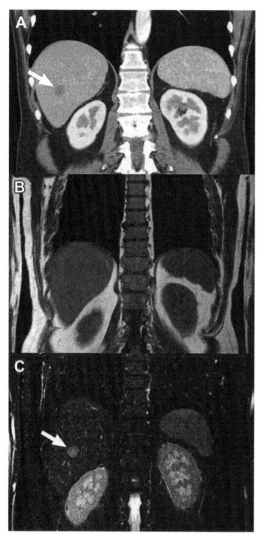

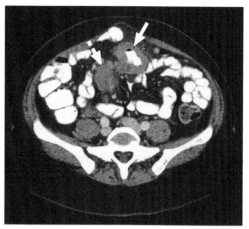

Fig. 10. Axial contrast-enhanced CT image in 44-year-old woman with diffuse large B-cell lymphoma shows moderate mural thickening of small bowel loop (*continuous arrow*) with surrounding infiltration of mesenteric fat, and enlarged mesenteric lymph node (*dashed arrow*), which were histologically proved to be lymphomatous.

narrowing or mural thickening, which is readily recognized by CT or MR imaging.[4]

All forms of renal lymphoma (seen in about 3% of patients undergoing abdominal staging scans) are well shown by CT, MR imaging, and US, including solitary or multiple renal masses, direct infiltration via the renal hilum, diffuse renal infiltration with renal enlargement, and perirenal masses surrounding the kidney. CT, MR imaging, and US can also document the presence and level of any ureteral obstruction.[4,42]

Although CT shows pelvic nodal disease and pelvic masses, MR imaging is the modality of choice for defining lymphoma of the pelvic viscera, whether primary or secondary.[4] The use of US for this purpose is again mainly limited to the pediatric population.

In evaluation of the testis, which may be involved primarily or secondarily with NHL in a focal or diffuse form, sometimes bilaterally, both MR imaging and US can be used for this purpose.[4]

Musculoskeletal System

Bone marrow involvement is found in 5% to 15% of patients with HL and in 20% to 40% of patients with NHL (**Fig. 11**).[58–61] Bone marrow biopsy (BMB) is considered as the reference standard for diagnosing bone marrow involvement, but is invasive and has a small but nonnegligible risk of hemorrhagic complications.[62] In addition, focal bone marrow involvement may be missed by BMB; previous studies showed that in patients with unilaterally proven bone marrow infiltration,

Fig. 9. Coronal contrast-enhanced CT image (*A*) in 47-year-old man with T-cell rich B-cell lymphoma shows hypoattenuating lymphomatous lesion in right hepatic lobe (*arrow*). The lesion cannot be seen on coronal T1-weighted MR image (*B*), but is clearly seen on coronal T2-weighted STIR MR imaging with hyperintense signal intensity relative to liver parenchyma and signal intensity similar to the spleen, which is characteristic of malignancy (*arrow*).

lymphoid tissue lymphomas, especially low-grade ones, typically result in minimal gastric wall thickening, which may not be identified by CT or MR imaging. In this instance, endoscopic US is of value. Multiorgan involvement can be seen in up to 25% of these patients and therefore extensive staging may be necessary. In the small bowel, CT and MR imaging can show the complications of lymphoma, such as bowel obstruction, perforation, and intussusception, in addition to mural thickening. Colonic lymphoma can cause luminal contralateral BMB of the iliac crest was negative in 10% to 60%.[58–61] Although CT is an excellent method to assess cortical bone (see **Fig. 11**), it is not suitable to evaluate the bone marrow, which is the location where lymphomatous bone involvement first occurs (**Fig. 12**). However, MR imaging allows for direct visualization of the bone marrow.[63] Lymphomatous bone marrow lesions typically have longer T1 and T2 relaxation times than normal yellow and red marrow (ie, low signal intensity on T1-weighted images and high signal intensity on fat-suppressed T2-weighted or STIR images) because they contain larger amounts of water and lesser amounts of fat (see **Fig. 12**). Despite its potential, MR imaging techniques are not sufficiently sensitive yet to (partially) replace BMB[64] (because false-negative results can occur where there is microscopic [<5%] infiltration[4]). Nevertheless, MR imaging and BMB can still be considered as complementary studies for improved bone marrow staging, especially given the often focal nature of bone marrow involvement. In addition, studies have shown that MR imaging-based assessment of the bone marrow has prognostic implications, independent of BMB

results. More specifically, patients with a positive MR imaging scan have a higher risk of relapse and a shorter survival compared with those with a negative MR imaging scan.[65,66] Future technical developments are expected to further increase the clinical usefulness of MR imaging in the evaluation of the bone marrow in lymphoma.

Muscles may occasionally be involved in HL and NHL.[42,67] In most HL cases, paravertebral masses are the result of invasion from retroperitoneal lymph nodes.[42] Intramuscular NHL mostly manifests as diffuse muscle enlargement.[67] Although CT and US may be used to evaluate the presence and extent of lymphomatous muscle involvement, MR imaging is the imaging modality of choice for this purpose (**Fig. 13**).

ADVANCED CT, MR IMAGING, AND US TECHNIQUES
Advanced CT Techniques: Dual-energy CT

CT is an important imaging modality that is routinely used for the evaluation of patients with lymphoma. Recently introduced dual-energy CT systems may further enhance the role of CT in

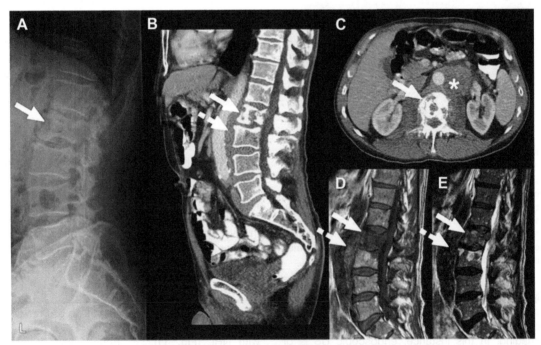

Fig. 11. Lateral radiograph of lumbar spine (*A*) in 67-year-old man with follicular lymphoma shows collapse of L2 vertebral body (*arrow*) and destruction of its pedicles, consistent with lymphomatous involvement. Sagittal (*B*) and axial contrast-enhanced CT images (*C*) show collapsed L2 vertebral body with mixed lytic-sclerotic appearance (*continuous arrow*). Also note prevertebral lymphomatous mass that displaces abdominal aorta anteriorly from spine (*B, dashed arrow; C, asterisk*). Sagittal T1-weighted (*D*) and T2-weighted MR images (*E*) also show same lesion, which is hypointense on T1-weighted MR imaging and mixed hypointense and hyperintense on T2-maging (*continuous arrow*) relative to skeletal muscle, with associated central canal stenosis. Prevertebral lymphomatous mass can also be seen (*D* and *E, dashed arrow*).

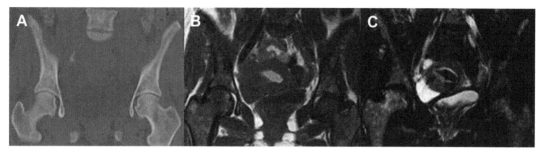

Fig. 12. Coronal CT image (*A*) in 40-year-old woman with HL does not reveal osseous or bone marrow lesions. However, coronal T1-weighted (*B*) and T2-weighted STIR MR images (*C*) show diffuse signal abnormalities in pelvic and femoral bone marrow, consistent with lymphomatous involvement.

lymphoma. Technologic advances in dual-energy CT systems have been triggered by the introduction of dual-source CT systems that were primarily developed to achieve a higher temporal resolution for cardiac imaging. Unlike conventional CT sys-only 1 radiograph energy source and 1 radiograph detector at 1 time, dual-energy CT systems can use 2 different radiograph energy sources (which can be operated at different voltage potentials) with 2 corresponding radiograph detectors at 1 It is possible to simultaneously acquire 2 data sets at 2 different photon energies during a single acquisition. By obtaining CT data at different photon energies and by using various dual-energy postprocessing algorithms that are based on 3-material decomposition principles, differences in material composition can be visualized and quantified based on differences in photon absorption. This system works especially well in materials with large atomic numbers such as iodine and calcium, because these materials show relatively large differences in photon absorption at different (low and high) photon energy settings.[68,69] A recent feasibility study[70] has indicated that it may be possible to use dual-energy CT for the assessment of the bone marrow. In this study, Pache and colleagues[70] reported a novel dual-energy CT postprocessing algorithm based on 3-material decomposition (bone mineral, yellow marrow, and red marrow), which was termed virtual noncalcium. The dual-energy CT virtual noncalcium technique subtracts calcium from trabecular bone, allowing for bone marrow assessment, and has shown promise for the detection of posttraumatic bone bruises of the knee in a small series of 21 patients.[70] This method may also allow for the detection of lymphomatous bone marrow involvement at an earlier stage than conventional single-source CT systems. However, clinical studies on the use of dual-energy CT in the assessment of the bone marrow in patients with cancer, including lymphoma, are still lacking.

Material characterization is not the only advantage of dual-energy CT scanning. With every dual-energy CT scan, both low and high tube voltage datasets can be separately evaluated. Scanning with a low tube voltage markedly increases attenuation of iodine (contrast enhancement) but image noise also increases. Higher tube voltage decreases image noise but at the expense of a lower enhancement level. Moreover, the data of a dual-energy CT scan can be mixed, generating the so-called weighted-average (WA) image dataset that combines the image data from the low and high peak voltage acquisitions according to the applied weighting factor. Any desired WA

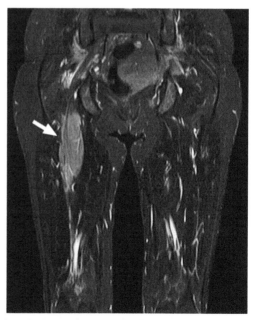

Fig. 13. Coronal T2-weighted STIR MR image in 65-year-old woman with extranodal marginal zone lymphoma shows high signal intensity of right biceps femoris muscle (*arrow*), consistent with lymphomatous involvement.

mixture from the 2 acquisitions can be generated, which can be used to improve lesion contrast/noise ratio compared with a standard single-source 120-kVp dataset, as has been shown in pancreatic adenocarcinoma, hepatocellular carcinoma, (hypovascular) liver metastases, and head and neck cancer.[71–74] The usefulness of this approach still has to be investigated in lymphoma, but it can be foreseen that it may improve image quality and the evaluation of lymphomatous lesions in different body regions.

Advanced MR Imaging Techniques: DWI, Dynamic Contrast-enhanced MR imaging, MR Imaging Spectroscopy, and Ultrasmall Superparamagnetic Iron Oxide-enhanced MR Imaging

The limitations of conventional (T1-weighted and T2-weighted) MR imaging are well recognized given the continuing pursuit for MR imaging sequences that allow a more functional assessment of normal and abnormal tissues, which, in turn, may improve the characterization and follow-up of lesions in patients with cancer or at risk for cancer.[10]

DWI is one of the advanced MR imaging techniques that is under active investigation, especially for body oncological imaging. DWI allows noninvasive visualization and quantification of the random microscopic movement of water molecules (ie, Brownian motion) within biologic tissues.[75] Pathologic processes that lead to changes in the diffusivity of water molecules can be evaluated using DWI. One of the main advantages of DWI over conventional MR imaging sequences is its ability to highlight lesions (which often have a prolonged T2 relaxation time and decreased diffusivity, and therefore high signal intensity at DWI), while suppressing signal from many unwanted background structures such as fat, flowing blood, cerebrospinal fluid, and gastrointestinal contents. This situation, in turn, may improve lesion detectability and staging accuracy, and reduce image interpretation time. Furthermore, the ability of DWI to quantify diffusion in biologic tissue by means of diffusion coefficient measurements may aid in the characterization and treatment response assessment of cancerous lesions.[75] The promising role of DWI in lymphoma is discussed in more detail by Kwee and colleagues elsewhere in this issue.

Dynamic contrast-enhanced (DCE)-MR imaging is another advanced MR imaging technique that allows (quantitative) assessment of functional aspects of tumor neovascularity in vivo in a noninvasive and repeatable way.[76,77] DCE-MR imaging is performed by obtaining sequential MR images before, during, and after the injection of a contrast agent (most often a small molecular weight gadolinium-containing compound such as gadopentetate dimeglumine).[76,77] DCE-MR imaging can be performed using dynamic T2* methods or dynamic T1-weighted methods. Dynamic T2* methods use the fact that the first pass of a contrast agent through a tissue causes a transient signal decrease because of local magnetic susceptibility (T2*) effects. Dynamic T2* methods can provide information about tumor perfusion, which may pathologically be related to tumor grade and vessel density.[76,77] On the other hand, dynamic T1-weighted methods use the T1 shortening effects of the contrast agent that cause an increase in signal intensity as it passes from the blood into the extracellular space of tissues. Dynamic T1 methods can provide information about blood vessel permeability, capillary surface area, and leakage space, which may pathologically be related to tumor grade, microvessel density, and levels of vascular endothelial growth factor expression.[76,77] DCE-MR imaging may be used for tumor detection, characterization, grading, and staging, determining prognosis, monitoring treatment, and detecting tumor relapse, as was shown in many types of cancer, including those involving the brain, breast, prostate, cervix, liver, lung, and rectum.[76,77] Furthermore, DCE-MR imaging may be used to measure the effects of antiangiogenic therapies. Research on the applications of this advanced MR imaging technique in lymphoma is still limited. Nevertheless, preliminary data have shown that DCE-MR imaging may be used to detect, grade, and assess response to therapy in patients with hematological malignancies (including lymphoma) as well as diffuse bone marrow involvement.[78,79]

Magnetic resonance spectroscopy (MRS) is a method that allows for separation of the MR imaging signal from a given tissue into its different chemical components. This situation is possible because the magnetic field experienced by an atomic nucleus is minutely shielded or modified by the fields produced by neighboring atoms on the same molecule. This phenomenon produces a chemical shift or small variation in the nuclear resonance frequency. A display of MR imaging signal amplitude as a function of nuclear resonance frequency forms a spectrum, with different chemical environments of a particular type of atomic nucleus within and between molecules forming peaks at characteristic chemical shift positions. It is possible to quantitatively assess the amount, type, and location of small molecular compounds within a tissue or organ of interest at the same time conventional MR imaging is performed.[80] The data are typically displayed as a grid of spectra of chemical compound abundances obtained at either single or multiple locations in a tissue or organ of interest. These spectra are collected from spinning nuclei (spins), most often ^{1}H given the abundance of water in tissue. ^{1}H MRS enables accurate quantitative assessment of the spatial distribution of tissue metabolites such as creatinine, choline, amino acids, nucleotides, lactate, and lipids.[81] Phosphorus is another element that has attracted a lot of attention for in vivo MRS, because it is fundamental to several cellular processes, including energy metabolism and membrane construction. MRS of phosphorus offers insight into processes such as cell energy metabolism, tissue oxygenation state, pH, and membrane turnover; furthermore, the ^{31}P MRS signal can be collected with relative technical ease.[80] Because NHL is a prevalent form of cancer that shows approximately 50% response to therapy and often presents with large superficial lesions easily accessible to multinuclear MRS measurements, it is an ideal test bed for development of MRS methods to predict and detect early response. A multicenter study has already shown that pretreatment ^{31}P MRS measurement of the phosphate monoester/nucleoside triphosphate ratio can identify about two-thirds of the patients who are destined not to show a complete clinical response to a variety of therapeutic agents.[82] Because ^{31}P MRS is limited to relatively large superficial tumors, ^{1}H MRS methods have also been explored for early detection of therapeutic response in lymphoma. Using xenografts of diffuse large B-cell lymphoma, therapeutic response could be detected within 1 cycle of therapy with CHOP (cyclophosphamide, doxorubicin, vincristine, prednisone), rituximab plus CHOP (RCHOP) or radiation (15 Gy) through detection of a decrease in lactic acid (Lac) or total choline (tCho).[82] ^{1}H MRS has also been performed in patients with NHL in a clinical scanner. It has been reported that 1 of the patients showed a 70% decrease in Lac within 48 hours of treatment with RCHOP.[82]

The discrimination between normal-sized nonmalignant lymph nodes and normal-sized lymphomatous lymph nodes is essentially impossible with structural imaging. Ultrasmall superparamagnetic iron oxide (USPIO)-enhanced MR imaging was introduced in the early 1990s as a promising imaging modality for evaluating lymph nodes,[83] allowing for the identification of malignant nodal infiltration independent of lymph node size. Intravenously administered USPIO particles are taken up by macrophages in the reticuloendothelial system, predominantly within the lymph nodes but also in the Waldeyer ring, spleen, and bone marrow. Normal homogeneous uptake of USPIO particles in nonmetastatic lymph nodes shortens the T2 and T2* values, making these lymph nodes hypointense on T2-weighted and T2*-weighted images, whereas malignant lymph nodes lack uptake and remain hyperintense.[83] USPIO-enhanced MR imaging has been shown to achieve higher diagnostic precision than conventional, unenhanced MR imaging for the detection of lymph node metastases of various tumors.[84] However, USPIO-enhanced MR imaging indirectly reveals cancer sites in lymph nodes. Therefore, the specificity of this method may prove to be suboptimal in lymph nodes that are involved by nonneoplastic processes. Besides its potential usefulness for lymph node imaging, another possible advantage of USPIO-enhanced MR imaging is the suppression of the normal Waldeyer ring, spleen, and normal or hyperplastic red bone marrow, whereas lymphomatous lesions in these organs can theoretically be highlighted.[85] The value of this method in lymphoma still has to be investigated. USPIO contrast agents are not approved by the US Food and Drug Administration for these applications in humans.

Advanced US Techniques: Compound, Tissue Harmonic, and Contrast-enhanced US

Novel techniques have opened new prospects for US. Compound US generates an image from multiple scanning lines that strike the target from different angles, thus reducing artifacts and noise. Tissue harmonic US is based on the nonlinear interaction of an acoustic signal as it propagates through tissues, and also reduces image noise and artifacts and improves SNR, contrast, and lateral resolution.[86] Injected gas-filled microbubbles rapidly reach the capillary bed in the parenchymal phase and enhance the vessel texture because they do not leak out of the vessels. The results of contrast-enhanced US are higher-resolution examinations and improved detection of malignant nodules compared with those at conventional US.[87] A recent study of 100 patients with HL has shown that harmonic compound US with contrast enhancement for the characterization of possible nodules provides a higher sensitivity than does CT or FDG-PET in the detection of splenic involvement.[87] However, another study of 250 patients with lymphoma (both HL and NHL) reported that contrast-enhanced US has no clear advantage over standard B-mode US for diagnosis of splenic involvement.[88] More studies are required to support the use of contrast-enhanced US as an adjunct to standard staging procedures (CT and FDG-PET/CT) for the evaluation of the spleen in the staging workup of patients with lymphoma.

SUMMARY

Of all cross-sectional structural imaging modalities available, CT is the mainstay for evaluating lymphoma, particularly because of its whole-body imaging capability, high spatial resolution, high scan speed, and successful hardware integration of CT with PET. MR imaging is emerging as a radiation-free alternative to CT for staging and follow-up of patients with lymphoma, currently capable of whole-body imaging with high soft tissue contrast resolution within a clinically acceptable scan time. Because MR imaging is a versatile imaging tool that can be used to extract both anatomic and functional information from tumors, its role in the management of patients with lymphoma is expected to further increase. The role of US in the evaluation of lymphoma is still limited, mainly because of its inability to accurately evaluate the chest, deep retroperitoneum, and most organs in obese patients, as well as its operator-dependency, although it is cheap and easy to perform and is useful for guidance of tissue sampling. CT, MR imaging, and US each have advantages and disadvantages, and it is important to understand these to maximize their usefulness in the management of patients with lymphoma. Advanced CT, MR imaging, and US techniques such as dual-energy CT, DWI, DCE-MR imaging, MRS, USPIO-enhanced MR imaging, and contrast-enhanced US may improve the detection, characterization, and response assessment of lymphomatous lesions in the body.

REFERENCES

1. Jemal A, Siegel R, Xu J, et al. Cancer statistics, 2010. CA Cancer J Clin 2010;60(5):277–300.
2. Armitage JO. Staging non-Hodgkin lymphoma. CA Cancer J Clin 2005;55(6):368–76.
3. Connors JM. State-of-the-art therapeutics: Hodgkin's lymphoma. J Clin Oncol 2005;23(26):6400–8.
4. Vinnicombe SJ, Reznek RH. Computerised tomography in the staging of Hodgkin's disease and non-Hodgkin's lymphoma. Eur J Nucl Med Mol Imaging 2003;30(Suppl 1):S42–55.
5. Murphy SB. Classification, staging and end results of treatment of childhood non-Hodgkin's lymphomas: dissimilarities from lymphomas in adults. Semin Oncol 1980;7(3):332–9.
6. Murphy SB, Fairclough DL, Hutchison RE, et al. Non-Hodgkin's lymphomas of childhood: an analysis of the histology, staging, and response to treatment of 338 cases at a single institution. J Clin Oncol 1989;7(2):186–93.
7. Cheson BD, Pfistner B, Juweid ME, et al. International Harmonization Project on Lymphoma. Revised response criteria for malignant lymphoma. J Clin Oncol 2007;25(5):579–86.
8. Seam P, Juweid ME, Cheson BD. The role of FDG-PET scans in patients with lymphoma. Blood 2007; 110(10):3507–16.
9. Van der Molen AJ, Schaefer-Prokop C, Leppert A. Lymphatic system. In: Prokop M, Galanski M, editors. Spiral and multislice computed tomography of the body. New York: Georg Thieme Verlag; 2003. p. 755–7.
10. Torigian DA, Huang SS, Houseni M, et al. Functional imaging of cancer with emphasis on molecular techniques. CA Cancer J Clin 2007;57(4):206–24.
11. Delbeke D, Stroobants S, de Kerviler E, et al. Expert opinions on positron emission tomography and computed tomography imaging in lymphoma. Oncologist 2009;14(Suppl 2):S30–40.
12. Rosenberg SA, Boiron M, DeVita VT Jr, et al. Report of the Committee on Hodgkin's Disease Staging Procedures. Cancer Res 1971;31(11):1862–3.
13. Kreel L. The EMI whole body scanner in the demonstration of lymph node enlargement. Clin Radiol 1976;27(4):421–9.
14. Lucey BC, Stuhlfaut JW, Soto JA. Mesenteric lymph nodes: detection and significance on MDCT. AJR Am J Roentgenol 2005;184(1):41–4.
15. Brenner DJ, Hall EJ. Computed tomography–an increasing source of radiation exposure. N Engl J Med 2007;357(22):2277–84.
16. Namasivayam S, Kalra MK, Torres WE, et al. Adverse reactions to intravenous iodinated contrast media: a primer for radiologists. Emerg Radiol 2006; 12(5):210–5.
17. Hopper KD, Diehl LF, Cole BA, et al. The significance of necrotic mediastinal lymph nodes on CT in patients with newly diagnosed Hodgkin disease. AJR Am J Roentgenol 1990;155(2):267–70.
18. Apter S, Avigdor A, Gayer G, et al. Calcification in lymphoma occurring before therapy: CT features and clinical correlation. AJR Am J Roentgenol 2002;178(4):935–8.
19. Rodriguez M, Rehn SM, Nyman RS, et al. CT in malignancy grading and prognostic prediction of non-Hodgkin's lymphoma. Acta Radiol 1999;40(2):191–7.
20. Pombo F, Rodriguez E, Caruncho MV, et al. CT attenuation values and enhancing characteristics of thoracoabdominal lymphomatous adenopathies. J Comput Assist Tomogr 1994;18(1):59–62.
21. Damadian R. Field focusing n.m.r. (FONAR) and the formation of chemical images in man. Philos Trans R Soc Lond B Biol Sci 1980;289(1037):489–500.
22. Lauterbur PC. Progress in n.m.r. zeugmatography imaging. Philos Trans R Soc Lond B Biol Sci 1980; 289(1037):483–7.

23. Kirchin MA, Runge VM. Contrast agents for magnetic resonance imaging: safety update. Top Magn Reson Imaging 2003;14(5):426–35.

24. Kellenberger CJ, Miller SF, Khan M, et al. Initial experience with FSE STIR whole-body MR imaging for staging lymphoma in children. Eur Radiol 2004; 14(10):1829–41.

25. Brennan DD, Gleeson T, Coate LE, et al. A comparison of whole-body MRI and CT for the staging of lymphoma. AJR Am J Roentgenol 2005;185(3):711–6.

26. Kwee TC, van Ufford HM, Beek FJ, et al. Whole-body MRI, including diffusion-weighted imaging, for the initial staging of malignant lymphoma: comparison to computed tomography. Invest Radiol 2009;44(10):683–90.

27. Punwani S, Taylor SA, Bainbridge A, et al. Pediatric and adolescent lymphoma: comparison of whole-body STIR half-Fourier RARE MR imaging with an enhanced PET/CT reference for initial staging. Radiology 2010;255(1):182–90.

28. Lin C, Luciani A, Itti E, et al. Whole-body diffusion-weighted magnetic resonance imaging with apparent diffusion coefficient mapping for staging patients with diffuse large B-cell lymphoma. Eur Radiol 2010;20(8):2027–38.

29. Abdulqadhr G, Molin D, Aström G, et al. Whole-body diffusion-weighted imaging compared with FDG-PET/CT in staging of lymphoma patients. Acta Radiol 2011;52(2):173–80.

30. Schick F. Whole-body MRI at high field: technical limits and clinical potential. Eur Radiol 2005;15(5):946–59.

31. Schmidt GP, Wintersperger B, Graser A, et al. High-resolution whole-body magnetic resonance imaging applications at 1.5 and 3 Tesla: a comparative study. Invest Radiol 2007;42(6):449–59.

32. Nagendank WG, Al-Katib AM, Karanes C, et al. Lymphomas: MR imaging contrast characteristics with clinical-pathologic correlations. Radiology 1990;177(1):209–16.

33. Glazer GM, Orringer MB, Chenevert TL, et al. Mediastinal lymph nodes: relaxation time/pathologic correlation and implications in staging of lung cancer with MR imaging. Radiology 1988;168(2):429–31.

34. Ranade SS, Trivedi PN, Bamane VS. Mediastinal lymph nodes: relaxation time/pathologic correlation and implications in staging of lung cancer with MR imaging. Radiology 1990;174(1):284–5.

35. Vassallo P, Wernecke K, Roos N, et al. Differentiation of benign from malignant superficial lymphadenopathy: the role of high-resolution US. Radiology 1992;183(1):215–20.

36. Mende U, Zierhut D, Ewerbeck V, et al. Ultrasound criteria for staging and follow-up of malignant lymphoma. Radiologe 1997;37(1):19–26 [in German].

37. Ahuja AT, Ying M. Evaluation of cervical lymph node vascularity: a comparison of colour Doppler, power Doppler and 3-D power Doppler sonography. Ultrasound Med Biol 2004;30(12):1557–64.

38. Giovagnorio F, Galluzzo M, Andreoli C, et al. Color Doppler sonography in the evaluation of superficial lymphomatous lymph nodes. J Ultrasound Med 2002;21(4):403–8.

39. Steinkamp HJ, Wissgott C, Rademaker J, et al. Current status of power Doppler and color Doppler sonography in the differential diagnosis of lymph node lesions. Eur Radiol 2002;12(7):1785–93.

40. Tang YZ, Booth TC, Bhogal P, et al. Imaging of primary central nervous system lymphoma. Clin Radiol 2011;66(8):768–77.

41. Nagpal S, Glantz MJ, Recht L. Treatment and prevention of secondary CNS lymphoma. Semin Neurol 2010;30(3):263–72.

42. Guermazi A, Brice P, de Kerviler E, et al. Extranodal Hodgkin disease: spectrum of disease. Radiographics 2001;21(1):161–79.

43. Chamberlain MC, Fink J. Neurolymphomatosis: a rare metastatic complication of diffuse large B-cell lymphoma. J Neurooncol 2009;95(2):285–8.

44. Kermarrec E, Demondion X, Khalil C, et al. Ultrasound and magnetic resonance imaging of the peripheral nerves: current techniques, promising directions, and open issues. Semin Musculoskelet Radiol 2010;14(5):463–72.

45. Chisin R, Weber AL. Imaging of lymphoma manifestations in the extracranial head and neck region. Leuk Lymphoma 1994;12(3–4):177–89.

46. Dooms GC, Hricak H, Crooks LE, et al. Magnetic resonance imaging of the lymph nodes: comparison with CT. Radiology 1984;153(3):719–28.

47. Bonomo L, Ciccotosto C, Guidotti A, et al. Staging of thoracic lymphoma by radiological imaging. Eur Radiol 1997;7(8):1179–89.

48. Frericks BB, Meyer BC, Martus P, et al. MRI of the thorax during whole-body MRI: evaluation of different MR sequences and comparison to thoracic multidetector computed tomography (MDCT). J Magn Reson Imaging 2008;27(3):538–45.

49. Tesoro-Tess JD, Balzarini L, Ceglia E, et al. Magnetic resonance imaging in the initial staging of Hodgkin's disease and non-Hodgkin lymphoma. Eur J Radiol 1991;12(2):81–90.

50. Bergin CJ, Healy MV, Zincone GE, et al. MR evaluation of chest wall involvement in malignant lymphoma. J Comput Assist Tomogr 1990;14(6):928–32.

51. Carlsen SE, Bergin CJ, Hoppe RT. MR imaging to detect chest wall and pleural involvement in patients with lymphoma: effect on radiation therapy planning. AJR Am J Roentgenol 1993;160(6):1191–5.

52. Stomper PC, Cholewinski SP, Park J, et al. Abdominal staging of thoracic Hodgkin disease: CT-lymphangiography-Ga-67 scanning correlation. Radiology 1993;187(2):381–6.

53. Kadin ME, Glatstein EJ, Dorfman RE. Clinicopatho-logic studies in 117 untreated patients subject to laparotomy for the staging of Hodgkin's disease. Cancer 1977;27(6):1277–94.

54. Castellino RA, Goffinet DR, Blank N, et al. The role of radiography in the staging of non-Hodgkin's lymphoma with laparotomy correlation. Radiology 1974;110(2):329–38.

55. De Jong PA, van Ufford HM, Baarslag HJ, et al. CT and 18F-FDG PET for noninvasive detection of splenic involvement in patients with malignant lymphoma. AJR Am J Roentgenol 2009;192(3):745–53.

56. Veronesi U, Spinelli P, Bonadonna G, et al. Laparos-copy and laparotomy in staging Hodgkin's and non-Hodgkin's lymphoma. AJR Am J Roentgenol 1976; 127(3):501–3.

57. Greene FL. Laparoscopy in malignant disease. Surg Clin North Am 1992;72(5):1125–37.

58. Brunning RD, Bloomfield CD, McKenna RW, et al. Bilateral trephine bone marrow biopsies in lym-phoma and other neoplastic diseases. Ann Intern Med 1975;82(3):365–6.

59. Coller BS, Chabner BA, Gralnick HR. Frequencies and patterns of bone marrow involvement in non-Hodgkin lymphomas: observations on the value of bilateral biopsies. Am J Hematol 1977;3:105–19.

60. Haddy TB, Parker RI, Magrath IT. Bone marrow involvement in young patients with non-Hodgkin's lymphoma: the importance of multiple bone marrow samples for accurate staging. Med Pediatr Oncol 1989;17(5):418–23.

61. Wang J, Weiss LM, Chang KL, et al. Diagnostic utility of bilateral bone marrow examination: significance of morphologic and ancillary technique study in malignancy. Cancer 2002;94(5):1522–31.

62. Bain BJ. Morbidity associated with bone marrow aspiration and trephine biopsy–a review of UK data for 2004. Haematologica 2006;91(9):1293–4.

63. Vogler JB 3rd, Murphy WA. Bone marrow imaging. Radiology 1988;168(3):679–93.

64. Kwee TC, Fijnheer R, Ludwig I, et al. Whole-body magnetic resonance imaging, including diffusion-weighted imaging, for diagnosing bone marrow involvement in malignant lymphoma. Br J Haematol 2010;149(4):628–30.

65. Tsunoda S, Takagi S, Tanaka O, et al. Clinical and prognostic significance of femoral marrow magnetic resonance imaging in patients with malignant lymphoma. Blood 1997;89(1):286–90.

66. Varan A, Cila A, Büyükpamukçu M. Prognostic importance of magnetic resonance imaging in bone marrow involvement of Hodgkin disease. Med Pediatr Oncol 1999;32(4):267–71.

67. Surov A, Holzhausen HJ, Arnold D, et al. Intramus-cular manifestation of non-Hodgkin lymphoma and myeloma: prevalence, clinical signs, and computed tomography features. Acta Radiol 2010;51(1):47–51.

68. Johnson TR, Krauss B, Sedlmair M, et al. Material differentiation by dual energy CT: initial experience. Eur Radiol 2007;17(6):1510–7.

69. Graser A, Johnson TR, Chandarana H, et al. Dual energy CT: preliminary observations and potential clinical applications in the abdomen. Eur Radiol 2009;19(1):13–23.

70. Pache G, Krauss B, Strohm P, et al. Dual-energy CT virtual noncalcium technique: detecting posttrau-matic bone marrow lesions–feasibility study. Radi-ology 2010;256(2):617–24.

71. Macari M, Spieler B, Kim D, et al. Dual-source dual-energy MDCT of pancreatic adenocarcinoma: initial observations with data generated at 80 kVp and at simulated weighted-average 120 kVp. AJR Am J Roentgenol 2010;194(1):W27–32.

72. Kim KS, Lee JM, Kim SH, et al. Image fusion in dual energy computed tomography for detection of hyper-vascular liver hepatocellular carcinoma: phantom and preliminary studies. Invest Radiol 2010;45(3): 149–57.

73. Robinson E, Babb J, Chandarana H, et al. Dual source dual energy MDCT: comparison of 80 kVp and weighted average 120 kVp data for conspicuity of hypo-vascular liver metastases. Invest Radiol 2010;45(7):413–8.

74. Tawfik AM, Kerl JM, Bauer RW, et al. Dual-energy CT of head and neck cancer: average weighting of low- and high-voltage acquisitions to improve lesion delineation and image quality – initial clinical experience. Invest Radiol 2011. DOI:10.1097/ RLI.0b013e31821e3062.

75. Padhani AR, Liu G, Koh DM, et al. Diffusion-weighted magnetic resonance imaging as a cancer biomarker: consensus and recommendations. Neoplasia 2009; 11(2):102–25.

76. Padhani AR. Dynamic contrast-enhanced MR imaging. Cancer Imaging 2000;1:52–63.

77. Hylton N. Dynamic contrast-enhanced magnetic re-sonance imaging as an imaging biomarker. J Clin Oncol 2006;4(20):3293–8.

78. Rahmouni A, Montazel JL, Divine M, et al. Bone marrow with diffuse tumor infiltration in patients with lymphoproliferative diseases: dynamic gadolinium-enhanced MR imaging. Radiology 2003;229(3): 710–7.

79. Zha Y, Li M, Yang J. Dynamic contrast enhanced magnetic resonance imaging of diffuse spinal bone marrow infiltration in patients with hematolog-ical malignancies. Korean J Radiol 2010;11(2): 187–94.

80. Aisen AM, Chenevert TL. MR spectroscopy: clinical perspective. Radiology 1989;173(3):593–9.

81. Mountford C, Lean C, Malycha P, et al. Proton spec-troscopy provides accurate pathology on biopsy and in vivo. J Magn Reson Imaging 2006;24(3): 459–77.

82. Lee SC, Poptani H, Delikatny EJ, et al. NMR metabolic and physiological markers of therapeutic response. Adv Exp Med Biol 2011;701:129–35.

83. Weissleder R, Elizondo G, Wittenberg J, et al. Ultrasmall superparamagnetic iron oxide: an intravenous contrast agent for assessing lymph nodes with MR imaging. Radiology 1990;175(2):494–8.

84. Will O, Purkayastha S, Chan C, et al. Diagnostic precision of nanoparticle-enhanced MRI for lymph-node metastases: a meta-analysis. Lancet Oncol 2006;7(1):52–60.

85. Senéterre E, Weissleder R, Jaramillo D, et al. Bone marrow: ultrasmall superparamagnetic iron oxide for MR imaging. Radiology 1991;179(2):529–33.

86. Oktar SO, Yücel C, Ozdemir H, et al. Comparison of conventional sonography, real-time compound sonography, tissue harmonic sonography, and tissue harmonic compound sonography of abdominal and pelvic lesions. AJR Am J Roentgenol 2003;181(5):1341–7.

87. Picardi M, Soricelli A, Pane F, et al. Contrast-enhanced harmonic compound US of the spleen to increase staging accuracy in patients with Hodgkin lymphoma: a prospective study. Radiology 2009;251(2):574–82.

88. Görg C, Faoro C, Bert T, et al. Contrast enhanced ultrasound of splenic lymphoma involvement. Eur J Radiol 2011;80(2):169–74.

FDG-PET in Lymphoma: Nuclear Medicine Perspective

Juliano Julio Cerci, MD, PhD[a,b,*], Lucia Zanoni, MD[c],
José C. Meneghetti, MD, PhD[b], Stefano Fanti, MD, PhD[c]

KEYWORDS

- Positron emission tomography • ^{18}F-Fluorodeoxyglucose
- Lymphoma • Staging

PET is a sectional molecular imaging procedure that allows evaluation of the metabolism at a molecular and cellular level. For a PET scan, the patient is injected with a radiotracer, such as ^{18}F-fluorodeoxyglucose (FDG). Based on Warburg's observations, the increased glucose metabolism of malignant cells is the rationale behind common use of the glucose analog FDG as a radiotracer in PET oncologic studies. Tumor cells present increased glucose uptake through increased expression of glucose transporters on the cell surface and upregulation of hexokinase production and activity. The uptake of the tracer FDG is similarly enhanced by cell membrane transporters, and then trapped within the cell by phosphorylation.

The PET scanner is composed of an array of detectors that detect radiation emitted by the radiotracer. Using these signals, the PET scanner detects the amount of metabolic activity while a computer reassembles the signals into images. The metabolism might be quantified by the standardized uptake value (SUV), which represents an estimate of the relative concentration of the tracer in the structure of interest compared with the average throughout the entire body.

Although the incidence of Hodgkin lymphoma (HL) and non-Hodgkin lymphoma (NHL) is only 8% of all malignancies, they are potentially curable. The extent of the disease is the most important factor in the definition of treatment.[1–4] Paul[2] presented the first study of PET in patients with lymphoma in 1987, demonstrating FDG-avid lesions in four of five patients with NHL using a conventional scynthigraphy gamma camera. Early PET studies by Okada and colleagues[5,6] showed the correlation between FDG uptake, the malignancy grade, and proliferative activity in lymphomas: the higher grade of lymphoma, the higher uptake of FDG. Lapela and coworkers[7] and Rodriguez and coworkers[8] later confirmed this demonstrating the correlation between FDG uptake and the malignancy grade. Newman and colleagues[9] investigated a mixed population of five patients with HL and 11 patients with NHL, confirming the excellent accuracy of FDG-PET for imaging NHL and HL, showing that PET detected all disease sites seen at computerized tomography (CT) in all five patients with HL. All of these early studies were performed on a relatively small number of patients with NHL.

In 2005, Schöder and colleagues[10] evaluated in 97 patients with NHL if the intensity of FDG uptake measured using the SUV could differentiate between indolent and aggressive NHL. They concluded that the SUV is lower in indolent than

Disclosure statement: The authors have no conflict of interest.
[a] Quanta – Diagnóstico Nuclear, R. Almirante Tamadaré, 1000, CEP 80045-170, Curitiba, Brazil
[b] Heart Institute (InCor), University of São Paulo Medical School, Av. Dr Enéas de Carvalho Aguiar, 44 - 05403-900, São Paulo, Brazil
[c] Policlinico S. Orsola, University of Bologna, Azienda Ospedaliero-Universitaria di Bologna Policlinico S. Orsola-Malpighi, Via Massarenti, 9, 40138 Bologna, Italy
* Corresponding author. Division of PET/CT, Quanta – Diagnóstico Nuclear, R. Almirante Tamadaré, 1000, CEP 80045-170, Curitiba (PR), Brazil.
E-mail address: cercijuliano@hotmail.com

PET Clin 7 (2012) 21–33
doi:10.1016/j.cpet.2011.12.001

in aggressive NHL, that patients with an SUV greater than 10 have a high likelihood of aggressive NHL, and that this information may be helpful if there is discordance between biopsy and clinical behavior. These findings might be helpful when suspecting cell transformation from indolent to aggressive subtypes, and clearly have implications in prognosis. However, similar to those previous studies, there is a considerable overlap in the SUVs between indolent and aggressive NHL, with a relatively wide range of SUVs observed even within the same histologic subtype.

FDG-PET frequently detected nodal and extranodal disease sites that were missed by conventional staging methods, including CT, and improved the characterization of lesions that were equivocal on other types of imaging. Taking that into account, in the last two decades FDG-PET and now more routinely combined PET and CT (PET-CT) have been introduced into major steps of lymphoma management including initial staging, posttherapy evaluation, interim treatment monitoring, and restaging in suspected relapse.[11–18] The advantage of combined PET-CT scanning with its better disease localization and attenuation correction is now reflected by the widespread adoption of this combined modality scanning.

INITIAL STAGING

A precise staging of patients with lymphoma is essential for selection of appropriate treatment and determining prognosis. Since 1970, staging of lymphoma has been based on the Ann Arbor classification.[19] In 1989, these criteria were modified.[20] Conventional staging procedures include a physical examination, CT, and a bone marrow biopsy (BMB). Although CT provides important anatomic details, it cannot reliably distinguish between malignant and benign lesions because the definition of nodal or organ involvement is based only on morphologic criteria (Fig. 1). The correlation of CT findings with pathologic staging demonstrated that the size of the lymph nodes was not always associated with the presence of lymphomatous involvement. In addition, CT has a limited sensitivity for the detection of extranodal disease including splenic, hepatic, and bone marrow involvement. Therefore, the clinical staging

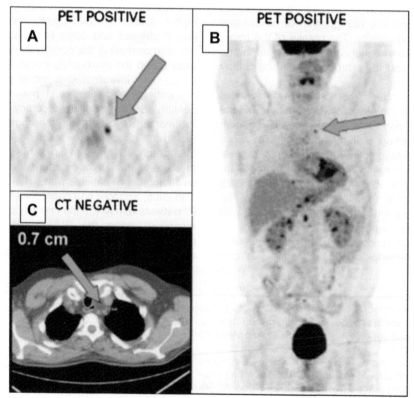

Fig. 1. (A, B) Hypermetabolic superoanterior mediastinal lymph node (arrow) related to lymphomatous disease. (C) The small diameter (0.7 mm) does not reach morphologic CT criteria for positivity confirming PET scan's major accuracy.

of patients may be underestimated and thus lead to inappropriate therapy, or clinical staging may overestimate the severity and lead to overtreatment. CT and ^{67}Ga in initial staging imaging have several limitations in determining lymphomatous disease. FDG-PET has a higher diagnostic sensitivity and accuracy for the detection of lymph nodes and also extranodal disease.[9,21–24] Taking this into account, several studies showed that FDG-PET presents a higher accuracy than CT in the clinical staging definition.[11–16,25]

BMB is the standard procedure for depicting bone marrow involvement; however, it explores only a limited part of the bone marrow. A meta-analysis involving a mixed population of different lymphoma showed distinct patterns of bone marrow infiltration and FDG avidity according to histologic type, with a good correlation of FDG-PET results and BMB in the detection of bone marrow involvement in patients with malignant lymphoma.[26] However, Moulin-Romsee and colleagues[27] retrospectively evaluated 83 patients with newly diagnosed HL; of those, seven had lymphomatous involvement on BMB. All patients with bone and bone marrow lesions at conventional staging were also diagnosed on FDG PET-CT scan. Nonetheless, PET-CT depicted FDG-avid bone and bone marrow foci in nine additional patients. Cerci and coworkers[25] evaluated FDG-PET in initial staging in 210 patients with HL; FDG-PET failed to identify only two patients with a positive BMB. However, 12 patients presented commitment of bone and bone marrow by PET with negative results in the BMB, with only two of these discordant cases considered as a false-positive FDG-PET. Further studies are necessary to clarify these differences in literature results.

From a practical standpoint of defining treatment, the detection of more affected sites is relevant only when it modifies the clinical stage of disease. FDG-PET in initial staging results in considerable modification in stage of disease compared with conventional staging, most commonly upstaging patients. In the published series,[28–32] FDG-PET changes stage in 10% to 40% of patients with NHL, leading to a change in treatment strategy in approximately half. Clearly, FDG-PET upstages more patients than it downstages. The impact of this upstaging reflects the "Will Rogers phenomenon," with anticipated improved treatment for patients using PET-CT–defined staging at diagnosis.[33]

A recent meta-analysis included 20 studies to evaluate the diagnostic performance of FDG-PET in the staging of patients with lymphoma.[34] The median sensitivity was 90.3% and the median specificity was 91.1%. The pooled sensitivity was 90.9% (95% confidence interval [CI]) and the pooled false-positive rate was 10.3%. The pooled sensitivity and false-positive rate seemed to be higher in patients with Hodgkin disease compared with those with NHL. Also, 14.5% of patients with HL were upstaged by PET (range, 11%–55%) and 7% downstaged (range, 0%–28%), with change in treatment strategy in a median of 14% of patients (range, 0%–25%).

For the heterogeneous group of low-grade or indolent lymphomas, there have been greater variations in the reported specificity and sensitivity and the reported impact on staging and treatment strategy, but the results are generally encouraging; FDG-PET seems to be a valuable addition to existing staging tools. For the staging of indolent lymphomas, FDG PET-CT is still used more sporadically.[35]

A major drawback of all studies that analyze FDG-PET in the initial staging of lymphoma is the absence of a histologic confirmation of all the FDG-avid lesions, which then requires the use of a reference standard instead of the gold standard. Concordant findings on PET and CT usually are regarded as either true-positive or true-negative. This is one limitation, because CT and PET can provide concordant false results. This approach biases results in favor of the least specific test, making it seem to be more accurate.

Because of possibility of false-positive results, when a PET result determines that treatment modification is recommended, further biopsy is needed in cases of equivocal lesions. However, to date, no study has cross-validated the best treatment based in PET staging. The exact impact of staging with PET and PET-CT in treatment outcome requires further studies.

According to the Revised Response Criteria for Malignant Lymphoma,[36] FDG-PET in the initial staging is not mandatory for assessment of response after treatment of patients with HL, diffuse large B cell lymphoma (DLBCL), follicular lymphoma, or mantle-cell lymphoma because these lymphomas routinely are FDG avid. However, initial staging PET is strongly recommended for these subtypes because it can facilitate the interpretation of posttherapy PET. In contrast, initial staging PET is mandatory for variably FDG-avid lymphomas if PET is planned to be used to assess their response to treatment. These include aggressive NHL subtypes, such as T-cell lymphomas, and all subtypes of indolent NHL other than follicular lymphoma, such as extranodal marginal zone lymphoma of mucosa associated lymphoid tissue and small lymphocytic lymphoma reportedly exhibiting modest FDG avidity (**Fig. 2**).[10,37,38] If PET is to be used for response assessment of patients with these histologic subtypes, there needs to be documentation that PET was positive at all disease sites greater than 1.5 cm in diameter noted by CT.

Very few studies have evaluated costs and accuracy of FDG-PET initial staging. Klose and coworkers[39] investigated the inclusion of FDG-PET in a mixed population of 20 malignant patients with lymphoma. The incremental cost-effective ratio was €3100 per patient for PET compared with CT, considered within an acceptable range. Cerci and coworkers[40] found that the incremental cost-effective ratio of PET-CT in initial and at the end of treatment was very cost effective. Also,

PET-CT costs in initial and in the end of treatment increase only 2% of total costs of HL staging and first-line treatment.

In the staging of lymphoma, PET can provide complementary information to conventional procedures, such as CT and BMB, with potential modification of stage (usually upstaging) and impact on management. There are data that suggest that the number of patients for whom PET alters stage sufficiently to alter therapy is smaller.

FDG-PET IN END-TREATMENT RESPONSE ASSESSMENT

Response assessment is an important guide in decisions regarding therapy and also carries

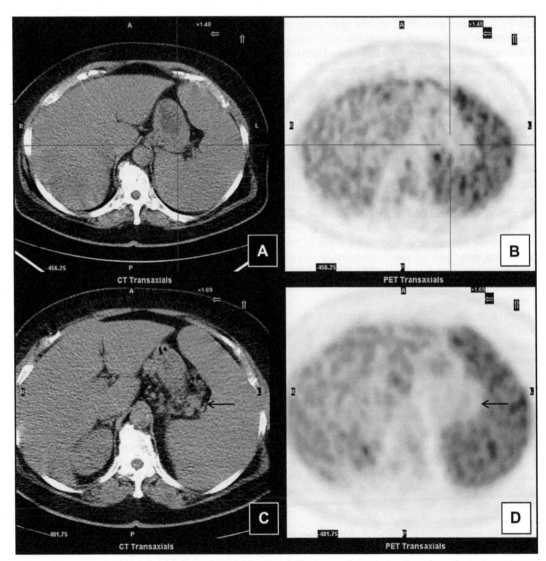

Fig. 2. False-negative PET case in mantle cell lymphoma of the stomach (*cross* in A) with pathologic perigastric adenopathies (*arrow* in C), non–FDG-avid (*cross* in B, *arrow* in D).

important information regarding overall survival and event-free survival (EFS). Before 1999, response assessment for lymphomas varied widely including the criteria of the size of a normal lymph node, the time and frequency assessment was made, the methods used to assess response, and the percentage increase required for disease progression. It is known that even relatively small differences in the definition of normal size of a lymph node can have a major impact on response rates.[41] In 1999, an international working group of clinicians, radiologists, and pathologists with expertise in the evaluation and management of patients with NHL published guidelines for response assessment.[42] These criteria were based mainly on morphologic changes, with a reduction in tumor size on CT being the most important factor, and were rapidly incorporated into clinician practice and also used in the approval process for a number of new modalities of therapy. However, these criteria were subject to considerable interobserver and intraobserver variation and several points were subject to misinterpretation, notably the application of the "complete remission unconfirmed" category. Assessing response by measuring the change in tumor volume on CT is limited because reduction in size alone is not a reliable sign of treatment effectivenes.[43]

Approximately two-thirds of patients with HL patients present residual mass after first treatment and 40% are considered in partial remission. However, CT is generally unable to differentiate between viable tumor and fibrosis in residual masses with a very poor positive predictive value.[44–49] The advantage of PET over anatomic imaging techniques, such as CT or magnetic resonance imaging, is its ability to distinguish between viable tumor and necrosis or fibrosis in residual masses. FDG-PET has the ability, at least to some extent, to distinguish between viable lymphoma cells and necrosis or fibrosis in residual masses after treatment (**Figs. 3–5**).

In the meta-analysis of Zijlstra and colleagues,[50] even though several methodologic deficiencies were identified, the study results consistently show that FDG-PET has a very high specificity in this setting for a pooled sensitivity (vs the gold standard of tumor-positive biopsy and clinical follow-up of at least 1 year) for HL and in aggressive NHL. Pooled sensitivity and specificity for detection of residual disease in HL were 84% (95% CI, 71%–92%) and 90% (95% CI, 84%–94%), respectively. For NHL, pooled sensitivity and specificity were 72% (95% CI, 61%–82%) and 100% (95% CI, 97%–100%), respectively. FDG-PET showed reasonable sensitivity and high specificity for evaluation of first-line therapy in HL and in aggressive NHL. FDG-PET is now the noninvasive imaging technique of choice for the detection of residual disease after treatment,[51] consistently shown to have a very high negative predictive value, over 90%, and exceeding 80% in virtually all reported studies.[13,30,52] However, false-positive results might occur, mainly because of inflammatory or infectious disease. Castellucci and colleagues[53] in a study of 1000 consecutive PET scans in patients with lymphoma demonstrated a 3% prevalence of false-positive PET results. Because of the false-positive results, FDG-positive lesions need to be confirmed by biopsy.

Kobe and coworkers[54] evaluated FDG-PET results of 311 patients with HL with residual mass measuring greater than or equal to 2.5 cm in diameter after bleomycin, etoposide, adriamicyn, cyclophosphamide, vincristin, procarbazine, prednisone

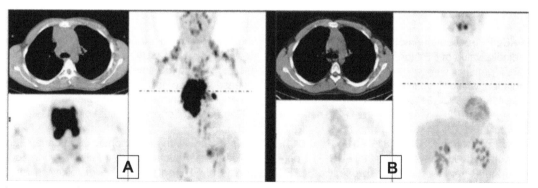

Fig. 3. Transaxial CT, transaxial PET, and maximum intensity projection images, respectively. (*A*) Staging scan of a patient affected by nodular sclerosis HL with supradiaphragmatic and subdiaphragmatic adenopathies (stage III) showing in particular pathologic uptake at the level of a mediastinal bulky and fisiologic brown fat uptake in cervical supraclavicular chain region. (*B*) End-treatment scan. Evidence of residual tissue in the anterior mediastinum at CT correction images showing complete metabolic response to therapy at PET images.

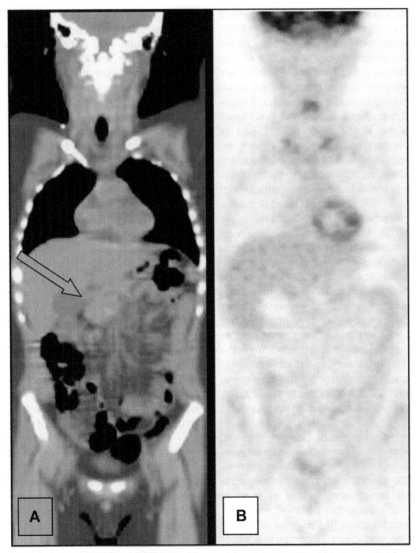

Fig. 4. Coronal CT (*A*) and PET (*B*) images of a patient treated for abdominal Burkitt disease. Evidence of a residual mass in the abdomen (*arrow*) without any pathologic uptake of FDG.

(BEACOPP)-based chemotherapy. The negative predictive value of PET (defined as the proportion of PET patients without progression, relapse, or irradiation within 1 year after PET review panel) was 94% (95% CI, 91%–97%). The progression-free survival (PFS) was 96% for PET-negative patients (95% CI, 94%–99%) and 86% for PET-positive patients (95% CI, 78%–95%; $P = .011$). Many other studies have shown that FDG-PET performed after treatment is highly predictive of PFS and overall survival in HL and aggressive NHL with or without residual masses on CT.[16,17,48,55–78]

The impact of FDG-PET is less clear for indolent NHL, but recent articles reported a clear correlation between posttherapy FDG-PET results and

short-term clinical outcomes.[79,80] Semiquantitative analysis with SUV is not superior to visual assessment to detect the presence of residual disease and so far cannot reliably differentiate between lymphoma and inflammation.[40,62]

Regarding economic evaluations of healthcare technologies, and cost-effectiveness of PET in patients with lymphoma, Remonnay and colleagues[81] evaluated the clinical and cost effects of PET on the choice of following radiotherapy (RT) treatment in 97 stage I and II patients with HL and 112 unresectable non–small cell lung cancer, two treatment decisions made on the basis of only CT or CT associated with PET. Treatment changes were defined as modification of the

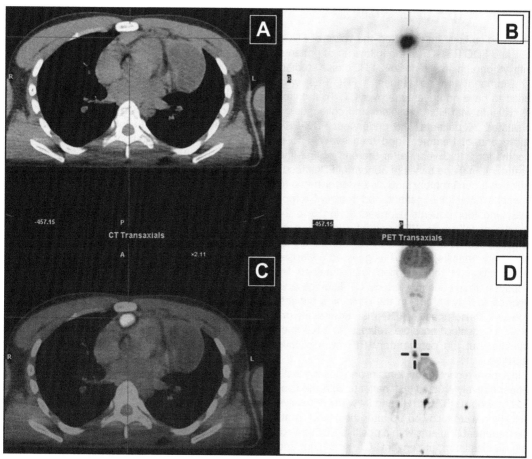

Fig. 5. End-treatment scan of a patient affected by a composite lymphoma (NHL and HL). Evidence of hypermetabolic activity (*B*) PET transaxial, (*C*) fused PET-CT transaxial, (*D*) MIP at the level of a residual tissue in the anterior mediastinum, and (*A*) CT transaxial (*cross sign*) related to persistence of disease.

target volume and the dose to be delivered, or even RT cancellation. The costs of new tests and the costs and savings associated with changes in the chosen treatment were calculated on the basis of reimbursement rates. With a PET cost of approximately €800 per patient, RT treatments were modified in 10% of patients with HL. Overall, the use of PET induced increase of €931 in the mean cost per stage I and II patients with HL. However, PET might be more beneficial for stages III and IV, because the disease is more progressive and therapeutic uncertainties may have more serious consequences than in stages I and II. Unfortunately, these stages were not included in the study because of the heterogeneity of practices among the participating centers. Also, the impact of RT changes on patients' health in the medium to long term was not evaluated.

Cerci and colleagues[40] in a prospective study, sponsored by the Health Ministry of Brazil, investi-

gated the healthcare costs of including FDG-PET imaging in the evaluation of patients with HL with unconfirmed complete remission or partial remission after first-line therapy. Of the 127 patients evaluated after first-line therapy, complete and partial remission was observed in 50 patients; FDG-PET demonstrated 95.9% accuracy in this scenario, compared with 77.7% of CT. The restaging costs strategy with CT in all patients and also PET in complete and partial remission patients showed 19% decrease in costs in relation to the restaging without PET, mainly related to saving patients from further biopsies and hospital procedures, with incremental cost-effectiveness ratio of $3268. PET costs represented only 1% of total costs of HL first-line treatment including restaging procedures. The authors concluded that from clinical and economic points of view, FDG-PET should be included in public and private healthcare programs in Brazil because of its cost-effective profile.

PET FOR FOLLOW-UP OF LYMPHOMA

Few studies have investigated the value of FDG-PET and FDG PET-CT in the follow-up of patients with lymphoma. In a series of 21 HL cases studied by Dittmann and colleagues,[62] FDG-PET was found to have no advantage over CT. To monitor 36 patients with HL, Jerusalem and colleagues[82] evaluated 36 patients who underwent FDG-PET at the end of treatment and then every 4 to 6 months for 2 to 3 years after the end of first-line treatment. In those cases of abnormal FDG accumulation a confirmatory study was performed 4 to 6 weeks later. One patient had residual tumor cells, and four patients relapsed during 5 to 24 months of follow-up. PET correctly identified all five relapses before clinical symptoms or signs, laboratory results, or CT-suggested relapse. Confirmation of the relapses was obtained by biopsy in four patients and by CT findings and clear clinical symptoms in the remaining patient. However, false-positive FDG-PET studies incorrectly suggested possible relapse in six other patients, but the confirmatory PET was always negative.

In a more recent study, Zinzani and colleagues[83] retrospectively studied 151 patients with mediastinal lymphoma (57 with HL and 94 with aggressive NHL) who were followed-up after the end of front-line treatment. Patients with a positive PET scan of the mediastinum underwent CT scanning and surgical biopsy. The follow-up program for each patient included FDG-PET every 6 months for the first 2 years and then every 12 months for a further 3 years, along with standard follow-up procedures. In 30 of 151 patients (21 HL and 9 NHL) a suspicion of lymphoma relapse was raised based on positive mediastinal PET scanning. Histology confirmed this suspicion in 17 (10 HL and 7 NHL) out of 30 patients (57%), whereas either benign (nine fibrosis and three sarcoid-like granulomatosis) or unrelated neoplastic conditions (one thymoma) were demonstrated in the remaining 13 patients (43%). They concluded that a positive PET in the mediastinum of a patient followed-up for a mediastinal lymphoma (hence after front-line treatment) should not be considered sufficient for final diagnostic purposes and that histologic confirmation should always be made.

More studies should be performed with the purpose of evaluating the role for FDG-PET in the detection of preclinical relapse, theoretically allowing patients to enter salvage therapy with minimal disease rather than overt relapse. It is also important to analyze the cost-effectiveness of FDG-PET in the follow-up setting.

PET FOR RESPONSE PREDICTION BEFORE HIGH-DOSE SALVAGE THERAPY

Despite progress in the treatment of lymphoma, considerable proportions of patients remain refractory to or relapse after standard first-line chemotherapy. These patients should receive salvage chemotherapy followed by high-dose consolidation chemotherapy with autologous hematopoietic stem cell transplantation (ASCT).[84] Moreover, relapse after high-dose therapy is not uncommon and is associated with substantial short-term morbidity and mortality. Therefore, it is important to identify prognostic factors to guide risk-oriented management.

For the past two decades, response to salvage therapy was determined by CT imaging and transplant eligibility was based on CT-defined response.[20] It is currently standard practice to proceed to transplantation with the presence of chemosensitive disease. Several studies have recently evaluated the prognostic value of FDG-PET when performed between salvage and consolidation high-dose therapy with stem cell transplantation. Terasawa and coworkers[85] published a systematic review and meta-analysis of the scientific literature from inception through January 2010. The eligible studies numbered 12 including a total of 630 patients. FDG-PET had a summary sensitivity of 0.69 (range, 0.56–0.81) and specificity of 0.81 (range, 0.73–0.87). Moreover, a positive scan was significantly associated with a shorter PFS interval. There is some evidence that PET may be a good replacement for CT-based conventional restaging for identifying patients most likely to fail in this invasive and costly treatment (**Fig. 6**). Moskowitz and colleagues[86] confirmed a poor outcome for functional imaging-positive patients with HL with a median EFS of 11 months and 5-year EFS of 31% (vs 75% in patients who were PET-negative). The status before ASCT was the only factor significant for EFS and overall survival by multivariate analysis. Similar results were provided by the cohort of Smeltzer and colleagues[87] (3-year EFS 41% vs 82% and 3-year overall survival 64% vs 91% in FDG-PET–positive and –negative group, respectively).

For patients who are chemoresistant, additional alternative regimens to cytoreduce disease burden and obtain a negative FDG-PET pre-ASCT or additional maintenance therapy after-ASCT may be required to improve long-term outcomes.[88] PET seemed to be useful for selecting those patients eligible for novel consolidation strategies after salvage therapies.[89] This topic is definitely less relevant for indolent subtypes and, at present,

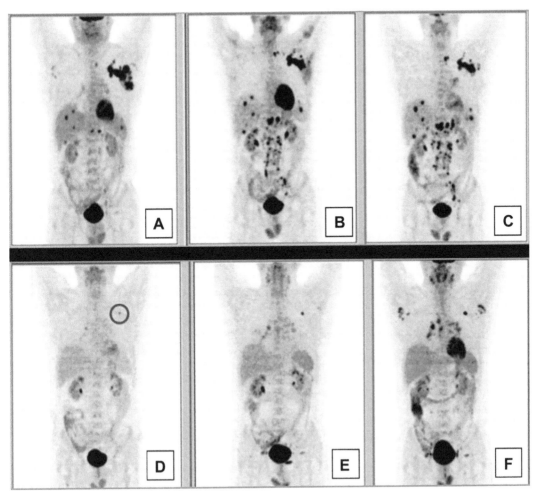

Fig. 6. Consecutive PET scans of a patient affected by aggressive NHL, stage IV (supradiaphragmatic and subdiaphragmatic adenopathies, spleen and liver). (A) Staging. The patient presented treatment failure to first-line standard therapy showing progressive disease at interim (B) and end-treatment (C) evaluation. The persistence of a hypermetabolic finding at pretransplant scanning (circle in D) represents a strong predictor of poor outcome. Indeed, the patient revealed early progression after transplant (E) and worsened in 3 months (F).

follow-up periods are too short to evaluate their PFS.

Limited studies[90] have evaluated posttransplant FDG-PET scans as correlated to outcome. Patients with positive results would likely be candidates for early intervention including ASCT.[91]

However, there are only studies with small sample size resulting in imprecise estimates of the test's prognostic value, particularly with respect to specific lymphoma subtypes other than DLBCL and classical HL. Literature is clinically and methodologically heterogeneous including different treatment settings, regimens, imaging technologies, and PET interpretation criteria. Prospective studies with standardized methodologies are needed to confirm and refine these promising results.

SUMMARY

FDG PET-CT has become an established modality for metabolic staging and plays an important role in the major steps of evaluation and treatment of most lymphoma subtypes, with significant impact in the initial staging, posttherapy evaluation, and suspect of relapse of disease. However, whenever the information of PET results is translated to changing treatment, especially in cases of further treatment, biopsy confirmation should always be made when possible.

REFERENCES

1. Warburg O. Über den stoffwechsel der tumoren: arbeiten aus dem kaiser wilhelm-institut für biologie, berlin-dahlem. Berlin: Springer; 1926.

2. Paul R. Comparison of fluorine-18-2-fluorodeoxy-glucose and gallium-67 citrate imaging for detection of lymphoma. J Nucl Med 1987;28:288–92.

3. Joth G, Bonadonna G. Prognostic factors in Hodgkin's disease: implications for modern treatment. Anticancer Res 1988;8:749–60.

4. Leskinen-Kallio S, Ruotsalainen U, Nagren K, et al. Uptake of carbon-11-methionine and fluorodeoxy-glucose in non-Hodgkin's lymphoma: a PET study. J Nucl Med 1991;32:1211–8.

5. Okada J, Yoshikawa K, Imazeki K, et al. The use of FDG-PET in the detection and management of malignant lymphoma: correlation of uptake with prognosis. J Nucl Med 1991;32:686–91.

6. Okada J, Yoshikawa K, Itami M, et al. Positron emission tomography using fluorine-18-fluorode-oxyglucose in malignant lymphoma: a comparison with proliferative activity. J Nucl Med 1992;33: 325–9.

7. Lapela M, Leskinen S, Minn HR, et al. Increased glucose metabolism in untreated non-Hodgkin's lymphoma: a study with positron emission tomog-raphy and fluorine-18-fluorodeoxyglucose. Blood 1995;86:3522–7.

8. Rodriguez M, Rehn S, Ahlstrom H, et al. Predicting malignancy grade with PET in non-Hodgkin's lymphoma. J Nucl Med 1995;36:1790–6.

9. Newman JS, Francis IR, Kaminski MS, et al. Imaging of lymphoma with PET with 2-[F-18]-fluoro-2-deoxy-d-glucose: correlation with CT. Radiology 1994;190: 111–6.

10. Schöder H, Noy A, Gonen M, et al. Intensity of 18-flurorodeoxyglucose uptake in PET distinguishes between indolent and aggressive non-Hodgkin's lymphomas. J Clin Oncol 2005;23:4643–51.

11. Hoh CK, Gaspy J, Rosen P, et al. Whole body FDG-PET imaging for staging of Hodgkin's disease and lymphoma. J Nucl Med 1997;38:343–8.

12. Moog F, Bangerter M, Diedrichs CG, et al. Lymphoma: role of whole-body 2-deoxy-2-[F-18]flu-oro-D-glucose (FDG) PET in nodal staging. Radi-ology 1997;203:795–800.

13. Moog F, Bangerter M, Diedrichs CG, et al. Extrano-dal malignant lymphoma: detection with FDG-PET versus CT. Radiology 1998;206:475–81.

14. Carr R, Barrington SF, Madan B, et al. Detection of lymphoma in bone marrow by whole-body positron emission tomography. Blood 1998;91:3340–6.

15. Moog F, Bangerter M, Kotzerke J, et al. 18-F-fluoro-deoxyglucose-positron emission tomography as a new approach to detect lymphomatous bone marrow. J Clin Oncol 1998;16:603–9.

16. Stumpe KD, Urbinelli M, Steinert HC, et al. Whole-body positron emission tomography using fluorodeoxyglucose for staging of lymphoma: effec-tiveness and comparison with computed tomog-raphy. Eur J Nucl Med 1998;25:721–8.

17. de Wit M, Bumann D, Beyer W, et al. Whole-body positron emission tomography (PET) for diagnosis of residual mass in patients with lymphoma. Ann On-col 1997;8(Suppl 1):57–60.

18. Romer W, Hanauske AR, Ziegler S, et al. Positron emission tomography in non-Hodgkin's lymphoma: assessment of chemotherapy with fluorodeoxyglu-cose. Blood 1998;91:4464–71.

19. Carbone PP, Kaplan HS, Musshoff K, et al. Report of the committee on Hodgkin's disease staging classi-fication. Cancer Res 1971;31:1860–1.

20. Lister TA, Crowther D, Sutcliffe SB, et al. Report of a committee convened to discuss the evalua-tion and staging of patients with Hodgkin's dis-ease: Cotswold meeting. J Clin Oncol 1989;7: 1630–6.

21. Castellino RA, Blank N, Hoppe RT, et al. Hodgkin's disease: contribution of chest CT in the initial staging evaluation. Radiology 1986;160:603–5.

22. Neumann CH, Robert NJ, Canellos G, et al. Computed tomography of the abdomen and pelvis in non-Hodgkin lymphoma. J Comput Assist Tomogr 1983;7:846–50.

23. Munker R, Stengel A, Stabler A, et al. Diagnostic accuracy of ultrasound and computed tomography in the staging of Hodgkin's disease. Cancer 1995; 76:1460–6.

24. Front D, Bar-Shalom R, Epelbaum R, et al. Early detection of lymphoma recurrence with gallium-67 scintigraphy. J Nucl Med 1993;34:2101–4.

25. Cerci JJ, Pracchia LF, Soares Junior J, et al. Positron emission tomography with 2-[18F]-fluoro-2-deoxy-D-glucose for initial staging of hodgkin lymphoma: a single center experience in Brazil. Clinics (Sao Paulo) 2009;64(6):491–8.

26. Pakos EE, Fotopoulos AD, Ioannidis JP. 18F-FDG PET for evaluation of bone marrow infiltration in staging of lymphoma: a meta-analysis. J Nucl Med 2005;46:958–63.

27. Moulin-Romsee G, Hindié E, Moretti JL. (18)F-FDG PET/CT bone/bone marrow findings in Hodgkin's lymphoma may circumvent the use of bone marrow trephine biopsy at diagnosis staging. Eur J Nucl Med Mol Imaging 2010;37(6):1095–105.

28. Buchmann I, Reinhardt M, Elsner K, et al. 2-(Fluo-rine-18)fluoro-2-deoxy-D-glucose positron emission tomography in the detection and staging of malig-nant lymphoma. A bicenter trial. Cancer 2001;91: 889–99.

29. Hutchings M, Eigtved AI, Specht L. FDG-PET in the clinical management of Hodgkin lymphoma. Crit Rev Oncol Hematol 2004;52:19–32.

30. Jerusalem G, Beguin Y, Fassotte MF, et al. Persistent tumor 18F-FDG uptake after a few cycles of poly-chemotherapy is predictive of treatment failure in non-Hodgkin's lymphoma. Haematologica 2000;85: 613–8.

31. Kostakoglu L, Leonard JP, Coleman M, et al. The role of FDG-PET imaging in the management of lymphoma. Clin Adv Hematol Oncol 2004;2:115–21.

32. Weihrauch MR, Re D, Bischoff S, et al. Whole-body positron emission tomography using 18F-fluoro-deoxyglucose for initial staging of patients with Hodgkin's disease. Ann Hematol 2002;81:20–5.

33. Michallet AS, Trotman J, Tychyj-Pinel C. Role of early PET in the management of diffuse large B-cell lymphoma. Curr Opin Oncol 2010;22(5):414–8.

34. Isasi CR, Lu P, Blaufox MD. A metaanalysis of 18F-2-deoxy-2-fluoro-D-glucose positron emission tomography in the staging and restaging of patients with lymphoma. Cancer 2005;104(5):1066–74.

35. Hutchings M, Specht L. PET/CT in the management of haematological malignancies. Eur J Haematol 2008;80:369–80.

36. Juweid ME, Stroobants S, Hoekstra OS, et al. Use of positron emission tomography for response assessment of lymphoma: consensus recommendations of the imaging subcommittee of the International harmonization project in lymphoma. J Clin Oncol 2007;25:571–8.

37. Elstrom R, Guan L, Baker G, et al. Utility of FDG-PET scanning in lymphoma by WHO classification. Blood 2003;101:3875–6.

38. Hoffmann M, Kletter K, Diemling M, et al. Positron emission tomography with fluorine-18-2- fluoro-2-deoxy-D-glucose (F18-FDG) does not visualize extranodal B-cell lymphoma of the mucosa-associated lymphoid tissue (MALT)-type. Ann Oncol 1999;10:1185–9.

39. Klose T, Leidl R, Buchmann I, et al. Primary staging of lymphomas: cost-effectiveness of FDG-PET versus computed tomography. Eur J Nucl Med 2000;27:1457–64.

40. Cerci JJ, Trindade E, Pracchia LF, et al. Cost effectiveness of positron emission tomography in patients with Hodgkin's lymphoma in unconfirmed complete remission or partial remission after first-line therapy. J Clin Oncol 2010;28:1415–21.

41. Grillo-López AJ, Cheson BD, Horning SJ, et al. Response criteria for NHL: importance of "normal" lymph node size and correlations with response rates. Ann Oncol 2000;11:399–408.

42. Cheson BD, Horning SJ, Coiffier B, et al. Report of an international workshop to standardize response criteria for non-Hodgkin's lymphomas. J Clin Oncol 1999;17:1244–53.

43. Castagna L, Bramanti S, Balzarotti M, et al. Predictive value of early 18F-fluorodeoxyglucose positron emission tomography (FDG-PET) during salvage chemotherapy in relapsing/refractory Hodgkin lymphoma (HL) treated with high-dose chemotherapy. Br J Haematol 2009;145:369–72.

44. Oza AM, Ganesan TS, Leahy M, et al. Patterns of survival in patients with Hodgkin's disease: long follow up in a single centre. Ann Oncol 1993;4:385–92.

45. Hasenclever D, Diehl V. A prognostic score for advanced Hodgkin's disease: international prognostic factors project on advanced Hodgkin's disease. N Engl J Med 1998;339:1506–14.

46. Juweid ME, Cheson BD. Role of positron emission tomography in lymphoma. J Clin Oncol 2005;23:4577–80.

47. Juweid ME, Cheson BD. Positron emission tomography and assessment of cancer therapy. N Engl J Med 2006;354:496–507.

48. Canellos GP. Residual mass in lymphoma may not be residual disease. J Clin Oncol 1988;6:931–3.

49. Jerusalem G, Beguin Y, Fassotte MF, et al. Whole-body positron emission tomography using 18Ffluorodeoxyglucose for posttreatment evaluation in Hodgkin's disease and non-Hodgkin's lymphoma has higher diagnostic and prognostic value than classical computed tomography scan imaging. Blood 1999;94:429–33.

50. Zijlstra JM, Lindauer-van der Werf G, Hoekstra OS, et al. 18F-fluoro-deoxyglucose positron emission tomography for post-treatment evaluation of malignant lymphoma: a systematic review. Haematologica 2006;91:522–9.

51. Jerusalem G, Hustinx R, Beguin Y, et al. Evaluation of therapy for lymphoma. Semin Nucl Med 2005;35:186–96.

52. Poulou LS, Karianakis G, Ziakas PD. FDG PET scan strategies and long-term outcomes after first-line therapy in Hodgkin's disease. Eur J Radiol 2009;70(3):499–506.

53. Castellucci P, Nanni C, Farsad M, et al. Potential pitfalls of 18F-FDG PET in a large series of patients treated for malignant lymphoma: prevalence and scan interpretation. Nucl Med Commun 2005;26:689–94.

54. Lister TA, Crowther D, Sutcliffe SB, et al. Report of a committee convened to discuss the evaluation and staging of patients with Hodgkin's disease: Cotswolds meeting. J Clin Oncol 1989;7:1630–6.

55. Bangerter M, Kotzerke J, Griesshammer M, et al. Positron emission tomography with 18-fluorodeoxyglucose in the staging and follow-up of lymphoma in the chest. Acta Oncol 1999;38:799–804.

56. Juweid ME, Wiseman GA, Vose JM, et al. Response assessment of aggressive non-Hodgkin's lymphoma by integrated international workshop criteria and fluorine-18-fluorodeoxyglucose positron emission tomography. J Clin Oncol 2005;23:4652–61.

57. Becherer A, Jaeger U, Szabo M, et al. Prognostic value of FDG-PET in malignant lymphoma. Q J Nucl Med 2003;47:14–21.

58. Brepoels L, Stroobants S, Verhoef G. PET and PET/CT for response evaluation in lymphoma: current practice and developments. Leuk Lymphoma 2007;48:270–82.

59. Cremerius U, Fabry U, Neuerburg J, et al. Positron emission tomography with ^{18}F-FDG to detect residual disease after therapy for malignant lymphoma. Nucl Med Commun 1998;19:1055–63.

60. de Wit M, Bohuslavizki KH, Buchert R, et al. [18]FDG-PET following treatment as valid predictor for disease-free survival in Hodgkin's lymphoma. Ann Oncol 2001;12:29–37.

61. Freudenberg LS, Antoch G, Schutt P, et al. FDG-PET/CT in re-staging of patients with lymphoma. Eur J Nucl Med Mol Imaging 2004;31:325–9.

62. Dittmann H, Sokler M, Kollmannsberger C, et al. Comparison of [18]FDG-PET with CT scans in the evaluation of patients with residual and recurrent Hodgkin's lymphoma. Oncol Rep 2001;8:1393–9.

63. Guay C, Lepine M, Verreault J, et al. Prognostic value of PET using ^{18}F-FDG in Hodgkin's disease for posttreatment evaluation. J Nucl Med 2003;44: 1225–31.

64. Hueltenschmidt B, Sautter-Bihl ML, Lang O, et al. Whole body positron emission tomography in the treatment of Hodgkin disease. Cancer 2001;91: 302–10.

65. Jerusalem G, Warland V, Najjar F, et al. Whole-body ^{18}F-FDG PET for the evaluation of patients with Hodgkin's disease and non-Hodgkin's lymphoma. Nucl Med Commun 1999;20:13–20.

66. Kazama T, Faria SC, Varavithya V, et al. FDG PET in the evaluation of treatment for lymphoma: clinical usefulness and pitfalls. Radiographics 2005;25: 191–207.

67. Lang O, Bihl H, Hultenschmidt B, et al. Clinical relevance of positron emission tomography (PET) in treatment control and relapse of Hodgkin's disease. Strahlenther Onkol 2001;177:138–44.

68. Maisey NR, Hill ME, Webb A, et al. Are [18]fluorodeoxyglucose positron emission tomography and magnetic resonance imaging useful in the prediction of relapse in lymphoma residual masses? Eur J Cancer 2000;36:200–6.

69. Lavely WC, Delbeke D, Greer JP, et al. FDG PET in the follow-up management of patients with newly diagnosed Hodgkin and non-Hodgkin lymphoma after first-line chemotherapy. Int J Radiat Oncol Biol Phys 2003;57:307–15.

70. Mikhaeel NG, Timothy AR, Hain SF, et al. 18-FDG-PET for the assessment of residual masses on CT following treatment of lymphomas. Ann Oncol 2000;11(Suppl 1):147–50.

71. Naumann R, Vaic A, Beuthien-Baumann B, et al. Prognostic value of positron emission tomography in the evaluation of post-treatment residual mass in patients with Hodgkin's disease and non-Hodgkin's lymphoma. Br J Haematol 2001;115:793–800.

72. Panizo C, Perez-Salazar M, Bendandi M, et al. Positron emission tomography using ^{18}F-fluorodeoxyglucose for the evaluation of residual Hodgkin's disease mediastinal masses. Leuk Lymphoma 2004;45: 1829–33.

73. Rahmouni A, Luciani A, Itti E. Quantitative CT analysis for assessing response in lymphoma (Cheson's criteria). Cancer Imaging 2005;5(Spec No A): S102–6.

74. Reinhardt MJ, Herkel C, Altehoefer C, et al. Computed tomography and ^{18}F-FDG positron emission tomography for therapy control of Hodgkin's and non-Hodgkin's lymphoma patients: when do we really need FDG-PET? Ann Oncol 2005;16:1524–9.

75. Reske SN. PET and restaging of malignant lymphoma including residual masses and relapse. Eur J Nucl Med Mol Imaging 2003;30(Suppl 1):S89–96.

76. Rigacci L, Castagnoli A, Dini C, et al. [18]FDG-positron emission tomography in post treatment evaluation of residual mass in Hodgkin's lymphoma: long-term results. Oncol Rep 2005;14:1209–14.

77. Spaepen K, Stroobants S, Dupont P, et al. Can positron emission tomography with [^{18}F]-fluorodeoxyglucose after first-line treatment distinguish Hodgkin's disease patients who need additional therapy from others in whom additional therapy would mean avoidable toxicity? Br J Haematol 2001;115:272–8.

78. Spaepen K, Stroobants S, Dupont P, et al. Prognostic value of positron emission tomography (PET) with fluorine-18 fluorodeoxyglucose ([^{18}F] FDG) after first-line chemotherapy in non-Hodgkin's lymphoma: is [^{18}F]FDG-PET a valid alternative to conventional diagnostic methods? J Clin Oncol 2001;19:414–9.

79. Zinzani PL, Musuraca G, Alinari L, et al. Predictive role of positron emission tomography in the outcome of patients with follicular lymphoma. Clin Lymphoma Myeloma 2007;7:291–5.

80. Bishu S, Quigley JM, Bishu SR, et al. Predictive value and diagnostic accuracy of F-18-fluorodeoxy-glucose positron emission tomography treated grade 1 and 2 follicular lymphoma. Leuk Lymphoma 2007;48:1548–55.

81. Remonnay R, Morelle M, Pommier P, et al. Assessing short-term effects and costs at an early stage of innovation: the use of positron emission tomography on radiotherapy treatment decision making. Int J Technol Assess Health Care 2008;24(2):212–20.

82. Jerusalem G, Beguin Y, Fassotte MF, et al. Early detection of relapse by whole-body positron emission tomography in the follow-up of patients with Hodgkin's disease. Ann Oncol 2003;14:123–30.

83. Zinzani PL, Tani M, Trisolini R, et al. Histological verification of positive positron emission tomography findings in the follow-up of patients with mediastinal lymphoma. Haematologica 2007;92: 771–7.

84. Brusamolino E, Bacigalupo A, Barosi G, et al. Classical Hodgkin's lymphoma in adults: guidelines of the Italian Society of Hematology, the Italian Society

of Experimental Hematology, and the Italian Group of Bone Marrow Transplantation on initial work-up, management, and follow-up. Haematologica 2009; 94(4):550–65.

85. Terasawa T, Dahabreh IJ, Nihashi T. 18F-FDG PET in response assessment before high-dose chemotherapy for lymphoma: a systematic review and meta-analysis. Oncologist 2010;15:750–9.

86. Moskowitz AJ, Yahalom J, Kewalramani T, et al. Pre-transplantation functional imaging predicts outcome following autologous stem cell transplantation for relapsed or refractory Hodgkin lymphoma. Blood 2010;116(23):4934–7.

87. Smeltzer JP, Cashen AF, Zhang Q, et al. Prognostic significance of FDG-PET in relapsed or refractory classical Hodgkin lymphoma treated with standard salvage chemotherapy and autologous stem cell transplantation. Biol Blood Marrow Transplant 2011;17(11):1646–52.

88. Moskowitz CH, Yahalom J, Zelenetz AD, et al. High-dose chemo-radiotherapy for relapsed or refractory Hodgkin lymphoma and the significance of pre-transplant functional imaging. Br J Haematol 2010; 148:890–7.

89. Dickinson M, Hoyt R, Roberts AW, et al. Improved survival for relapsed diffuse large B cell lymphoma is predicted by a negative pre-transplant FDG-PET scan following salvage chemotherapy. Br J Haematol 2010;150(1):39–45.

90. Johnston PB, Wiseman GA, Micallef IN. PET using F-18 FDG pre- and post-autologous stem cell transplant in non-Hodgkin's lymphoma. Bone Marrow Transplant 2008;41:919–25.

91. Sucak GT, Özkurt ZN, Suyani E, et al. Early post-transplantation positron emission tomography in patients with Hodgkin lymphoma is an independent prognostic factor with an impact on overall survival. Ann Hematol 2011;90(11):1329–36.

The Evolving Role of Medical Imaging in Lymphoma Management: The Clinician's Perspective

Jakub Svoboda, MD*, Stephen J. Schuster, MD

KEYWORDS

• Lymphoma • Imaging • FDG-PET scan • Management

INTRODUCTION TO LYMPHOMAS

Lymphoma is a general term encompassing a heterogeneous group of hematologic malignancies arising from lymphocytes. The malignant lymphocytes accumulate in lymph nodes, causing enlargement and appearance of solid masses. In some cases, the lymphocytes infiltrate extranodal tissues such as bone marrow and various organs (eg, gastrointestinal tract, lung, skin, central nervous system). Some forms of lymphoma may also involve peripheral blood.

In the United States, it is estimated that about 75,000 patients are diagnosed annually and that 22,000 patients die of lymphoma.[1] Hodgkin lymphoma (HL) accounts for only about 10% of cases and is more common in younger patients.[1] Non-Hodgkin lymphomas (NHLs) are a diverse group of diseases and the incidence increases with age.[1]

The current classification of lymphomas is complex. The diagnosis of lymphoma is based on tissue biopsy, usually by excision of an enlarged lymph node. The pathologic criteria for assigning a specific lymphoma subtype continues to evolve with advances in laboratory techniques and understanding of lymphoma biology. The initial classification systems distinguished between Hodgkin disease (later renamed as HL) and other lymphomas (grouped as NHL).[2,3] These systems were based on the morphology of the tumors and malignant lymphocytes. The most recent World Health Organization (WHO) classification system from 2008 incorporates information about morphology, cell origin (B cell vs T cell/NK cells), immunohistochemical markers, genetic features, and clinical features to define more than 50 lymphoma subtypes.[4] In addition, some lymphomas (eg, follicular) are assigned a grade (1, 2, or 3) depending on the percentage of large malignant cells within a lymph node area.

Once the diagnosis of lymphoma is established by tissue biopsy, the patient undergoes staging to determine the extent of disease. Accurate staging is important for clinicians to assess prognosis and determine optimal management. A unified staging system is also essential for conducting clinical trials and objectively comparing results.

Although staging in solid malignancies often uses the TNM (tumor, nodes, and metastasis) classification system, this is not applicable in most hematological malignancies, including lymphomas. Current lymphoma staging is based on the modified Ann Arbor system, which was originally developed for patients with HL.[5,6] This system has some limitations when applied to patients with NHL, because these lymphomas do not spread in the contiguous fashion characteristic of HL. However, the general principles of staging are identical. Stages I to IV are assigned according to the number and location of lymph node groups involved, the presence or absence of extranodal disease, B symptoms (fevers, night sweats, weight loss), and bulky disease (**Table 1**).

Division of Hematology/Oncology, Department of Medicine, The University of Pennsylvania School of Medicine, Philadelphia, PA 19104, USA
* Corresponding author.
E-mail address: jakub.svoboda@uphs.upenn.edu

PET Clin 7 (2012) 35–46
doi:10.1016/j.cpet.2011.12.004
1556-8598/12/$ – see front matter © 2012 Elsevier Inc. All rights reserved.

Table 1
Lymphoma staging (based on Ann Arbor classification)

Stage	Description
I	Localized disease within a single lymph node region or an involvement of a single extranodal site (IE)[a]
II	Involvement of 2 or more lymph node regions on the same side of the diaphragm with or without involvement of limited, contiguous extranodal site
III	Involvement of lymph node regions on both sides of the diaphragm, which may include the spleen or limited, contiguous extranodal organ
IV	Diffuse involvement of 1 or more extranodal organs or tissue (including bone marrow) with or without associated nodal involvement

Notes: A (absence) or B (presence) of B symptoms including fever greater than 38°C (100.4°F), night sweats, or 10% weight loss.

[a] E designates contiguous extranodal extension that can be encompassed within a radiation field (as opposed to diffuse or disseminated foci of organ involvement).

Data from Lister TA, Crowther D, Sutcliffe SB, et al. Report of a committee convened to discuss the evaluation and staging of patients with Hodgkin's disease: Cotswolds meeting. J Clin Oncol 1989;7(11):1630–6.

Historically, the Ann Arbor staging system for HL recommended that patients undergo pathologic staging that included exploratory laparotomy and splenectomy.[5,6] This invasive surgical intervention was thought to be justified given the poor accuracy of imaging techniques. Because of limited systemic chemotherapy and effective local therapy with radiation at that time, ruling out abdominal disease with certainty by surgical exploration was important.[7,8] With advances in imaging techniques in 1990s, clinical staging based on tissue biopsy, physical examination, radiologic imaging, and usually bone marrow biopsy has been considered sufficient for most patients with lymphoma.[9]

There are prognostic indices for specific lymphomas that help clinicians estimate prognosis at the time of diagnosis. These indices are based on clinical and laboratory factors at presentation and differ slightly for specific subtypes of lymphoma. Examples include the International Prognostic Index (IPI) for diffuse large B-cell lymphoma (DLBCL), the Follicular Lymphoma International Prognostic Index (FLIPI) for follicular lymphoma (FL), and the International Prognostic Score (IPS) for HL.[10–12] These scoring systems have limited accuracy and might not reflect the recent advances in the therapeutic options. New prognostic factors, including results of interim imaging during therapy, are being investigated.[13–15]

Clinically, patients with NHL are divided into 3 groups based on the natural history of the disease: indolent, aggressive, and highly aggressive (**Fig. 1**). Indolent or low-grade lymphomas (eg, grade 1 and 2 FL, marginal zone lymphoma, chronic lymphocytic leukemia/small lymphocytic lymphoma) are usually slow-growing malignancies that can present as asymptomatic lymphadenopathy and might not require treatment for years after diagnosis. Aggressive NHL (eg, DLBCL, peripheral T-cell lymphoma, most forms of mantle cell lymphoma, grade 3 FL) usually present with fast-growing lymphadenopathy (over a period of months or weeks) and are frequently associated with lymphoma-related symptoms such as fevers, night sweats, and weight loss. Highly aggressive

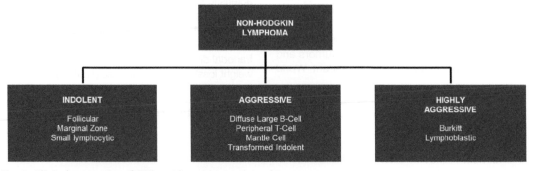

Fig. 1. Clinical categories of NHLs with representative subtypes.

lymphomas, such as Burkitt lymphoma or lympho-blastic lymphoma, usually present with rapidly growing lymphadenopathy and bulky masses that may cause mechanical obstruction of various organs. Treatment of patients with highly aggres-sive lymphomas is often administered on an emer-gent basis. Some low-grade lymphomas transform into aggressive lymphomas with an annual fre-quency about 3% in patients with FL.[16]

In contrast with solid malignancies, most patients with HL and many patients with NHL are considered curable even in advanced stages. Patients with advanced indolent (low-grade) lym-phomas cannot be cured with current treatment modalities, but they may enjoy long-term progres-sion-free periods. For example, the estimated 10-year overall survival for patients with advanced low-grade FL and low FLIPI score is 71%.[12]

Clinicians treating patients with lymphoma have several management options. Patients with low-grade NHL might be observed initially without active treatment until they develop lymphoma-related symptoms. This strategy is based on several randomized clinical trials that did not show clear survival benefit for immediate chemo-therapy treatment compared with initial observa-tion in asymptomatic patients with advanced FL.[17,18] Most patients with HL or aggressive and highly aggressive NHL are treated with cytotoxic chemotherapy and/or monoclonal antibodies. Chemotherapy agents cause cell death by nonse-lective inhibition of cell division and DNA synthesis affecting both the dividing malignant and nonma-lignant cells.[19] Antibody-based agents such as rit-uximab attach directly to antigens expressed on malignant lymphocytes and cause cell death by apoptosis, complement-mediated lysis, and antibody-dependent cellular cytotoxicity.[20] For localized therapy in patients with limited disease or residual masses after systemic treatment, radiation can be effective.[19] Some patients with low-grade NHL are treated with radioimmunother-apy.[21] This technique uses a monoclonal antibody labeled with a radionuclide to deliver targeted radi-ation directly to the tumor site.

Patients with recurrent disease or those refrac-tory to primary therapy can also be cured with salvage chemotherapy followed by autologous stem cell transplant.[22–24] Various novel treatments (ie, monoclonal antibodies, histone deacetylase inhibitors, immunomodulatory drugs, small-molecule tyrosine kinase inhibitors) are currently being investigated for treatment of lymphoma.[25,26] After completion of therapy, patients with lymphoma are followed closely for relapse and development of treatment-related secondary malignancies, but the optimal frequency of visits, laboratory tests, and radiographic studies remains to be determined.[27]

Imaging plays an important part in management of patients with lymphoma. Traditionally, it was used to assess the extent of disease as part of staging and response after completion of therapy. However, with advancing technology, novel im-aging approaches are being used for detection of extranodal disease, early relapse, and transforma-tion from low-grade lymphoma to aggressive disease. Imaging could also be a factor in deter-mining prognosis more accurately and developing individualized therapeutic strategies as part of risk-adapted management. This article provides an overview of the evolving role of imaging in lymphoma from clinician's perspective. It serves as an introduction to the other articles in this publi-cation that focus in greater detail on specific areas of lymphoma imaging.

DIAGNOSIS: THE ROLE OF IMAGING

Patients who are suspected to have lymphoma clinically with palpable lymphadenopathy on physical examination typically undergo surgical excisional lymph node biopsy to establish the diagnosis. However, for patients without palpable lymphadenopathy, image-guided needle biopsies may be necessary. Ultrasound or computed to-mography (CT)–guided needle biopsy can be a safe and efficient alternative to excisional biopsy in the evaluation of lymphomas at presentation or relapse.[28,29]

Functional imaging using 2-deoxy-2-[^{18}F] fluo-ro-D-glucose positron emission tomography (FDG-PET) scan can determine the optimal site to biopsy, especially in patients with low-grade lymphomas that might be transforming into aggressive disease. Bodet-Milin and colleagues[30] showed that, in their cohort of 38 patients with low-grade lymphomas, all patients with lesions of standardized uptake value (SUV) greater than 17 had transformed disease on biopsy. In another study of 33 patients with biopsy-proven transfor-mation, most of the transformed lesions had SUV greater than 10.[31] Because documenting transformation to aggressive lymphoma by tissue biopsy is essential for selecting the appropriate therapy, targeting the lesion with the highest SUV on FDG-PET scan should be preferentially pursued.

STAGING: IMAGING OPTIONS

Imaging studies used in the staging process allow clinicians to assess the location and volume of disease objectively and also to detect disease not identified by examination. The evolving imaging options available to clinicians for staging reflect the advances in imaging technology.

Standard chest radiographs can be used to estimate lymph node size in the mediastinum and were primarily used in the older staging systems.[5,9] Lymphography could detect abnormal lymph nodes in the abdomen and pelvis by injecting radiopaque contrast into the lymphatic system, but it had limited ability to visualize lymph nodes outside of retroperitoneum. By the late 1980's it was shown that lymphography did not add any more information to technologically improved CT scans.[32]

Ultrasound has several advantages compared with traditional CT imaging, but it is rarely used in initial lymphoma staging. Although it is less expensive and not associated with radiation exposure, it cannot accurately image deep lymph nodes in the pelvis, abdomen, and mediastinum.[33–35]

Magnetic resonance (MR) imaging is used in staging various malignancies, including lymphomas.[36] The excellent soft-tissue contrast allows MR imaging to detect extranodal disease and also osseous disease. Its radiofrequency energy and magnetic fields have not been associated with any significant biologic risk to the patient.[37] When using MR imaging, the presence of nodal disease is based on size criteria and involvement of extranodal tissues is determined by signal abnormalities. However, because of the cost and demand on patients, MR imaging is currently used mostly for limited organ or site assessment (eg, involvement of central nervous system). New technology is being developed and studies are being conducted in various settings using whole-body MR imaging.[38,39]

CT scans have been the core imaging technique in lymphoma staging for the past 2 decades. Current CT technology using multisection CT scanners allows improved resolution, increased concentration of intravascular contrast material, and decreased image noise.[40] These factors substantially improve the diagnostic accuracy of the examination compared with single-section helical CT scans. The determination of nodal involvement is based on anatomic size.[41] Complete response (CR) is defined by all lymph nodes decreasing to less than or equal to 1.5 cm in their greatest transverse diameter (for lymph nodes >1.5 cm before therapy). Previously involved nodes that were 1.1 to 1.5 cm before treatment should decrease to less than or equal to 1 cm after treatment, or by more than 75% in the sum of the products of the greatest diameters.[41]

Functional imaging technology has added valuable information to CT scans during initial staging because it can identify malignant lymph nodes of normal or borderline anatomic size. It can also identify extranodal disease not seen by anatomic imaging.[42] Gallium-67 accumulates within lymphoma cells by binding to the transferrin receptor, and this property was used in lymphoma imaging in the past.[43,44] However, gallium scans had several limitations, including inability to clearly detect abdominal lymphoma because of gallium uptake by the bowel, obscuring smaller lesions.[45] These scans were shown to be inferior to FDG-PET technology for both staging and assessment of residual masses.[46,47]

FDG-PET scanning has replaced gallium scanning as the most commonly used functional imaging technique in lymphoma imaging. Although several isotopes have been evaluated in PET imaging, the radiolabeled glucose analog FDG is the only isotope widely used commercially. After injecting FDG intravenously into the patient, the isotope is transported into the cells and phosphorylated similarly to glucose. FDG preferentially accumulates in some tissues (eg, brain, kidney) and also in metabolically active tumors.[48] As the radioisotope decays, it emits a positron that, after encountering an electron, produces annihilation photons. These photons are then detected on the scintillator in the scanning device.[49] Tumor cells in most lymphoma subtypes take up the FDG and the involved lymph nodes appear as hypermetabolic on FDG-PET scans.[50] As per the revised criteria for malignant lymphomas (**Table 2**), a positive scan is defined as focal or diffuse FDG uptake greater than background in a location incompatible with normal anatomy or physiology, without a specific SUV cutoff.[51] Sites that have FDG uptake less than or equal to the mediastinal blood pool or the surrounding liver/spleen uptake are usually not considered positive.[51]

FDG-PET scanning is now usually combined with low-dose, noncontrast, nonenhanced CT scan as a fusion FDG-PET/CT scan. The CT scan, which is obtained just before the FDG-PET scan, is used for better anatomic localization. Images from the 2 scans are then fused together.

Multiple studies have shown that FDG-PET and FDG-PET/CT scans are superior in detecting active lymphoma compared with anatomic imaging with CT scan alone in most settings.[42,52–57] Although there are no convincing data that functional imaging at staging affects the outcome, upstaging affects treatment recommendations. Patridge and colleagues[58] reviewed data on 44 patients with HL from a single institution who had both FDG-PET scan and CT before starting treatment. They found that 40% of patients were upstaged and 25% had treatment modified by the FDG-PET scan.

Table 2
Revised response criteria for malignant lymphoma incorporating FDG-PET

	Definition	Lymph Nodes	Spleen/Liver
CR	Disappearance of all evidence of disease	FDG-PET positive before therapy; mass of any size permitted if PET negative Variably FDG avid or PET negative; regression to normal size on CT	Not palpable; nodules disappeared
PR	Regression of measurable disease and no new sites	$\geq$50% decrease in SPD of up to 6 largest dominant masses; no increase in size of other nodes FDG-PET positive before therapy; 1 or more PET positive at previously involved site Variably FDG avid or PET negative; regression on CT	$\geq$50% decrease in SPD of nodules (for single nodule in greatest transverse diameter); no increase in size of liver or spleen
SD	Failure to attain CR/PR or PD	FDG-PET positive before therapy; PET positive at prior sites of disease and no new sites on CT or PET Variably FDG avid or PET negative; no change in size of previous lesions on CT	—
RP PD	Any new lesion or increase by $\geq$50% of previously involved sites from nadir	Appearance of a new lesion(s) >1.5 cm in any axis, $\geq$50% increase in SPD of more than 1 node, or $\geq$50% increase in longest diameter of a previously identified node >1 cm in short axis Lesions PET positive if FDG-avid lymphoma or PET positive before therapy	>50% increase from nadir in the SPD of any previous lesions

Abbreviations: PD, progressive disease; PR, partial remission; RP, relapsed disease; SD, stable disease; SPD, sum of the product of the diameters.

Data from Cheson BD, Pfistner B, Juweid ME, et al. Revised response criteria for malignant lymphoma. J Clin Oncol 2007;25(5):579–86.

There is an ongoing controversy whether oncologists need to expose patients with lymphoma to both an FDG-PET/CT and dedicated contrast-enhanced CT scan during staging process. There have been some studies suggesting that FDG-PET/CT is adequate and the contrast-enhanced CT scan does not add any further information.[59,60] The optimal choice of imaging modality probably depends on the underlying lymphoma subtype. A recent report from Chong and colleagues[61] compared the sensitivity of detection of specific lymphomas by FDG-PET/CT versus contrast-enhanced CT in 56 patients. For patients with DLBCL and FL, FDG-PET/CT was superior to contrast-enhanced CT scan in detecting active disease. However, dedicated contrast-enhanced CT scan was superior to FDG-PET/CT imaging in a small group of patients with chronic lymphocytic leukemia/small lymphocytic lymphoma and marginal zone lymphomas.[61] Although the data on FDG-PET imaging in patients with T-cell lymphoma are limited, it seems that many aggressive subtypes of T-cell lymphomas are FDG avid.[50,62]

In 2007, an attempt to unify recommendations on the use of FDG-PET scans in patients with lymphoma, especially in the context of clinical trials, was made by the International Harmonization Project.[51] Pretreatment staging FDG-PET or FDG-PET/CT scans were strongly recommended for patients with FDG-avid, curable lymphomas (ie,

DLBCL or HL) to better delineate the extent of disease. However, for patients with incurable lymphomas or variably FDG-avid lymphomas, FDG-PET scan was not recommended before treatment unless response rate was a major end point of the trial.[51] Currently, the general practice of using pretreatment staging FDG-PET/CT versus contrast-enhanced CT scan versus both for lymphoma staging varies among institutions and individual clinicians.

There are several issues with FDG-PET scan results aside from cost and limited availability compared with traditional CT-based anatomic imaging. Inflammation, infection, and other non-malignant processes (eg, thymic rebound, brown fat, sarcoidosis) might result in increased FDG uptake and false-positive findings. Clinicians using FDG-PET or FDG-PET/CT in initial lymphoma staging often need to determine whether the FDG uptake (especially when borderline) reflects a true site of disease or another process. There are no large studies to determine the rate of false-positive findings in patients with lymphoma with FDG-avid lymph nodes. For patients with certain comorbidities (eg, human immunodeficiency virus [HIV]) or from geographic areas with high prevalence of some infections, the FDG-PET results might be especially challenging to interpret. A group from India correlated biopsy results of 35 patients with FDG-avid mediastinal lymph nodes without known malignancy or lung abnormality.[63] Pathology of the lymph nodes revealed that 12 patients had tuberculosis, 8 had sarcoidosis, and 15 had lymphoma. The overall SUV of the nonmalignant lymph nodes was lower than those with lymphoma. The investigators suggested that, in countries where tuberculosis and other granulomatous diseases are endemic, an SUV cutoff value of 2.5 (used by some institutions as consistent with malignancy) has low specificity.[63] In HIV-positive patients with a history of lymphoma who were found to have FDG-avid lymph nodes of normal anatomic size by CT criteria, high viral load was associated with benign cause.[64]

ASSESSMENT OF BONE MARROW INVOLVEMENT BY IMAGING

Bone marrow involvement by lymphoma is an important part of staging and requires invasive bone marrow aspiration and core biopsy that is usually performed under local anesthesia from the posterior iliac crest. This procedure may be associated with discomfort to the patient and risks such as bleeding, injury, or infection. There have been efforts to use MR imaging and FDG-PET technology to determine bone marrow involve-

ment.[52,65,66] This way, patients might be spared an invasive procedure. In addition, full body imaging might detect focal osseous involvement that could be missed on a biopsy sample from a single area.

Pelosi and colleagues[67] correlated FDG-PET scan with bone marrow biopsy results and concluded that the sensitivity is similar in both modalities and that they are complementary. In pediatric patients with lymphoma for whom invasive bone marrow biopsies might be especially traumatic, FDG-PET/CT had high sensitivity of detecting bone marrow involvement (92%).[68] In meta-analysis of 13 studies focusing on the evaluation of bone marrow infiltration in staging of lymphoma (with the total of 587 patients), FDG-PET scans had good, but not excellent, concordance with results of bone marrow biopsy for the detection of bone marrow infiltration.[69] Subgroup analyses showed better sensitivity in patients with HL and in aggressive subtypes of NHL.[69] Most clinicians continue to use traditional invasive bone marrow biopsy as a standard part of lymphoma staging.

INTERIM IMAGING DURING THERAPY

Traditionally, clinicians have been using imaging to assess response after the therapy was completed. However, the usefulness of interim imaging in lymphomas (during active chemotherapy treatment) is being studied both for prognosis and for developing risk-adapted strategies.

It has been shown that results of interim FDG-PET imaging could estimate prognosis in several settings. In HL and aggressive NHL, such as DLBCL, it has been shown that interim FDG-PET scan results after 2 cycles of chemotherapy might identify patients with a poor prognosis independently of pretreatment prognostic scores such as IPS or IPI.[14,15] In patients with DLBCL with a positive FDG-PET after 4 cycles of therapy, the 5-year event-free survival was 36% as opposed to 80% for those with a negative examination.[70] However, data from other studies do not concur with those results. In 97 patients with DLBCL treated with R-CHOP (rituximab, cyclophosphamide, doxorubicin, vincristine, and prednisone) chemotherapy, the progression-free survival (PFS) was similar for patients with either positive or a negative FDG-PET scan after cycle 4 of initial chemotherapy.[71] It has been suggested that the change in maximal SUV based on pretreatment and interim FDG-PET is a better predictor of outcome in DLBCL.[13]

In the near future, results of interim functional imaging might also help clinicians to develop risk-adapted strategies for lymphoma treatment. Several clinical studies have used interim FDG-PET scans to escalate or de-escalate therapy.[72,73] However, changing therapy based on interim FDG-PET scan results cannot be considered the standard of care outside a clinical trial. Currently, the definition of positive FDG-PET is vague and correlation with active lymphoma remains controversial. In a study of patients with DLBCL undergoing first-line treatment, only 5 of the 38 patients with positive interim FDG-PET had viable lymphoma when the lesion was biopsied.[71]

In patients with relapsed/refractory lymphoma, our previously reported data and similar studies from other institutions indicate that patients with FDG-PET–positive lesions after salvage chemotherapy and prior autologous stem cell transplantation (ASCT) have poor outcomes.[74,75] In our study, patients with residual FDG-PET–positive lesions before ASCT had a median PFS of 5 months with only 7% of patients without progression at 12 months after ASCT (**Fig. 2**).

ASSESSMENT OF RESIDUAL MASSES

Patients who completed therapy for lymphoma might have anatomic abnormalities and residual masses on follow-up imaging, especially those with initial bulky lymphadenopathy. CT scans cannot distinguish between active disease and residual scar tissue. Several groups determined that functional imaging with FDG-PET scans is more reliable in this setting.[76–78] In 2007, the new response assessment criteria for lymphoma incorporated FDG-PET as part of the assessment and eliminated the previous category CR unconfirmed (see **Table 2**).

FOLLOW-UP AFTER FINISHING TREATMENT AND MONITORING FOR RELAPSE

Posttreatment surveillance in patients with lymphoma is a matter of controversy and the guidelines for imaging are not clearly established or evidence based. Similarly, there are not sufficient data to determine the frequency of imaging in patients with indolent lymphomas who are being clinically observed without treatment.

Because a subset of patients with relapsed lymphoma can be cured (as opposed to most relapsed solid tumors), there may be an advantage to detecting relapse early. It has been shown by several groups that more than 80% of patients with relapsed lymphoma presented with symptoms or new findings on physical examination rather than abnormalities on routine imaging.[79–82] However, it is likely that the numbers vary depending on underlying histology, modality, and imaging frequency. In one study, the relapse was usually associated with symptoms in aggressive NHL, but less so in HL.[83]

There are valid concerns regarding the long-term risks associated with radiation exposure and cost-effectiveness. There is also concern that frequent imaging, especially with FDG-PET, results in unnecessary procedures to determine the cause of false-positive findings. In a retrospective analysis of 192 patients with HL in first remission, 7.8% of FDG-PET/CT scans were designated as false-positive and clinicians usually pursued invasive procedures for tissue diagnosis or secondary imaging.[84]

The current guidelines, especially from Europe, are conservative in terms of surveillance imaging in patients with lymphoma. The 2010 National Cancer Center Network (NCCN) guidelines for

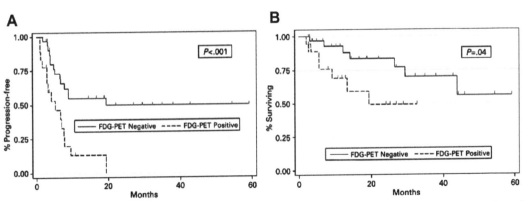

Fig. 2. (A) PFS for the FDG-PET–negative group (median PFS, 19 months; range, 2–59 months) and FDG-PET–positive group (median PFS, 5 months; range: 1–19 months). (B) Overall survival (OS) for the FDG-PET–negative group (median OS not reached) and FDG-PET–positive group (median OS, 19 months; range: 1–34 months). (*From* Svoboda J, Andreadis C, Elstrom R, et al. Prognostic value of FDG-PET scan imaging in lymphoma patients undergoing autologous stem cell transplantation. Bone Marrow Transplant 2006;38(3):211–6; with permission.)

DLBCL and FL, which are followed by most oncologists in the United States, recommend repeating all positive studies at the end of treatment. Follow-up imaging every 3 to 6 months is recommended for 5 years and then annually, or as clinically indicated.[85] In contrast, the European Society of Medical Oncology (ESMO) recommends against routine follow-up imaging except for evaluation of residual disease.[86] The International Working Group also advises against routine imaging for surveillance in lymphomas.[51] For HL, the 2010 NCCN guidelines recommend chest imaging (chest radiograph or CT) every 6 to 12 months for the first 2 to 5 years. Abdominal and pelvic CT scans are recommended every 6 to 12 months for the first 2 to 3 years. These guidelines also specifically advise against using surveillance FDG-PET scans in patients with HL. Annual chest imaging after 5 years is recommended in patients at increased risk for lung cancer, such as those who received radiography to the chest.[85] The ESMO guidelines recommend an FDG-PET scan only at end of treatment (if available) and no routine CT scans in patients with HL.[86]

Because of the lack of evidence-based data, most clinicians in the United States determine the frequency of imaging and the specific modality according to the underlying subtype of lymphoma (ie, curative vs noncurative lymphoma), the estimated risk of relapse (based on prognostic factors), the presence of residual lesions after completing therapy, and patient age or other clinical factors.

FUTURE ROLE OF IMAGING IN MANAGEMENT OF LYMPHOMAS

Many novel imaging technologies are being developed for patients with lymphoma and are covered in detail elsewhere in this issue. New isotopes used for PET scans could improve the ability to distinguish between benign lesions and lymphomas compared with FDG.[87] The thymidine analog 3-deoxy-3-[^{18}F] fluorothymidine (FLT) may be a superior tracer for detection of malignant lymphoma in organs with high physiologic FDG uptake, and also in early detection of transformation.[88]

Studies using functional MR imaging technology also seem promising and could spare patients radiation exposure. Diffusion-weighted MR imaging is a noninvasive technique that examines the motion of water molecules within biologic tissues and may be used to better characterize malignant lymphomas.[89–91] In a recent pilot study, results of diffusion-weighted MR imaging in combination with whole-body MR imaging were comparable with FDG-PET/CT results in patients with DLBCL who were imaged before treatment,

after 1 week, and after 2 cycles of chemotherapy.[92] Novel contrast agents such as superparamagnetic iron oxide might also enhance MR imaging findings.[93]

Biologic therapies such as monoclonal antibodies and immunomodulatory drugs, which are being increasingly used in the management of patients with lymphoma, pose new challenges in lymphoma imaging and response assessment. Because the novel biologic agents work by different mechanisms of action than cytotoxic chemotherapy, traditional response criteria using size or even FDG avidity might need to be revised. In a recent clinical trial, more than 50% of patients with a subtype of low-grade B-cell lymphoma treated with the immunomodulatory drug lenalidomide experienced a tumor flare reaction presenting clinically with tender enlargement of involved lymph nodes or spleen within several days of starting the drug.[94] This immune-mediated phenomenon, which can be managed by antiinflammatory agents, seems to correlate with clinical response.[95] Patients with other subtypes of lymphoma might also experience transient lymph node enlargement after initiating biologic therapy, and the radiographic picture can be mistaken for progression of disease.[96] It is likely that functional imaging is better suited for assessing response to the novel biologic agents compared with anatomic imaging.

This is an exciting time in lymphoma research, and progress in imaging techniques is an important part of it. In the near future, the ability of clinicians to diagnose, accurately stage, determine prognosis, and detect residual/relapsed lymphoma will continue to improve with innovations in imaging. Patients will be spared invasive procedures and exposed to less radiation. Together with advances in therapeutic options, imaging technology might allow clinicians to design risk-adapted treatment strategies, which should greatly benefit patients with lymphoma and ultimately improve their clinical outcome.

REFERENCES

1. Howlader N, Noone AM, Krapcho M, et al, editors. SEER cancer statistics review, 1975-2008. Bethesda (MD): National Cancer Institute; 2011.
2. Hicks EB, Rappaport H, Winter WJ. Follicular lymphoma; a re-evaluation of its position in the scheme of malignant lymphoma, based on a survey of 253 cases. Cancer 1956;9(4):792–821.
3. Rappaport H, Berard CW, Butler JJ, et al. Report of the committee on histopathological criteria contributing to staging of Hodgkin's disease. Cancer Res 1971;31(11):1864–5.

4. Swerdlow SH, editor. WHO classification of tumours of haematopoietic and lymphoid tissues. 4th edition. Lyon Cedex (France): International Agency for Research on Cancer (IARC); 2008.

5. Carbone PP, Kaplan HS, Musshoff K, et al. Report of the committee on Hodgkin's disease staging classification. Cancer Res 1971;31(11):1860–1.

6. Rosenberg SA, Boiron M, DeVita VT Jr, et al. Report of the committee on Hodgkin's disease staging procedures. Cancer Res 1971;31(11):1862–3.

7. Cannon WB, Kaplan HS, Dorfman RF, et al. Staging laparotomy with splenectomy in Hodgkin's disease. Surg Annu 1975;7:103–14.

8. Jonsson K, Karp W, Landberg T, et al. Radiologic evaluation of subdiaphragmatic spread of Hodgkin's disease. Acta Radiol Diagn (Stockh) 1983;24(2):153–9.

9. Lister TA, Crowther D, Sutcliffe SB, et al. Report of a committee convened to discuss the evaluation and staging of patients with Hodgkin's disease: Cotswolds meeting. J Clin Oncol 1989;7(11):1630–6.

10. Hasenclever D, Diehl V. A prognostic score for advanced Hodgkin's disease. International Prognostic Factors Project on Advanced Hodgkin's Disease. N Engl J Med 1998;339(21):1506–14.

11. Shipp MA, Harrington DP, Anderson JR, et al. A predictive model for aggressive non-Hodgkin's lymphoma. The International Non-Hodgkin's Lymphoma Prognostic Factors Project. N Engl J Med 1993;329(14):987–94.

12. Solal-Celigny P, Roy P, Colombat P, et al. Follicular Lymphoma International Prognostic Index. Blood 2004;104(5):1258–65.

13. Casasnovas RO, Meignan M, Berriolo-Riedinger A, et al. SUVmax reduction improves early prognosis value of interim positron emission tomography scans in diffuse large B-cell lymphoma. Blood 2011;118(1): 37–43.

14. Gallamini A, Hutchings M, Rigacci L, et al. Early interim 2-[18F]fluoro-2-deoxy-D-glucose positron emission tomography is prognostically superior to International Prognostic Score in advanced-stage Hodgkin's lymphoma: a report from a joint Italian-Danish study. J Clin Oncol 2007;25(24):3746–52.

15. Haioun C, Itti E, Rahmouni A, et al. [18F]fluoro-2-deoxy-D-glucose positron emission tomography (FDG-PET) in aggressive lymphoma: an early prognostic tool for predicting patient outcome. Blood 2005;106(4):1376–81.

16. Al-Tourah AJ, Gill KK, Chhanabhai M, et al. Population-based analysis of incidence and outcome of transformed non-Hodgkin's lymphoma. J Clin Oncol 2008;26(32):5165–9.

17. Ardeshna KM, Smith P, Norton A, et al. Long-term effect of a watch and wait policy versus immediate systemic treatment for asymptomatic advanced-stage non-Hodgkin lymphoma: a randomised controlled trial. Lancet 2003;362(9383):516–22.

18. Brice P, Bastion Y, Lepage E, et al. Comparison in low-tumor-burden follicular lymphomas between an initial no-treatment policy, prednimustine, or interferon alfa: a randomized study from the Groupe d'Etude des Lymphomes Folliculaires. Groupe d'Etude des Lymphomes de l'Adulte. J Clin Oncol 1997;15(3):1110–7.

19. Pazdur R, Coia LR, Hoskins WJ, et al, editors. Cancer management: a multidisciplinary approach. Jersey City (NJ): CMPMedica; 2007.

20. Cartron G, Watier H, Golay J, et al. From the bench to the bedside: ways to improve rituximab efficacy. Blood 2004;104(9):2635–42.

21. Kaminski MS, Tuck M, Estes J, et al. 131I-tositumomab therapy as initial treatment for follicular lymphoma. N Engl J Med 2005;352(5):441–9.

22. Philip T, Armitage JO, Spitzer G, et al. High-dose therapy and autologous bone marrow transplantation after failure of conventional chemotherapy in adults with intermediate-grade or high-grade non-Hodgkin's lymphoma. N Engl J Med 1987;316(24): 1493–8.

23. Philip T, Guglielmi C, Hagenbeek A, et al. Autologous bone marrow transplantation as compared with salvage chemotherapy in relapses of chemotherapy-sensitive non-Hodgkin's lymphoma. N Engl J Med 1995;333(23):1540–5.

24. Ferme C, Mounier N, Divine M, et al. Intensive salvage therapy with high-dose chemotherapy for patients with advanced Hodgkin's disease in relapse or failure after initial chemotherapy: results of the Groupe d'Etudes des Lymphomes de l'Adulte H89 Trial. J Clin Oncol 2002;20(2):467–75.

25. Reeder CB, Ansell SM. Novel therapeutic agents for B-cell lymphoma: developing rational combinations. Blood 2011;117(5):1453–62.

26. Re D, Thomas RK, Behringer K, et al. From Hodgkin disease to Hodgkin lymphoma: biologic insights and therapeutic potential. Blood 2005;105(12):4553–60.

27. Wagner-Johnston ND, Bartlett NL. Role of routine imaging in lymphoma. J Natl Compr Canc Netw 2011;9(5):575–84.

28. Ben-Yehuda D, Polliack A, Okon E, et al. Image-guided core-needle biopsy in malignant lymphoma: experience with 100 patients that suggests the technique is reliable. J Clin Oncol 1996;14(9):2431–4.

29. Pappa VI, Hussain HK, Reznek RH, et al. Role of image-guided core-needle biopsy in the management of patients with lymphoma. J Clin Oncol 1996;14(9):2427–30.

30. Bodet-Milin C, Kraeber-Bodere F, Moreau P, et al. Investigation of FDG-PET/CT imaging to guide biopsies in the detection of histological transformation of indolent lymphoma. Haematologica 2008;93(3): 471–2.

31. Noy A, Schoder H, Gonen M, et al. The majority of transformed lymphomas have high standardized

uptake values (SUVs) on positron emission tomography (PET) scanning similar to diffuse large B-cell lymphoma (DLBCL). Ann Oncol 2009;20(3):508–12.

32. North LB, Wallace S, Lindell MM Jr, et al. Lymphography for staging lymphomas: is it still a useful procedure? AJR Am J Roentgenol 1993;161(4):867–9.

33. Raskin MM. Combination of CT and ultrasound in the retroperitoneum and pelvis examination. Crit Rev Diagn Imaging 1980;13(3):173–228.

34. Vassallo P, Wernecke K, Roos N, et al. Differentiation of benign from malignant superficial lymphadenopathy: the role of high-resolution US. Radiology 1992;183(1):215–20.

35. Neumann CH, Robert NJ, Rosenthal D, et al. Clinical value of ultrasonography for the management of non-Hodgkin lymphoma patients as compared with abdominal computed tomography. J Comput Assist Tomogr 1983;7(4):666–9.

36. Lauenstein TC, Semelka RC. Emerging techniques: whole-body screening and staging with MRI. J Magn Reson Imaging 2006;24(3):489–98.

37. Budinger TF. Nuclear magnetic resonance (NMR) in vivo studies: known thresholds for health effects. J Comput Assist Tomogr 1981;5(6):800–11.

38. Kwee TC, Akkerman EM, Fijnheer R, et al. MRI for staging lymphoma: whole-body or less? J Magn Reson Imaging 2011;33(5):1144–50.

39. Brennan DD, Gleeson T, Coate LE, et al. A comparison of whole-body MRI and CT for the staging of lymphoma. AJR Am J Roentgenol 2005;185(3):711–6.

40. Rydberg J, Buckwalter KA, Caldemeyer KS, et al. Multisection CT: scanning techniques and clinical applications. Radiographics 2000;20(6):1787–806.

41. Cheson BD, Horning SJ, Coiffier B, et al. Report of an international workshop to standardize response criteria for non-Hodgkin's lymphomas. NCI Sponsored International Working Group. J Clin Oncol 1999;17(4):1244.

42. Buchmann I, Reinhardt M, Elsner K, et al. 2-(Fluorine-18)fluoro-2-deoxy-D-glucose positron emission tomography in the detection and staging of malignant lymphoma. A bicenter trial. Cancer 2001;91(5):889–99.

43. van Amsterdam JA, Kluin-Nelemans JC, van Eck-Smit BL, et al. Role of 67Ga scintigraphy in localization of lymphoma. Ann Hematol 1996;72(4):202–7.

44. Larcos G, Farlow DC, Antico VF, et al. The role of high dose 67-gallium scintigraphy in staging untreated patients with lymphoma. Aust N Z J Med 1994;24(1):5–8.

45. Friedberg JW, Chengazi V. PET scans in the staging of lymphoma: current status. Oncologist 2003;8(5):438–47.

46. Yamamoto F, Tsukamoto E, Nakada K, et al. 18F-FDG PET is superior to 67Ga SPECT in the staging of non-Hodgkin's lymphoma. Ann Nucl Med 2004;18(6):519–26.

47. Friedberg JW, Fischman A, Neuberg D, et al. FDG-PET is superior to gallium scintigraphy in staging and more sensitive in the follow-up of patients with de novo Hodgkin lymphoma: a blinded comparison. Leuk Lymphoma 2004;45(1):85–92.

48. Gallagher BM, Fowler JS, Gutterson NI, et al. Metabolic trapping as a principle of radiopharmaceutical design: some factors responsible for the biodistribution of [18F] 2-deoxy-2-fluoro-D-glucose. J Nucl Med 1978;19(10):1154–61.

49. Phelps ME. PET: the merging of biology and imaging into molecular imaging. J Nucl Med 2000;41(4):661–81.

50. Elstrom R, Guan L, Baker G, et al. Utility of FDG-PET scanning in lymphoma by WHO classification. Blood 2003;101(10):3875–6.

51. Cheson BD, Pfistner B, Juweid ME, et al. Revised response criteria for malignant lymphoma. J Clin Oncol 2007;25(5):579–86.

52. Pelosi E, Pregno P, Penna D, et al. Role of whole-body [18F] fluorodeoxyglucose positron emission tomography/computed tomography (FDG-PET/CT) and conventional techniques in the staging of patients with Hodgkin and aggressive non Hodgkin lymphoma. Radiol Med 2008;113(4):578–90.

53. Jerusalem G, Beguin Y, Najjar F, et al. Positron emission tomography (PET) with 18F-fluorodeoxyglucose (18F-FDG) for the staging of low-grade non-Hodgkin's lymphoma (NHL). Ann Oncol 2001;12(6):825–30.

54. Jerusalem G, Beguin Y, Fassotte MF, et al. Whole-body positron emission tomography using 18F-fluorodeoxyglucose compared to standard procedures for staging patients with Hodgkin's disease. Haematologica 2001;86(3):266–73.

55. Hoh CK, Glaspy J, Rosen P, et al. Whole-body FDG-PET imaging for staging of Hodgkin's disease and lymphoma. J Nucl Med 1997;38(3):343–8.

56. Moog F, Bangerter M, Diederichs CG, et al. Lymphoma: role of whole-body 2-deoxy-2-[F-18]fluoro-D-glucose (FDG) PET in nodal staging. Radiology 1997;203(3):795–800.

57. Stumpe KD, Urbinelli M, Steinert HC, et al. Whole-body positron emission tomography using fluorodeoxyglucose for staging of lymphoma: effectiveness and comparison with computed tomography. Eur J Nucl Med 1998;25(7):721–8.

58. Partridge S, Timothy A, O'Doherty MJ, et al. 2-Fluorine-18-fluoro-2-deoxy-D glucose positron emission tomography in the pretreatment staging of Hodgkin's disease: influence on patient management in a single institution. Ann Oncol 2000;11(10):1273–9.

59. Elstrom RL, Leonard JP, Coleman M, et al. Combined PET and low-dose, noncontrast CT scanning obviates the need for additional diagnostic contrast-enhanced CT scans in patients undergoing

staging or restaging for lymphoma. Ann Oncol 2008; 19(10):1770–3.

60. Rodriguez-Vigil B, Gomez-Leon N, Pinilla I, et al. PET/CT in lymphoma: prospective study of enhanced full-dose PET/CT versus unenhanced low-dose PET/CT. J Nucl Med 2006;47(10):1643–8.

61. Chong EA, Torigian DA, Alavi A, et al. Comparison of contrast-enhanced CT, PET/CT, PET, and low-dose non-contrast enhanced CT imaging of diffuse large B-cell (DLBCL), follicular (FL), small lymphocytic/CLL (CLL/SLL), and marginal zone lymphomas (MZL) [abstract]. J Clin Oncol 2010;28(Suppl 15): 8079.

62. Kako S, Izutsu K, Ota Y, et al. FDG-PET in T-cell and NK-cell neoplasms. Ann Oncol 2007;18(10): 1685–90.

63. Kumar A, Dutta R, Kannan U, et al. Evaluation of mediastinal lymph nodes using F-FDG PET-CT scan and its histopathologic correlation. Ann Thorac Med 2011;6(1):11–6.

64. Goshen E, Davidson T, Avigdor A, et al. PET/CT in the evaluation of lymphoma in patients with HIV-1 with suppressed viral loads. Clin Nucl Med 2008; 33(9):610–4.

65. Rahmouni A, Montazel JL, Divine M, et al. Bone marrow with diffuse tumor infiltration in patients with lymphoproliferative diseases: dynamic gadolinium-enhanced MR imaging. Radiology 2003; 229(3):710–7.

66. Moulin-Romsee G, Hindie E, Cuenca X, et al. (18) F-FDG PET/CT bone/bone marrow findings in Hodgkin's lymphoma may circumvent the use of bone marrow trephine biopsy at diagnosis staging. Eur J Nucl Med Mol Imaging 2010;37(6):1095–105.

67. Pelosi E, Penna D, Douroukas A, et al. Bone marrow disease detection with FDG-PET/CT and bone marrow biopsy during the staging of malignant lymphoma: results from a large multicentre study. Q J Nucl Med Mol Imaging 2011;55(4):469–75.

68. Cheng G, Chen W, Chamroonrat W, et al. Biopsy versus FDG PET/CT in the initial evaluation of bone marrow involvement in pediatric lymphoma patients. Eur J Nucl Med Mol Imaging 2011;38(8):1469–76.

69. Pakos EE, Fotopoulos AD, Ioannidis JP. 18F-FDG PET for evaluation of bone marrow infiltration in staging of lymphoma: a meta-analysis. J Nucl Med 2005;46(6):958–63.

70. Dupuis J, Itti E, Rahmouni A, et al. Response assessment after an inductive CHOP or CHOP-like regimen with or without rituximab in 103 patients with diffuse large B-cell lymphoma: integrating 18fluorodeoxyglucose positron emission tomography to the International Workshop Criteria. Ann Oncol 2009;20(3):503–7.

71. Moskowitz CH, Schoder H, Teruya-Feldstein J, et al. Risk-adapted dose-dense immunochemotherapy determined by interim FDG-PET in advanced-stage diffuse large B-Cell lymphoma. J Clin Oncol 2010; 28(11):1896–903.

72. Kasamon YL, Wahl RL, Ziessman HA, et al. Phase II study of risk-adapted therapy of newly diagnosed, aggressive non-Hodgkin lymphoma based on mid-treatment FDG-PET scanning. Biol Blood Marrow Transplant 2009;15(2):242–8.

73. Dann EJ, Bar-Shalom R, Tamir A, et al. Risk-adapted BEACOPP regimen can reduce the cumulative dose of chemotherapy for standard and high-risk Hodgkin lymphoma with no impairment of outcome. Blood 2007;109(3):905–9.

74. Svoboda J, Andreadis C, Elstrom R, et al. Prognostic value of FDG-PET scan imaging in lymphoma patients undergoing autologous stem cell transplantation. Bone Marrow Transplant 2006;38(3):211–6.

75. Spaepen K, Stroobants S, Dupont P, et al. Prognostic value of pretransplantation positron emission tomography using fluorine 18-fluorodeoxyglucose in patients with aggressive lymphoma treated with high-dose chemotherapy and stem cell transplantation. Blood 2003;102(1):53–9.

76. Jerusalem G, Beguin Y, Fassotte MF, et al. Whole-body positron emission tomography using 18F-fluorodeoxyglucose for posttreatment evaluation in Hodgkin's disease and non-Hodgkin's lymphoma has higher diagnostic and prognostic value than classical computed tomography scan imaging. Blood 1999;94(2):429–33.

77. Spaepen K, Stroobants S, Dupont P, et al. Prognostic value of positron emission tomography (PET) with fluorine-18 fluorodeoxyglucose ([18F]FDG) after first-line chemotherapy in non-Hodgkin's lymphoma: is [18F]FDG-PET a valid alternative to conventional diagnostic methods? J Clin Oncol 2001;19(2):414–9.

78. Cerci JJ, Trindade E, Pracchia LF, et al. Cost effectiveness of positron emission tomography in patients with Hodgkin's lymphoma in unconfirmed complete remission or partial remission after first-line therapy. J Clin Oncol 2010;28(8):1415–21.

79. Guppy AE, Tebbutt NC, Norman A, et al. The role of surveillance CT scans in patients with diffuse large B-cell non-Hodgkin's lymphoma. Leuk Lymphoma 2003;44(1):123–5.

80. Elis A, Blickstein D, Klein O, et al. Detection of relapse in non-Hodgkin's lymphoma: role of routine follow-up studies. Am J Hematol 2002;69(1):41–4.

81. Radford JA, Eardley A, Woodman C, et al. Follow up policy after treatment for Hodgkin's disease: too many clinic visits and routine tests? A review of hospital records. BMJ 1997;314(7077):343–6.

82. Mocikova H, Obrtlikova P, Vackova B, et al. Positron emission tomography at the end of first-line therapy and during follow-up in patients with Hodgkin lymphoma: a retrospective study. Ann Oncol 2010; 21(6):1222–7.

83. Goldschmidt N, Or O, Klein M, et al. The role of routine imaging procedures in the detection of relapse of patients with Hodgkin lymphoma and aggressive non-Hodgkin lymphoma. Ann Hematol 2011;90(2):165–71.

84. Lee AI, Zuckerman DS, Van den Abbeele AD, et al. Surveillance imaging of Hodgkin lymphoma patients in first remission: a clinical and economic analysis. Cancer 2010;116(16):3835–42.

85. Zelenetz AD, Abramson JS, Advani RH, et al. NCCN clinical practice guidelines in oncology: non-Hodgkin's lymphomas. J Natl Compr Canc Netw 2010; 8(3):288–334.

86. Jost L. Newly diagnosed large B-cell non-Hodgkin's lymphoma: ESMO clinical recommendations for diagnosis, treatment and follow-up. Ann Oncol 2007;18(Suppl 2):ii55–6.

87. Kumar R, Dhanpathi H, Basu S, et al. Oncologic PET tracers beyond [(18)F]FDG and the novel quantitative approaches in PET imaging. Q J Nucl Med Mol Imaging 2008;52(1):50–65.

88. Buck AK, Bommer M, Stilgenbauer S, et al. Molecular imaging of proliferation in malignant lymphoma. Cancer Res 2006;66(22):11055–61.

89. Le Bihan D. Molecular diffusion, tissue microdynamics and microstructure. NMR Biomed 1995;8(7–8):375–86.

90. Perrone A, Guerrisi P, Izzo L, et al. Diffusion-weighted MRI in cervical lymph nodes: differentiation between benign and malignant lesions. Eur J Radiol 2011; 77(2):281–6.

91. Holzapfel K, Duetsch S, Fauser C, et al. Value of diffusion-weighted MR imaging in the differentiation between benign and malignant cervical lymph nodes. Eur J Radiol 2009;72(3):381–7.

92. Wu X, Kellokumpu-Lehtinen PL, Pertovaara H, et al. Diffusion-weighted MRI in early chemotherapy response evaluation of patients with diffuse large B-cell lymphoma - a pilot study: comparison with 2-deoxy-2-fluoro-D-glucose-positron emission tomography/computed tomography. NMR Biomed 2011. [Epub ahead of print].

93. Mack MG, Balzer JO, Straub R, et al. Superparamagnetic iron oxide-enhanced MR imaging of head and neck lymph nodes. Radiology 2002;222(1): 239–44.

94. Chanan-Khan A, Miller KC, Musial L, et al. Clinical efficacy of lenalidomide in patients with relapsed or refractory chronic lymphocytic leukemia: results of a phase II study. J Clin Oncol 2006;24(34):5343–9.

95. Chanan-Khan A, Miller KC, Lawrence D, et al. Tumor flare reaction associated with lenalidomide treatment in patients with chronic lymphocytic leukemia predicts clinical response. Cancer 2011;117(10):2127–35.

96. Eve HE, Rule SA. Lenalidomide-induced tumour flare reaction in mantle cell lymphoma. Br J Haematol 2010;151(4):410–2.

Review of Clinical Applications of Fluorodeoxyglucose-PET/Computed Tomography in Pediatric Patients with Lymphoma

Gang Cheng, MD, PhD[a],*, Scott R. Akers, MD, PhD[a],
Hongming Zhuang, MD, PhD[b],
Abass Alavi, MD, PhD (Hon), DSc (Hon)[c]

KEYWORDS

• FDG-PET/CT • Lymphoma • Pediatrics • Diagnosis

Since being approved by the US Health Care Administration in the late 1990s as a diagnostic imaging tool for lymphoma, [18F]fluorodeoxyglucose (FDG)-positron emission tomography (PET) has played an ever-increasing role in the clinical management of patients with Hodgkin disease (HD) and non-Hodgkin lymphoma (NHL). In current clinical practice, hybrid FDG-PET/computed tomography (CT) imaging has replaced stand-alone PET devices and is routinely used in the initial diagnosis and response assessment during and immediately after therapy, as well as surveillance follow-up.[1] A lot of effort has been spent comparing the accuracy of FDG/PET or PET/CT versus conventional imaging modalities (CIM) such as CT, magnetic resonance imaging, bone scan, and bone biopsy in the evaluation of pediatric patients with lymphoma, with an accumulation of a wealth of experience.

PET/CT FOR INITIAL STAGING

PET/CT is the most important recent advance in imaging evaluation of lymphoma, with high accuracy with all HD and most subtypes of indolent and aggressive NHL. The higher accuracy of the PET/CT imaging over the conventional imaging is because of the ability of PET/CT to assess both anatomic and functional abnormalities (**Fig. 1**). CT is the most readily available study with high anatomic resolution and is often the first imaging tool for staging pediatric lymphoma. However, the accuracy of CT is limited because it is highly dependent on change in size, with poor detection of bone marrow (BM) and extranodal tissue involvement. PET and CT have concordant findings in approximately 70% of patients on initial diagnosis.[2] In patients with a discordant finding, PET typically detects additional lesions (often in a normal-sized lymph node or in extranodal

[a] Department of Radiology, Philadelphia VA Medical Center, 3900 Woodland Avenue, Philadelphia, PA 19104, USA
[b] Department of Radiology, Children's Hospital of Pennsylvania, 34th Street and Civic Center Boulevard, Philadelphia, PA 19104, USA
[c] Division of Nuclear Medicine, Department of Radiology, Hospital of the University of Pennsylvania, 3400 Spruce Street, Philadelphia, PA 19102, USA
* Corresponding author.
E-mail address: gangcheng99@yahoo.com

PET Clin 7 (2012) 47–56
doi:10.1016/j.cpet.2011.12.006
1556-8598/12/$ – see front matter Published by Elsevier Inc.

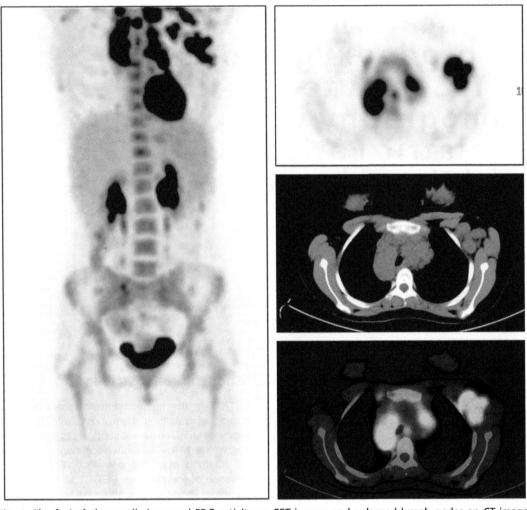

Fig. 1. The foci of abnormally increased FDG activity on PET images and enlarged lymph nodes on CT images matched well on the fusion images in a patient with HD.

lesions) and results in upstaging of disease. The superiority of PET/CT is more prominent in the detection of extranodal sites of disease, and it is a major contributing factor for upstaging by PET/CT. Miller and colleagues[2] reported that most additional lesions detected by PET/CT were in the bone and BM, the thymus, the spleen, and the liver, as well as normal-sized lymph nodes. The sensitivity, specificity, positive predictive value (PPV) and negative predictive value (NPV) of PET/CT in the evaluation of pediatric lymphoma were 99%, 100%, 100%, and 86%, respectively, in contrast to 80%, 23%, 92%, and 7%, respectively, for diagnostic CT. A prospective, blinded study comparing FDG/PET with conventional staging methods (CIM, including CT, ultrasonography, bone scanning, and BM examination) for initial staging of 55 children and adolescents with HD or NHL revealed that FDG/PET identified significantly more lesions

than CIM, PET detected 34% additional lesions that were negative on CIM, whereas CIM revealed only 5% additional lesions that were negative on PET. The sensitivity of PET and CIM for pretreatment staging was 96.5% and 87.5%, respectively; specificity was 100% and 60%, and accuracy, 96.7% and 85.2%, respectively.[3]

The increased accuracy in the initial staging has led to upstaging and downstaging in many pediatric patients with lymphoma ranging from 10% to 32.3%,[4–8] which in turn leads to modification of management in pediatric patients with lymphoma, approximately 10.5% of the cases at initial evaluation.[5] This finding is consistent with our own clinical experience reported in the literature.[9,10] Among 18 pediatric patients with HD and 15 patients with NHL who had a PET/CT scan at diagnosis with a diagnostic contrast CT within a week of PET/CT before any therapy, PET/CT scan detected more positive lesions than diagnostic CT scan. FDG-PET/CT led to upstaging in 1 of 3 pediatric patients with HD and NHL compared with the diagnostic CT scan.[9,10] More recent work by Riad and colleagues[7] showed that PET/CT upstaged 5 patients and downstaged 6 patients among 41 pediatric patients with lymphoma on initial evaluation. Equally important, FDG-PET findings can also help optimize the selection of biopsy site of active tumor tissues in patients with heterogeneous tumor masses or with BM involvement, to avoid sampling errors.[11]

PET/CT FOR INTERIM AND POSTTHERAPY STUDIES

In addition to its application on initial diagnosis, FDG-PET or PET/CT has been frequently used in the assessment of treatment response during and immediately after therapy, as well as surveillance follow-up.

Gallium-67 (^{67}Ga) citrate scintigraphy was traditionally used as a functional imaging of lymphoma but has low spatial resolution and low sensitivity and has essentially been replaced by FDG-PET/CT.[12,13] FDG-PET/CT also overcomes a major limitation of the posttherapy CT scan, which often has low PPV on posttherapy studies, because residual masses are common in these patients.

Interim Treatment Monitoring

Current standard therapeutic strategy of multiagent chemotherapy and selected field radiotherapy have excellent results in children and adolescents with HD and NHL, with the long-term disease-free survival rate of more than 90% for HD and more than 75% for NHL.[1,7] There is interest in differentiating patients who have a likely favorable response to therapy from those who will likely have a less favorable response to therapy, so that less aggressive treatment can be applied to patients with favorable prognosis to avoid many side effects, such as infections, gonad dysfunctions, secondary malignancies, and other late complications. FDG-PET provides an excellent early response indicator to guide therapeutic strategy in patients with lymphoma.

Early response assessment in the treatment of patients with lymphoma is often performed after 2 or 3 cycles of chemotherapy, with PET providing a reliable indicator of prognosis, allowing adjustment of therapeutic strategies accordingly if a tumor is FDG-avid on the baseline study. The value of early response assessment with FDG-PET in predicting clinical outcome is well established by numerous studies in the adult lymphoma population.[14,15] Many studies in this regard in

pediatric patients had only a few patients, making statistical analysis difficult.[1,16]

Recent data with greater statistical power provide stronger evidence of FDG-PET value in treatment of pediatric lymphoma. A prospective study performed in 40 pediatric patients with HD indicated that FDG-PET alone is superior to CIM in early response assessment, with an accuracy of 70% for PET versus only 8% for CIM (the sensitivity, specificity, PPV, and NPV of PET for the prediction of relapse were 100%, 68%, 14%, and 100%, respectively, and were 100%, 3%, 5%, and 100% for CIM, respectively).[17] Riad and colleagues[7] recently reported a study with the largest population of pediatric patients with lymphoma (51 children) and analyzed the performance of FDG-PET/CT versus CIM performed 12 to 14 days after the end of 2 to 3 courses of chemotherapy to evaluate early response. PET/CT and CIM were concordant in 34 of 51 (66.7%) patients. In the 17 cases with discordant findings, PET/CT was true-negative in 15 patients (which were false-positive in CT), true-positive in 1 case (which was false-negative in CT), and was false-positive in only 1 case with intense FDG uptake in the bowel wall associated with wall thickening in which open biopsy showed inflammation of the bowel wall with no evidence of lymphomatous infiltration. The sensitivity, specificity, accuracy, and PPVs and NPVs of PET/CT in the evaluation of early response to therapy after the end of 2 to 3 courses of chemotherapy were 100%, 97.7%, 98%, 85.7%, and 100%, respectively, compared with 83%, 66.6%, 68.6%, 25%, and 96.7% for CIM.

End of Therapy Evaluation

After completion of chemotherapy or chemoradiation therapy, it is critically important to determine if the residual mass contains viable tumor cells or just necrotic tissues to decide if additional treatment is required. CT alone has a limited role in the differentiation of necrotic tissue, fibrous tissue, or viable tumor tissue in patients after definitive treatment of HD or NHL (**Fig. 2**). For example, in a retrospective analysis of 256 pediatric patients with HD in which 38% of patients with a persistent mass at end of therapy had viable tumor, the sensitivity and specificity of CT scan was 67% and 8%, respectively, with high false-positive findings and a PPV of only 33%.[18] The sensitivity and specificity of gallium scan was 71% and 71%, respectively, with a PPV of 55%).[18] FDG-PET/CT has dramatically changed the way of clinical practice by providing a reliable method in the differentiation of residual resistant tumor tissues from nontumor tissues.

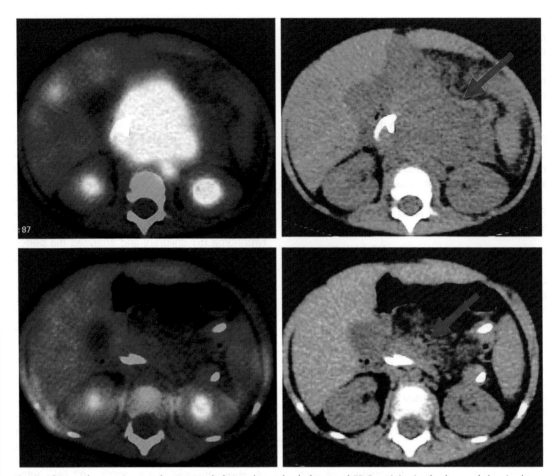

Fig. 2. The pretherapy images (*upper row*) showed matched abnormal FDG activity in the large abdominal mass (*arrow*) in a patient with Burkitt lymphoma. The posttherapy images (*lower row*) revealed normal FDG activity on PET. However, there was still residual soft tissue mass on CT although it was significantly smaller compared with the pretherapy scan.

In adult patients, FDG-PET has good sensitivity and high specificity for evaluation of posttherapy residual disease in HD and NHL, with an overall sensitivity and specificity of 84% and 90%, respectively, in patients with HD, and 72% and 100% respectively in patients with NHL.[19] Multiple retrospective studies have also shown that FDG-PET is highly accurate in assessing posttherapy residual masses in pediatric patients with HD and NHL.[5,13,20] Edeline and colleagues[21] reported in a prospective study of 16 pediatric patients with HD or NHL that FDG-PET had a high NPV in the evaluation of residual mediastinal disease after completion of therapy: none of the 11 patients with negative PET findings had relapse during their follow-up (in contrast, 14 of the 16 patients had residual masses on CT evaluation) although only 2 of 5 patients with positive PET findings were true-positive for malignancy. Furth and colleagues[17] reported in another prospective study

performed in 29 patients with HD that FDG-PET alone is superior to CIM in late response assessment, with an accuracy of 79% for PET versus only 14% for CIM (the sensitivity, specificity, PPV, and NPV of PET for the prediction of relapse were 100%, 78%, 25%, and 100%, respectively, and 50%, 11%, 4%, and 75% for CIM, respectively). More recently, Riad and colleagues[7] compared the performance of FDG-PET/CT versus CIM (performed 3–8 weeks after end of therapy) in the evaluation of late response to therapy in 42 pediatric patients with lymphoma. PET/CT and CIM were concordant in 22 of 42 (52.4%) patients. One study was false-positive in both PET/CT and CIM. In the remaining 19 cases with discordant findings, PET/CT was true-negative in 13 cases (which were false-positive in CT), true-positive in 4 cases (which were false-negative in CT), and false-positive in 2 cases (which were true-negative on CT). The sensitivity, specificity, accuracy, and

PPVs and NPVs of PET/CT in the evaluation of early response to therapy after the end of 2 to 3 courses of chemotherapy were 100%, 90.9%, 92.8%, 75%, and 100%, respectively, compared with 55.5%, 57.5%, 57.1%, 26.3%, and 82.6% for CIM.

Surveillance Imaging After Treatment

Surveillance studies are necessary in patients with complete remission after successful completion of treatment, and these patients are typically followed up for another 5 years with imaging to exclude recurrence. Several earlier studies reported that FDG-PET had a low PPV for surveillance of lymphoma recurrence in pediatric patients, although PET was reported as highly sensitive with a strong NPV.[22,23] In early studies of posttherapy PET scan, especially performed with FDG-PET alone without CT correlation, false-positive findings were common. For example, Levine and colleagues[22] found false-positive PET findings in 25 of 28 positive PET studies performed in 34 pediatric patients with HD, with a PPV of only 11%. Identifiable causes of false-positive scans included abdominal wall hernia, appendicitis, thymus uptake, and human immunodeficiency virus-associated lymphadenopathy. Similarly, only 2 of 11 patients who had a positive FDG-PET scan within 6 to 9 months after the end of therapy had relapsed HD confirmed by biopsy, with a PPV of 18.2%.[23]

With routine use of an integrated PET/CT system, false-positive studies seem minimized, as reflected on more recent PET/CT studies.[24] Riad and colleagues[7] compared the performance of FDG-PET/CT versus CIM in the surveillance follow-up studies in 18 pediatric patients with lymphoma. These imaging studies were performed after 3 to12 months during follow-up of patients in complete clinical remission. PET/CT and CIM were concordant in 13 of 18 (72.2%) patients (concordantly true-negative in 8 of 18 of patients and concordantly true-positive in 5 of 18 of patients). PET/CT was true-negative in the remaining 5 cases with discordant findings, which was confirmed by another follow-up study after 6 months. PET/CT had 100% sensitivity, specificity, accuracy, and PPVs and NPVs, whereas CIM had 100% sensitivity, 38.4% specificity, 72.2% accuracy, 50% PPV, and 100% NPV. The consensus is that FDG-PET has a very good NPV, although more studies are needed to determine the PPV of PET. Increased FDG uptake on posttherapy studies solely at sites other than the original tumor sites at initial diagnosis rarely indicates relapsed HD, and pathologic correlation should be considered for positive PET/CT findings before any therapeutic decisions.[23]

PET/CT FOR EVALUATION OF NODAL AND EXTRANODAL DISEASE

A recent study of FDG-PET/CT versus CIM performed within 4 weeks of the PET/CT study (the largest analysis in pediatric patients with lymphoma) reported a lesion-based analysis of 209 PET/CT scans with a valid CIM comparator (16 nodal and 8 extranodal regions, a total of 3342 lymph nodal regions and 1672 extranodal regions).[24] This study provided new evidence of better performance of FDG-PET/CT compared with CIM in the detection of malignant lesions both on initial evaluation and on posttherapy studies. FDG-PET/CT was more accurate with fewer false-positive findings than CIM. When there were discordant findings, FDG-PET/CT findings were correct in 86% of cases, whereas CIM was correct in only 14% of cases.[24] PET/CT had a very high NPV: PET/CT was the correct modality in 74% of cases with positive PET/CT findings but negative CIM findings, and correct in 94% of cases with negative PET/CT findings but positive CIM findings. Lesion-based regional analysis of 4246 regions on initial diagnosis in 177 pediatric patients with HD and NHL indicated that, for the detection of malignant lesions, the sensitivity and specificity were 95.9% and 99.7%, respectively for PET/CT, and 70.1% and 99.0%, respectively, for conventional imaging. Lesion-based regional analysis of 768 regions in 32 pediatric patients with HD and NHL to evaluate lesion response during therapy concluded that PET/CT had fewer false-positive findings than CIM: PET/CT had 6 false-positive lesions, whereas CIM had 24 false-positive lesions, with a specificity of 99.2% (95% confidence interval [CI]: 98.2–99.7) for PET/CT versus 96.9% (95% CI: 95.3–97.9) for CIM.[24]

FDG-PET/CT IN EVALUATION OF NODAL LESIONS

FDG-PET or PET/CT is superior to other CIM in detecting nodal lesions in patients with lymphoma partly because FDG-PET or PET/CT is able to detect lymphoma involvement of small lymph nodes that likely would be interpreted as normal on CT images.[2,3,13,25,26] From our own experience, per lesion analysis in 18 pediatric patients with HD and 14 pediatric patients with NHL on initial evaluation showed that, among 174 total lesions, 39 were detected only by FDG-PET/CT, whereas diagnostic CT detected an additional 14 lesions not detected on PET/CT.[9,10]

Detection of more nodal lesions on PET on initial diagnosis has limited clinical significance, because detecting a few more nodal lesions often does not change staging significantly enough to modify the treatment plan or even does not change staging at all (most upstaging by FDG-PET is caused by detection of additional extranodal lesions, especially BM lesions, an indicator of stage IV disease).[9,10] However, detection of additional nodal lesions on posttherapy studies is often critically important because it is the most important indicator of viable malignancy. Different criteria should be used when interpreting PET studies in posttherapy patients, because both chemotherapy and radiation therapy may cause significant FDG uptake even in nonmalignancy tissues, and should be carefully differentiated from true malignancy. In 2007, the International Harmonization Project proposed guidelines for performing and interpreting FDG-PET imaging for treatment assessment in patients with lymphoma both in clinical practice and in clinical trials.[27,28] The importance of a pretherapeutic baseline PET study has been emphasized in all FDG-avid lymphoma and is regarded as mandatory for variably FDG-avid lymphomas if FDG-PET is used to assess their response to therapy. For response assessment at the conclusion of therapy, FDG-PET should be performed at least 3 weeks (preferably at 6–8 weeks) after chemotherapy, and at 8 to 12 weeks after radiation or chemoradiotherapy, to minimize nonspecific FDG uptake secondary to posttherapy inflammatory changes rather than lymphoma, which may be present several weeks after completion of chemotherapy. Mild and diffusely increased FDG uptake in a soft tissue mass with a diameter of 2 cm or greater should not be considered positive for viable residual lymphoma if the uptake intensity is lower than or equal to that of mediastinal blood pool structures. However, stricter criteria are used in the evaluation of smaller residual tissues (<2 cm in diameter), in which any increased uptake above surrounding background should be considered positive for lymphoma.

FDG-PET/CT IN EVALUATION OF EXTRANODAL LESIONS
BM Involvement

BM involvement is common in patients with lymphoma and often advances the staging. CT has a low sensitivity for evaluation of BM infiltration by lymphoma, because BM involvement causes minimal structural/morphologic changes on CT scans (**Fig. 3**). In the initial evaluation of BM involvement in patients with lymphoma, FDG-PET significantly outperforms diagnostic CT, which is a major contributing factor for upstaging lymphoma by PET or PET/CT.[29] FDG-PET/CT

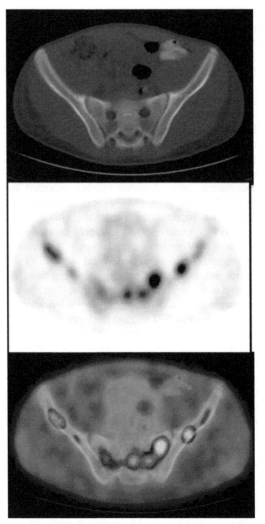

Fig. 3. Despite normal morphology on CT (*upper*) image, tumor involvement is clearly visualized on PET (*middle*) and fusion (*lower*) image.

also outperforms bone scan for the assessment of osseous involvement in pediatric patients with lymphoma for both initial diagnosis and suspected recurrence evaluation[30]: PET detected all osseous metastases identified on bone scan, plus many additional sites of bony involvement missed by bone scan. In current practice, FDG-PET/CT has essentially replaced bone scan in the assessment of BM involvement in patients with lymphoma.

Data in the adult population also suggest that FDG-PET or PET/CT outperforms BM biopsy (BMB) regarding BM infiltration, with more additional positive findings in the initial diagnosis of HD or NHL patients.[31–33] FDG-PET/CT is superior to CT alone and to CT in combination with BMB for detection of BM involvement by lymphoma. In 50 consecutive patients with HD and NHL with bone lesions, FDG-PET was superior to CT alone or in combination with unilateral BMB, with multiple additional findings leading to upstaging in 42% patients with regards to unifocal or multifocal BM involvement.[31] In contrast, CT had no additional positive findings of bone lesion in these 50 patients compared with FDG-PET, and most BMBs performed at the iliac crests were negative, although target BMBs were often positive.[31] Similar findings were noted in pediatric patients.[3] Recently, we evaluated the role of FDG-PET/CT versus BMB in the initial evaluation of BM involvement in 54 pediatric patients with lymphoma (31 HD, 23 NHL), and found that FDG-PET/CT has high sensitivity and accuracy and a substantial complementary value to BMB in the initial diagnosis of pediatric lymphoma.[11] All 54 patients had BMB and FDG-PET/CT scans within 2 weeks of biopsy. Among the 31 patients with HD, FDG-PET/CT studies were positive in all 4 cases with BM involvement, whereas BMBs were positive in only 2 of these 4 cases. Among the 23 patients with NHL, FDG-PET/CT scans were positive in 8 of 9 cases with positive BM involvement (4 of them were negative on BMB) and had 1 false-negative finding, whereas BMBs were positive in 5 of these 9 patients (with 1 additional positive case of BM involvement, missed by PET/CT, and 4 false-negative cases on initial studies). The sensitivity of detecting BM involvement by lymphoma was 92% and 54% ($P<.05$) for FDG-PET/CT and BMB, respectively. Bone lesions detected on PET provide important information to guide targeted biopsy, significantly decreasing false-negative findings of BMB.

Available data indicate that the presence of multiple foci of abnormal FDG uptake in BM on initial evaluation, even without biopsy, should strongly raise the suspicion of osseous lymphoma infiltration, and patients should subsequently be treated as having stage IV disease.[11,33] Rarely primary NHL may show as numerous osseous lesions without any lymph node involvement on FDG-PET/CT images.[34,35] However, the value of posttherapeutic FDG-PET/CT in patients with lymphoma remains unclear because chemotherapy and especially use of colony-stimulating factors such as granulocyte colony-stimulating factor (G-CSF) causes diffuse and intense BM uptake,[36] and may obscure any concurrent FDG-avid lesions. FDG uptake in BM is highest at cessation of chemotherapy, declines quickly during the first 6 months after completion of chemotherapy, and then declines more slowly thereafter.[37] For this reason, FDG-PET should be avoided immediately after chemotherapy for evaluation of bony involvement.

Splenic Lesions

There are limited data to determine the value of FDG-PET/CT versus diagnostic CT in the detection of splenic involvement at initial staging of lymphoma (including the pediatric population), although the sensitivity and specificity of PET/CT may be slightly better than diagnostic CT.[38] An abnormal PET finding is generally regarded as splenic uptake greater than hepatic uptake, which often indicates lymphoma involvement if the uptake is focal. The clinical significance of diffusely increased splenic uptake on FDG-PET is less clear and seems to vary in different clinical settings. Substantial FDG uptake is observed in the spleen during and after G-CSF treatment.[36] On a pretherapeutic scan for lymphoma without recent cytokine administration, diffuse splenic uptake (greater than hepatic uptake) is a relatively reliable indication of lymphomatous involvement of the spleen.[39,40] However, diffuse splenic uptake on posttherapy studies is often secondary to administration of G-CSF.[40]

Thymus

FDG uptake in the thymus is common and often physiologic in children and adolescents, and should generally not be regarded as anterior mediastinal lymphoma involvement. It is reported that increased FDG accumulation in the thymus is seen in 73% of children before and 75% after chemotherapy, whereas increased thymic uptake was observed in only 5% of postchemotherapy adult patients, with no increased thymic uptake in prechemotherapy adults.[41] Thymic hyperplasia or thymus rebound often occurs after chemotherapy and may cause a false-positive PET finding without anatomic correlation,[42] but is now a well-recognized postchemotherapy finding. It is important to be familiar with FDG uptake in the thymus during and after chemotherapy in children to avoid misinterpretation.[37,43] FDG uptake in the thymus is significantly lower during chemotherapy than that before chemotherapy in pediatric patients, reaching its lowest level at cessation of chemotherapy. A serial follow-up study of disease-free children and adolescent patients with malignant lymphoma (with a mean follow-up duration of 40 months) found that thymic regrowth occurred 1 to 12 months after chemotherapy.[44] The thymus uptake steadily increases in postchemotherapy pediatric patients until it reaches a peak on average 10 months after therapy, after which it slowly decreases.[37,43] In these patients with thymus rebound, the thymus often has diffusely enlarged parenchymatous tissues, with mildly increased but uniform FDG uptake (with a mean standardized uptake value of 2.7).[44]

Gastrointestinal Tract

It is challenging to evaluate the gastrointestinal (GI) tract involvement in pediatric patients with lymphoma. Diffuse and focal FDG uptake is commonly visualized in the colon, the stomach, and occasionally in the small bowel, often because of inflammation, or as a normal variant. Sometimes oral contrast produces an artifact that appears as FDG uptake in the GI tract. Diffusely increased uptake in the stomach is often physiologic, making diffuse lymphoma involvement of the stomach at an early stage difficult to evaluate by PET. Lymphoma may also be poorly appreciated by CT because of significant variation of normal morphology of the stomach. Primary gastric lymphoma, if focally located, may present as an isolated hypermetabolic gastric mass on PET/CT and lead to the diagnosis.[45] Abdominal Burkitt lymphoma in pediatric patients commonly involves the GI tract and abdominal lymph nodes, and a high suspicion is needed to make a correct diagnosis on a PET/CT. This situation can be problematic for postchemotherapy evaluation for inexperienced interpreters, as aggressive chemotherapy may lead to tumor necrosis complicated by acute inflammation, infections, perforation, or intestinal bleeding. These postchemotherapy findings commonly result in increased FDG uptake, which is sometimes difficult to differentiate from residual malignancy on PET/CT.[46] It seems that the value of PET lies not in the confirmation of residual malignancy in these patients but serves to point to suspected areas for further evaluation.

Pulmonary Lesions

CT remains the best imaging modality in detecting pulmonary involvement in patients with lymphoma. FDG-PET alone is inferior to CT for the detection of small lung metastases because of its limited spatial resolution.[3] The adoption of hybrid PET/CT systems in most clinical practices has significantly increased sensitivity of FDG-PET studies for small lung lesions. Still, small lung lesions may be missed on PET/CT, as noted in a recent study[24] on pediatric patients with HD and NHL, and correlation with CT images is essential for correct diagnosis.

In the assessment of response to therapy, new lung nodules that are 1.5 cm or greater by CT in patients with no evidence of pulmonary lymphoma before therapy should not be considered suggestive of lymphoma if their uptake does not exceed that of mediastinal blood pool structures. New lung nodules in patients without pulmonary lymphoma at baseline and who have evidence of complete response elsewhere should be considered negative for lymphoma regardless of their size or uptake. However, FDG uptake is regarded as unreliable for assessment of small, new lung lesions (<1.5 cm) because of partial volume effect and, therefore, residual lymphoma cannot be excluded.[27,28]

ASSOCIATED INFLAMMATORY/INFECTIOUS FINDINGS

Increased FDG uptake is not specific for lymphoma. Inflammatory/infectious cause is the most common cause of false-positive PET findings. Nonspecific FDG uptake is more common in posttherapy studies than on initial evaluation, because chemotherapy or radiation therapy can be a cause of secondary infection and other inflammatory reactions. Postradiation change is the most common cause of increased FDG uptake as a result of inflammatory reactions and is well recognized.[1] On initial staging studies of pediatric patients, who usually have a relatively simple medical history, the finding of increased FDG uptake on PET was highly accurate in providing correct staging in a patient with biopsy-proven lymphoma. However, accompanying medical conditions are occasionally present. Intussusception is common in pediatric patients and is occasionally detected by FDG-PET/CT in a pediatric lymphoma patient as increased FDG uptake.[47] Sarcoidosis, often characterized by multiple enlarged lymph nodes and mimicking lymphoma on FDG-PET/CT, is occasionally seen in pediatric patients and may represent a challenge to nuclear medicine physicians.[48,49]

SUMMARY

We are seeing wider application of FDG-PET/CT in current clinical practice. Diagnostic CT is often the first study in pediatric patients who are suspicious for lymphoma, but FDG-PET/CT offers more accurate staging and leads to upstaging, and sometimes downstaging, in many patients, because of the capability of PET to detect additional nodal lesions, and more importantly, in the detection of BM involvement and other extranodal lesions. FDG-PET/CT is more accurate than BMB in the evaluation of BM involvement and provides guidance in the selection of a biopsy site. FDG-PET/CT has essentially replaced bone scan for assessment of BM infiltration, and replaced the ^{67}Ga scan for assessment of lymphoma activity. FDG-PET/CT is more accurate than CT in the response assessment during and at the end of therapy in pediatric patients with lymphoma, because metabolic changes can happen independently of anatomic resolution in a patient who has a tumor.

These findings make PET/CT a valuable tool to guide further treatment in lymphoma.

REFERENCES

1. Cheng G, Servaes S, Alavi A, et al. FDG PET and PET/CT in the management of pediatric lymphoma patients. PET Clin 2008;3:621–34.

2. Miller E, Metser U, Avrahami G, et al. Role of 18F-FDG PET/CT in staging and follow-up of lymphoma in pediatric and young adult patients. J Comput Assist Tomogr 2006;30:689–94.

3. Kabickova E, Sumerauer D, Cumlivska E, et al. Comparison of 18F-FDG-PET and standard procedures for the pretreatment staging of children and adolescents with Hodgkin's disease. Eur J Nucl Med Mol Imaging 2006;33:1025–31.

4. Montravers F, McNamara D, Landman-Parker J, et al. [(18)F]FDG in childhood lymphoma: clinical utility and impact on management. Eur J Nucl Med Mol Imaging 2002;29:1155–65.

5. Depas G, De Barsy C, Jerusalem G, et al. 18F-FDG PET in children with lymphomas. Eur J Nucl Med Mol Imaging 2005;32:31–8.

6. Hermann S, Wormanns D, Pixberg M, et al. Staging in childhood lymphoma: differences between FDG-PET and CT. Nucl Med 2005;44:1–7.

7. Riad R, Omar W, Kotb M, et al. Role of PET/CT in malignant pediatric lymphoma. Eur J Nucl Med Mol Imaging 2010;37:319–29.

8. Hernandez-Pampaloni M, Takalkar A, Yu JQ, et al. F-18 FDG-PET imaging and correlation with CT in staging and follow-up of pediatric lymphomas. Pediatr Radiol 2006;36:524–31.

9. Cheng G, Servaes S, Chen W, et al. FDG PET/CT outperforms diagnostic CT in the initial staging of non Hodgkin's lymphoma (NHL) in pediatric patients. J Nucl Med 2009;50:641.

10. Cheng G, Servaes S, Li G, et al. Initial staging of Hodgkin's lymphoma in pediatric patients by PET/CT as compared to diagnostic CT. Clin Nucl Med 2009;34:969–70.

11. Cheng G, Chen W, Chamroonrat W, et al. Biopsy versus FDG PET/CT in the initial evaluation of bone marrow involvement in pediatric lymphoma patients. Eur J Nucl Med Mol Imaging 2011;38:1469–76.

12. Hines-Thomas M, Kaste SC, Hudson MM, et al. Comparison of gallium and PET scans at diagnosis and follow-up of pediatric patients with Hodgkin lymphoma. Pediatr Blood Cancer 2008;51:198–203.

13. Mody RJ, Bui C, Hutchinson RJ, et al. Comparison of (18)F fluorodeoxyglucose PET with Ga-67 scintigraphy and conventional imaging modalities in pediatric lymphoma. Leuk Lymphoma 2007;48:699–707.

14. Hampson FA, Shaw AS. Response assessment in lymphoma. Clin Radiol 2008;63:125–35.

15. Schoder H, Moskowitz C. PET imaging for response assessment in lymphoma: potential and limitations. Radiol Clin North Am 2008;46:225–41.

16. Shankar A, Fiumara F, Pinkerton R. Role of FDG PET in the management of childhood lymphomas–case proven or is the jury still out? Eur J Cancer 2008; 44:663–73.

17. Furth C, Steffen IG, Amthauer H, et al. Early and late therapy response assessment with [18F]fluorodeoxyglucose positron emission tomography in pediatric Hodgkin's lymphoma: analysis of a prospective multicenter trial. J Clin Oncol 2009;27:4385–91.

18. Nasr A, Stulberg J, Weitzman S, et al. Assessment of residual posttreatment masses in Hodgkin's disease and the need for biopsy in children. J Pediatr Surg 2006;41:972–4.

19. Zijlstra JM, Lindauer-van der Werf G, Hoekstra OS, et al. 18F-fluoro-deoxyglucose positron emission tomography for post-treatment evaluation of malignant lymphoma: a systematic review. Haematologica 2006;91:522–9.

20. Amthauer H, Furth C, Denecke T, et al. FDG-PET in 10 children with non-Hodgkin's lymphoma: initial experience in staging and follow-up. Klin Padiatr 2005;217:327–33.

21. Edeline V, Bonardel G, Brisse H, et al. Prospective study of 18F-FDG PET in pediatric mediastinal lymphoma: a single center experience. Leuk Lymphoma 2007;48:823–6.

22. Levine JM, Weiner M, Kelly KM. Routine use of PET scans after completion of therapy in pediatric Hodgkin disease results in a high false positive rate [see comment]. J Pediatr Hematol Oncol 2006;28:711–4.

23. Meany HJ, Gidvani VK, Minniti CP. Utility of PET scans to predict disease relapse in pediatric patients with Hodgkin lymphoma. Pediatr Blood Cancer 2007;48:399–402.

24. London K, Cross S, Onikul E, et al. 18F-FDG PET/CT in paediatric lymphoma: comparison with conventional imaging. Eur J Nucl Med Mol Imaging 2011; 38:274–84.

25. Furth C, Denecke T, Steffen I, et al. Correlative imaging strategies implementing CT, MRI, and PET for staging of childhood Hodgkin disease. J Pediatr Hematol Oncol 2006;28:501–12.

26. Lopci E, Burnelli R, Ambrosini V, et al. (18)F-FDG PET in pediatric lymphomas: a comparison with conventional imaging. Cancer Biother Radiopharm 2008;23:681–90.

27. Cheson BD, Pfistner B, Juweid ME, et al. Revised response criteria for malignant lymphoma. J Clin Oncol 2007;25:579–86.

28. Juweid ME, Stroobants S, Hoekstra OS, et al. Use of positron emission tomography for response assessment of lymphoma: consensus of the Imaging Subcommittee of International Harmonization Project in Lymphoma. J Clin Oncol 2007;25:571–8.

29. Buchmann I, Reinhardt M, Elsner K, et al. 2-(fluorine-18)fluoro-2-deoxy-D-glucose positron emission tomography in the detection and staging of malignant lymphoma. A bicenter trial. Cancer 2001;91:889–99.

30. Shulkin BL, Goodin GS, McCarville MB, et al. Bone and [18F]fluorodeoxyglucose positron-emission tomography/computed tomography scanning for the assessment of osseous involvement in Hodgkin lymphoma in children and young adults. Leuk Lymphoma 2009;50:1794–802.

31. Schaefer NG, Strobel K, Taverna C, et al. Bone involvement in patients with lymphoma: the role of FDG-PET/CT. Eur J Nucl Med Mol Imaging 2007;34:60–7.

32. Muslimani AA, Farag HL, Francis S, et al. The utility of 18-F-fluorodeoxyglucose positron emission tomography in evaluation of bone marrow involvement by non-Hodgkin lymphoma. Am J Clin Oncol 2008;31:409–12.

33. Moulin-Romsee G, Hindié E, Cuenca X, et al. 18F-FDG PET/CT bone/bone marrow findings in Hodgkin's lymphoma may circumvent the use of bone marrow trephine biopsy at diagnosis staging. Eur J Nucl Med Mol Imaging 2010;37:1095–105.

34. Sato TS, Ferguson PJ, Khanna G. Primary multifocal osseous lymphoma in a child. Pediatr Radiol 2008;38:1338–41.

35. Cheng G, Servaes S, Chamroonrat W, et al. Non-Hodgkin's lymphoma of the bone and the liver without lymphadenopathy revealed on FDG-PET/CT. Clin Imaging 2010;34:476–9.

36. Sugawara Y, Fisher SJ, Zasadny KR, et al. Preclinical and clinical studies of bone marrow uptake of fluorine-1-fluorodeoxyglucose with or without granulocyte colony-stimulating factor during chemotherapy. J Clin Oncol 1998;16:173–80.

37. Goethals I, Hoste P, De Vriendt C, et al. Time-dependent changes in 18F-FDG activity in the thymus and bone marrow following combination chemotherapy in paediatric patients with lymphoma. Eur J Nucl Med Mol Imaging 2010;37:462–7.

38. de Jong PA, van Ufford HM, Baarslag HJ, et al. CT and 18F-FDG PET for noninvasive detection of splenic involvement in patients with malignant lymphoma. AJR Am J Roentgenol 2009;192:745–53.

39. Salaun PY, Gastinne T, Bodet-Milin C, et al. Analysis of 18F-FDG PET diffuse bone marrow uptake and splenic uptake in staging of Hodgkin's lymphoma: a reflection of disease infiltration or just inflammation? Eur J Nucl Med Mol Imaging 2009;36:1813–21.

40. Liu Y. Clinical significance of diffusely increased splenic uptake on FDG-PET. Nucl Med Commun 2009;30:763–9.

41. Brink I, Reinhardt MJ, Hoegerle S, et al. Increased metabolic activity in the thymus gland studied with 18F-FDG PET: age dependency and frequency after chemotherapy. J Nucl Med 2001;42:591–5.

42. Weinblatt ME, Zanzi I, Belakhlef A, et al. False-positive FDG-PET imaging of the thymus of a child with Hodgkin's disease. J Nucl Med 1997;38:888–90.

43. Kawano T, Suzuki A, Ishida A, et al. The clinical relevance of thymic fluorodeoxyglucose uptake in pediatric patients after chemotherapy. Eur J Nucl Med Mol Imaging 2004;31:831–6.

44. Zhen Z, Sun X, Xia Y, et al. Clinical analysis of thymic regrowth following chemotherapy in children and adolescents with malignant lymphoma. Jpn J Clin Oncol 2010;40:1128–34.

45. Jacquemart C, Guidi O, Etienne I, et al. Pediatric gastric lymphoma: a rare entity. J Pediatr Hematol Oncol 2008;30:984–6.

46. Riad R, Omar W, Sidhom I, et al. False-positive F-18 FDG uptake in PET/CT studies in pediatric patients with abdominal Burkitt's lymphoma. Nucl Med Commun 2010;31:232–8.

47. Chamroonrat W, Cheng G, Servaes S, et al. Intussusception incidentally detected by FDG-PET/CT in a pediatric lymphoma patient. Ann Nucl Med 2010;24:555–8.

48. Alsultan A, Raddaoui E, Osman ME, et al. Sarcoidosis presenting with massive splenomegaly in a child with a history of iridocyclitis and sensorineural deafness. Pediatr Hematol Oncol 2010;27:490–5.

49. Li YJ, Zhang Y, Gao S, et al. Cervical and axillary lymph node sarcoidosis misdiagnosed as lymphoma on F-18 FDG PET-CT. Clin Nucl Med 2007;32:262–4.

Role of Positron Emission Tomography with Fludeoxyglucose F 18 in Personalization of Therapy in Patients with Lymphoma

Anthony R. Mato, MD, MSCE*, Andre Goy, MD, MS

KEYWORDS

- Positron emission tomography (PET) • Hodgkin lymphoma
- Diffuse large B-cell lymphoma • PET/CT

The widespread availability of functional imaging in clinical practice has revolutionized the care (staging, response assessment, surveillance) of patients with lymphoma. Using positron emission tomography/computed tomography (PET/CT) with fludeoxyglucose F 18 (FDG), the potential exists for prognostic risk stratification and therapeutic adjustment. The various possibilities include:

1. Identification of patients who are likely to derive definite benefit (cure or long-term disease-free control) from a particular treatment approach
2. Minimization of both short-term and long-term toxicity, without loss of efficacy, by identifying patients who may be overtreated (ie, in Hodgkin lymphoma (HL), de-escalation of therapy or reduction of number of cycles)
3. Identification of early chemoresistance in vivo, and defining early salvage strategies, although this last point is debated.

This review examines the current level evidence to support the use of PET/CT imaging as a means to personalize therapy in clinical lymphoma management. To achieve this goal, we searched recent literature in MEDLINE, Embase, BIOSIS and abstracts from the American Society of Hematology and the American Society of Clinical Oncology between the years 2008 and 2011.

Studies included in this review were required to identify the means of data collection (prospective vs retrospective); to identify the cohort by disease subtype (World Health Organization [WHO]), treatment regimens, and relevant disease-specific clinical characteristics; and to specify the response criteria or method used to review PET imaging. This review mainly focuses on 2 lymphoma subtypes: diffuse large B-cell lymphoma (DLBCL) and HL.

CURRENT LEVEL OF EVIDENCE
DLBCL

DLBCL is the most common subtype of non-Hodgkin lymphoma (NHL) and constitutes more than one-third of all NHLs. The addition of immunotherapy to cytotoxic combination chemotherapy (rituximab, cyclophosphamide, vincristine, doxorubicin (adriamycin), prednisone administered every 21 days [R-CHOP-21] being the current standard of care) has markedly improved patient outcomes in terms of disease-free progression (PFS) and overall survival (OS) compared with treatment approaches used in the prerituximab era. However, in about one-half of the patients, the condition still relapses, and two-thirds of the relapses occur in the first 18 months with then

John Theurer Cancer Center at Hackensack University Medical Center, 92 Second Street, Hackensack, NJ 07601, USA
* Corresponding author.
E-mail address: AMato@humed.com

PET Clin 7 (2012) 57–65
doi:10.1016/j.cpet.2011.12.003

a very poor outcome.[1,2] Several clinical and pathologic prognostic markers have been reported that correlate with poor outcome after standard dose R-CHOP.[3–6] These markers include high International Prognostic Index score; bulky disease; high β_2-microglobulin level; proliferation index Ki-67 (MIB-1) (>70%–80%); c-MYC rearrangement; and, more recently, the cell of origin (activated B-cell type vs germinal center subtype). The development of functional imaging, gallium initially (^{67}Ga citrate, which significantly improved the accuracy of response assessment of patients with lymphoma), has been largely replaced by PET scanning, particularly using FDG, a marker of glucose metabolism.

Beyond CT scan imaging, FDG-PET results in a modification of disease stage (usually upstaging) in about 15% to 20% of patients with an impact on management in about 5% to 15%. Pretreatment FDG-PET also facilitates the interpretation of post-therapy FDG-PET studies in patients with DLBCL.

At present, PET is used commonly as part of PET/CT evaluation in patients with lymphoma, especially in restaging or surveillance setting. FDG-PET/CT has been tested as a means to risk stratify patients with DLBCL in various treatment settings, including (1) early response assessment during front-line therapy, (2) after the completion of front-line therapy, (3) after chemotherapy to identify optimal candidates for consolidative radiotherapy, and (4) before autologous stem cell transplantation (ASCT) or allogeneic stem cell transplantation in the relapsed/refractory setting.

The use of PET/CT for early response assessment during front-line therapy is the most controversial and contested application of functional PET imaging in the management of lymphoma. The goal of this approach is to detect chemoresistance in vivo; it has been shown that PET scan can show negative results as early as after 1 cycle of chemotherapy.[7] The rationale is to detect early failures to switch to high-dose salvage therapy (HDT) to overcome chemoresistance, although the impact of earlier HDT remains controversial. Although earlier studies initially supported a role for interim therapy PET/CT to prognosticate patients with DLBCL in the front-line setting, more recent studies do not support its routine use and highlight some of the limitations of functional imaging in clinical practice.[8–11]

Moskowitz and colleagues[12] recently published their series of 98 newly diagnosed patients with DLBCL treated at Memorial Sloan-Kettering Cancer Center (MSKCC) (median follow-up, 44 months) with 4 cycles of dose-dense R-CHOP followed by an interim PET/CT, which was then used to risk stratify patients and determine post-PET consolidation therapy. PET/CT images were interpreted centrally using visual inspection, and the results were categorized as positive (with confirmatory biopsy–proven residual disease), false-positive (confirmatory biopsy with negative results), or negative. Patients with biopsy-proven PET-positive disease received consolidation therapy that included ASCT. Patients with positive PET scan results but biopsy-negative or negative PET imaging were treated with ifosfamide, carboplatin, etoposide (ICE × 3 cycles) followed by observation. In this series, FDG-PET did not correlate with PFS ($P = .146$). Surprisingly, most patients with PET-positive interim scans on visual inspection had a negative confirmatory biopsy (87%, 33/38 patients) and therefore a high false-positive rate when using this approach to identify sites of persistent disease. In an exploratory analysis, the investigators were unable to determine a cutoff point for maximum standardized uptake value (SUV_{max}) or change in standardized uptake value (ΔSUV) that could delineate FDG avidity secondary to malignancy compared with nonmalignant inflammation or infection (ie, some of the false-positive scan results had an $SUV_{max}>35$). A caveat to this study is that all patients had alteration of therapy after the PET scan (ie, switch to ICE), limiting the ability to extrapolate these findings to prediction with a single therapeutic approach.

Pregno and colleagues[13] reported their data on the prognostic value of interim PET imaging, dichotomized using visual inspection according to the International Harmonization Project (IHP) consensus conference criteria in 82 newly diagnosed patients with DLBCL treated with 6 to 8 cycles of R-CHOP.[14] In this retrospective series, in which confirmatory biopsies were not required, the investigators also found no correlation between the presence of FDG avidity on interim imaging and PFS. In contrast to these results, Safar and colleagues[15] also examined the prognostic value of interim PET imaging in 112 newly diagnosed patients with DLBCL treated with rituximab-anthracycline–based chemotherapy. PET results were again assessed using visual inspection and categorized as positive or negative; however, in this series, the interim PET (after 2 cycles of therapy, R-CHOP-21, R-CHOP regimen administered every 14 days [R-CHOP-14], or R-ACVBP) was strongly associated with a 5-year PFS (81% PET negative vs 47% PET positive, $P = .005$) and OS (88% vs 62%, $P<.0034$), particularly in the subset of patients treated with R-CHOP-21.[15] Casasnovas and colleagues[16] found interim PET imaging to be associated with PFS when using a quantitative approach in interpreting scans. Using a receiver operator characteristic curve

(ROC) analysis, the investigators determined that a reduction greater than 66% in FDG avidity in the SUV_{max} after 2 cycles of either R-CHOP-14 or R-ACVBP was associated with a superior outcome (1-year PFS). Visual inspection failed to identify patients at high risk for failure in this series (1-year PFS).[16] Moskowitz and colleagues[17] were unable to validate a decrease greater than 66% in SUV_{max} as the appropriate prognostic cut point for PFS in a series of 54 patients with primary mediastinal DLBCL treated with 4 cycles of R-CHOP-14 followed by ICE consolidation. A reduction greater than 66% in FDG avidity in the SUV_{max} after 4 cycles of R-CHOP-14 (interim PET) was not associated with PFS.

Overall, patients whose interim scan results are positive but turn negative by the end of treatment seem to do about as well as those with negative scan results at both times. The current literature does not support the use of midtherapy (interim) PET/CT imaging to prognosticate patients undergoing front-line therapy with DLBCL. The studies presented in this section highlight some of the major limitations of this imaging modality and its application in clinical practice. First, there is a lack of consistency among investigators in determining when these imaging techniques should be performed relative to a cycle of chemotherapy. Second, there is a need to select a validated model designed for the interpretation of interim PET imaging. Thus, it is extremely difficult to directly compare results between the reported studies because of differences in patient population, therapy, timing of PET imaging, methodologies used to perform/interpret the images, and lack of interrater reliability when interpreting PET imaging even in the most experienced hands. Recent data reported by Horning and colleagues[18] highlight a moderate (at best) reproducibility of PET interpretation among radiologists with nuclear medicine expertise in a clinical research setting (Eastern Cooperative Oncology Group 3404). In an intriguing, hypothesis-generating editorial published in the *Journal of Clinical Oncology*, Huttmann and colleagues[19] discuss possible explanations for why there may be such a disparity in results observed in studies that have questioned the prognostic role of a midtherapy PET/CT in lymphoma. Differences may be attributed in part to the use of granulocyte colony-stimulating factor (potentiation of FDG avidity and alteration of distribution), timing of scans relative to the last cycle of chemotherapy (posttreatment inflammatory response peaks at day 10, which may increase false-positive rate), use of rituximab (cell senescence), and lack of standard/appropriate response criteria used (IHP criteria were designed to examine PET images after the completion of therapy).[19,20]

Although the routine use of interim PET imaging to risk stratify patients with newly diagnosed DLBCL undergoing therapy in the front-line setting is not recommended in clinical practice, there is greater consensus on the prognostic role of PET imaging performed for risk stratification following the completion of front-line immunochemotherapy to identify patients with a favorable prognosis and those with a high likelihood of relapse.[13,21–23] These studies largely use visual inspection of posttherapy PET imaging performed 4 to 6 weeks after the completion of immunochemotherapy. The major advantage of posttherapy PET imaging seems to be a significant improvement in the positive predictive value (PPV) of scan results.

After the completion of chemotherapy, PET/CT may play a role in limiting toxicity due to exposure to consolidative radiotherapy in patients with newly diagnosed DLBCL with residual suspected sites of disease. The British Columbia Cancer Agency reported a retrospective series of 196 patients with newly diagnosed DLBCL treated with 6 to 8 cycles of R-CHOP.[24] Posttreatment CT scans were performed for all patients, and those with lesions larger than 2 cm were recommended to undergo PET imaging (categorized as negative, indeterminate, or positive by visual inspection). About 77% of patients with positive PET imaging underwent targeted radiotherapy to sites of FDG avidity. Patients with positive PET results who underwent consolidative radiotherapy had a similar 3-year PFS as those with negative PET results after R-CHOP and had a superior survival experience than those who had positive PET results and did not undergo elective radiotherapy. Because biopsies were not required or reported in this series, it is unknown how many of the radiated areas represented true lymphoma. The most important result from this series was that 62% of patients who would have normally been exposed to radiotherapy in this practice based on CT imaging were spared the exposure and potential toxicities of radiotherapy without any obvious loss of efficacy.[24] PET/CT delivers an effective radiation dose of 0.01 to 0.03 Gy (varying depending on the quality of the CT portion of the study). This is a negligible dose (.001%) when contrasted with effective doses from therapeutic radiation for lymphoma that ranges between 20 and 45 Gy (varying depending on stage, bulk, and histology).

PET imaging may also play a role in identifying patients with relapsed DLBCL at high risk for failure before consolidative ASCT or allogeneic stem cell transplantation. The (cardiovascular outcomes in renal atherosclerotic lesions) CORAL study group recently examined postsalvage preautotransplant

PET/CT as a predictor of long-term event-free survival (EFS).[2] Patients with relapsed DLBCL were treated with either R-ICE (ICE plus rituximab) or rituximab, dexamethasone, ara-C, and cisplatin (R-DHAP) (dexamethasone, cisplatin, cytarabine plus rituximab) in the salvage setting, with no difference observed between the treatment arms (response rates assessed by 1999 International Working Group [IWG] criteria).[25] PET was recommended but not required by the investigators, and PET results were not used to alter therapy. Of 394 patients, 123 underwent PET imaging after salvage therapy, and the results were reported by the investigators as positive (62/123 patients) or negative (61/123 patients) using 2007 IWG response criteria.[26] For the subset of patients with positive PET results (n = 26) who underwent ASCT, there was a marked difference in 3-year EFS but not PFS or OS (vs those with negative PET results). Having a positive PET after salvage therapy was associated with an inferior PFS (28% vs 43%), EFS (16% vs 40%), and OS (49% vs 66%). Hoppe and colleagues[27] recently examined the prognostic value of PET imaging before ASCT at MSKCC. In this series (positive PET was defined as $SUV_{max}>3$), 22% (18/83 patients who underwent auto transplant) had positive pretransplant PET results. Having positive scan results was associated with an inferior PFS, disease-specific survival, and OS. In a retrospective series of 80 patients (22 of whom had DLBCL) with chemosensitive disease before nonmyeloablative allogeneic stem cell transplantation, PET imaging was performed after salvage chemotherapy (median time, 30 days) and reviewed by 3 radiologists using the IHP consensus conference criteria.[28] Having a positive PET result before allogeneic stem cell transplantation was also associated with inferior 3-year PFS (31% vs 73%) and OS (33% vs 76%) and identified a patient population at high risk for failure. What remains unknown in DLBCL is whether the addition of alternative therapies to patients who remain PET positive after standard salvage chemotherapy can improve prognosis before ASCT or allogeneic stem cell transplantation.[9]

HL

The literature supports the use of both midtherapy and posttherapy PET imaging to risk stratify patients with HL. More recent data suggest that PET imaging may soon play an important role in response-adaptive approaches soon to be ready for clinical practice with the goals of (1) minimization of toxicity and overtreatment and (2) identification of high-risk patients destined to fail standard treatment approaches.

Zinzani and colleagues[29] reported their experience with interim PET imaging to prognosticate 304 patients after 2 cycles of adriamycin (doxorubicin), bleomycin, vincristine, dacarbazine (ABVD) and demonstrated a significant difference in 9-year PFS and 9-year OS between PET-negative and PET-positive groups (median follow-up, 31 months). Markova and colleagues[30] examined the value of midtreatment PET/CT imaging (assessed by visual inspection) performed after 4 cycles of bleomycin, etoposide, adriamycin (=doxorubicin), cyclophosphamide, vincristine, procarbazine, prednisone (BEACOPP) in a cohort of 50 patients treated in the German Hodgkin Study Group Hodgkin's Disease trial (HD15 for advanced stage Hodgkin's disease: Quality assurance protocol for reduction of toxicity and the prognostic relevance of fluorodeoxyglucose-positron-emission tomography (FDG-PET) in the first-line treatment of advanced stage Hodgkin's disease) trial. In this series, the negative predictive value (NPV) and PPV of PET/CT were calculated to be 100% and 22%, respectively. Using visual inspection of PET imaging, Furth and colleagues[31] explored the prognostic value of interim therapy and posttherapy PET/CT tested in a pediatric patient population (n = 40) undergoing polychemotherapy (Phase II Pilot Study of Combination Chemotherapy Comprising Vincristine, Etoposide, Cyclophosphamide, Vinblastine, Prednisone, and Doxorubicin Hydrochloride in Pediatric Males with Previously Untreated Intermediate or Advanced Hodgkin's Lymphoma [HD 2002P], GPOH-HD 2003 therapy study for pediatric Hodgkin's disease German Hodgkin Study Group [HD 2003]). Interim PET/CT imaging was associated with an NPV and a PPV of 100% and 14%, respectively. Posttherapy PET/CT imaging was associated with an NPV and a PPV of 100% and 25%, respectively. The investigators also performed an ROC analysis to determine a cut point for reduction in SUV_{max} to risk stratify patients based on interim PET/CT imaging and found a reduction greater than 58% in FDG avidity to be associated with a favorable outcome (NPV, 100%; PPV, 67%; sensitivity, 100%; specificity, 97%). The CALGB (Cancer and Leukemia Group B) examined the prognostic role of interim PET/CT imaging in patients with early-stage nonbulky HL treated with doxorubicin, gemcitabine, and vinblastine and found a significant difference in 2-year PFS based on interim therapy (88% vs 54%) and posttherapy (89% vs 27%) PET/CT status performed after 2 and 6 cycles of therapy.[32] The NPV of interim PET/CT was found to be 84% in this series. Using IHP criteria, interim PET was evaluated to prognosticate patients for PFS in 246 newly diagnosed patients after 2 cycles of ABVD with early-stage classical HL. In this series, treatment was not altered based on PET results. Interim PET was calculated to have an NPV of 99% and a PPV of 59% in nonbulky patients and an NPV and a PPV of 93% and 40%, respectively, in bulky patients. A positive PET result after 2 cycles of ABVD was associated with an inferior PFS (98% vs 29%, nonbulky; 99% vs 45%, bulky).[33]

An overriding theme observed from these results is the extremely high and consistent NPV associated with interim PET imaging in HL regardless of the method used to interpret the scans. Clearly achieving a negative PET result during or after therapy identifies a subset of patients with improved clinical outcomes. These results have led investigators to incorporate PET results into next generation of clinical trials using functional imaging to influence treatment decisions.

In a series of 45 patients with high-risk HL treated with 2 cycles escalated BEACOPP, Avigdor and colleagues[34] report that interim PET/CT imaging (assessed by visual inspection) was used to select patients with a favorable prognosis (defined as a negative PET result in the setting of responding disease by CT) to de-escalate therapy to ABVD with the goal of minimizing toxicity. Of 45 patients, 31 successfully converted their PET/CT to negative after 2 cycles of escalated BEACOPP and had a 4-year PFS of 87% (NPV, 87%). Patients with a positive PET/CT result went on to complete front-line escalated BEACOPP and were found to have a 4-year PFS of 53% (PPV, 45%; $P = .01$). Gallamini and colleagues[35] reported a retrospective international series of 165 patients with HL treated with a response-adapted approach. All patients received 2 cycles of ABVD and then underwent PET imaging with a plan to escalate to BEACOPP in the PET-positive subset of patients (categorized using a 5-point scale).[36] The 2-year failure-free survival was 95% and 62% for interim PET-negative versus PET-positive patient subsets, respectively, ($P = .00001$). The investigators concluded that achievement of a negative PET result after ABVD identifies a subset of patients who can do well clinically without the need for added toxicity associated with escalated BEACOPP. The HD0607 study is currently underway to prospectively validate these findings.

The role of postchemotherapy radiotherapy in patients with suspected residual disease is a remaining area of controversy in the management of HL. Undoubtedly, radiotherapy decreases the risk of local recurrence but at the cost of increased risk of both short-term and long-term toxicities. Studies have examined whether functional imaging can be used to identify patients with

a low risk for local recurrence and can therefore eliminate consolidative radiotherapy to residual areas of suspected disease. In HD15, patients with lesions at suspected sites of disease (>2.5 cm by CT) with concomitant FDG-avid lesions were scheduled to undergo radiotherapy to areas of residual disease (confirmatory biopsy not required).[37] A negative PET scan result was associated with a 3-year time to progression of 86% in 74% of patients who achieved a negative PET result after BEACOPP (NPV of 95%). As compared with previous studies with a similar patient population universally radiated based on CT results (randomized trial carried out by the German Hodgkin Study Group [GHSG] for elderly patients with advanced Hodgkin's disease comparing BEACOPP baseline and COPP-ABVD (study HD9elderly) [HD9]), the investigators concluded that most patients can be spared consolidative radiotherapy in the setting of postchemotherapy PET negativity. Recently, the second planned interim analysis of the a randomized phase III trial to determine the Role of FDG-PET Imaging in Clinical Stages IA/IIA Hodgkin's Disease (RAPID) trial has been reported.[38] This study is exploring the role of eliminating involved field radiation therapy in patients with stage 1a-2a supradiaphragmatic HL with negative PET results after 3 cycles of ABVD. Using a 5-point scale to assess PET imaging, 79% of patients are reported to be PET negative after ABVD. At present, 331 patients have enrolled in this study, and we await trial completion and efficacy results. Similarly, the European Organisation for the Research and Treatment of Cancer, GELA (Groupe d'Etude Des Lymphomes De l'Adulte), and IIL (Intergruppo Italiano Linfomi) are currently using interim PET imaging to prognosticate patients and modify therapy in H10. This study includes patients with early-stage HL with both a favorable and unfavorable risk profile with risk status–specific treatment arms.[39] At last report, 1097 patients have enrolled and interim results indicate that 76% (unfavorable risk) and 86% (favorable risk) of patients have negative PET/CT results with an acceptable level of agreement on interim PET status between expert central reviewers. Efficacy data have not yet been reported.

In the pretransplant setting, PET has been examined as a prognostic tool. In a series of 198 patients with relapsed/refractory HL before ASCT, patients were stratified into 3 groups based on PET and CT results: (1) both negative PET and CT results, (2) negative PET results/residual mass on CT, and (3) positive PET results. Patients with positive PET results before ASCT had an overall poor prognosis with both an inferior OS and EFS compared with groups 1 and 2.[40] The presence of a residual mass (PET negative) also had a significant impact on OS and EFS in this series. Building on this experience, Moskowitz and colleagues[41] have reported preliminary results of a phase II response-adapted study using PET/CT performed after 2 cycles of ICE salvage chemotherapy in 40 patients with relapsed/refractory HL. The goal of the study was to determine the added value of non–cross-resistant salvage chemotherapy before ASCT in high-risk patients defined by pretransplant PET positivity. Patients who achieved a negative PET result after ICE salvage underwent ASCT, whereas those who were PET positive after ICE received 4 cycles of GVD (gemcitabine, vinorelbine, liposomal doxorubicin) followed by a repeat PET/CT. In this series, 25 of 37 patients remained PET positive after ICE salvage and underwent GVD therapy, of whom 13 were able to normalize their PET scan result before ASCT. In terms of EFS, patients who were PET negative after ICE and those who were PET negative after GVD had a similar survival experience and were both superior to the subset of patients who underwent ASCT with PET-positive disease.

To help determine which response criteria are best for interpreting interim therapy PET/CT imaging in HL, Gastinne and colleagues[42] compared IHP criteria with both the Gallamini criteria and the London 5-point scale in 90 patients with HL after 2 cycles of ABVD. The results of this retrospective comparison suggest an improvement in test characteristics (in particular the PPV and specificity) when either the Gallamini criteria or the London 5-point scale criteria are compared with IHP criteria, with the 5-point scale demonstrating the best results (PPV, 55%; NPV, 96%, vs PPV, 16%; 95% NPV IHP).[42] Based on the current literature review, IHP criteria should be reserved for PET interpretation following the completion of planned therapy because they were intended when proposed by Juweid and colleagues.[14] This is especially true in the design of future research testing response-adaptive approaches in HL. A similar analysis would be quite useful in helping to determine which criteria should be included in future studies of interim PET/CT imaging in DLBCL and other lymphoma subtypes. The Gallamini Criteria, London Criteria, and IHP criteria are summarized in **Table 1**.

OTHER LYMPHOMA SUBTYPES: RECENT HIGHLIGHTS
Follicular Lymphoma

Although follicular center cell lymphoma is second only to DLBCL in terms of its incidence, limited data are available regarding the use of PET/CT imaging to risk stratify patients. Recently the Primary Rituximab and Maintenance (PRIMA) study group retrospectively explored the association between PET/CT status and patient outcomes in 160 patients with follicular lymphoma treated with chemotherapy with rituximab in the frontline setting.[44] Patients who had a positive PET/CT result after the completion of induction therapy

Table 1
PET imaging criteria

IHP Criteria[14]	London Criteria[35]	Gallamini Criteria[11,43]
• PET reviewed (attenuation corrected recommended) by visual assessment after completion of therapy • Results are interpreted as positive or negative • Lesions ≥2 cm: use mediastinal blood pool activity as reference background • Lesions <2 cm: positive if its activity is more than that of the surrounding background • Liver, spleen, lung, and bone marrow assessment by specific criteria	• PET scans with score 1–3 are considered negative • PET scans with a score 4–5 are considered positive • Score 1: no residual uptake • Score 2: <mediastinum blood pool • Score 3: <mediastinum blood pool and ≤liver • Score 4: uptake increased above liver at any site • Score 5: update increased markedly above liver at any site or new site of disease	• Pretreatment PET imaging required • Disease was evaluated site by site for the involved lymph nodes and organs • Negative result: no pathologic FDG uptake at any site (including sites of previously increased uptake) • Positive result: presence of a focal FDG concentration outside the physiologic uptake areas (increased activity relative to the background) • Patients with a PET scan showing minimal residual uptake are considered PET negative (SUV of 2.0–3.5)

had a more aggressive clinical course with an inferior PFS (hazard ratio [HR], 3.5; P<.0001), and thus PET/CT was useful to identify high-risk patients with inferior outcomes with conventional treatment strategies. This result was most pronounced in patients who were randomized to posttherapy observation. In addition, FDG-PET and 3-deoxy-3[18]fluorothymidine positron emission tomography (FLT-PET) scans may help to identify sites of transformed lymphoma in patients with indolent NHL.[16]

Mantle Cell Lymphoma

Although mantle cell lymphoma (MCL) is reported to be an FDG-avid NHL subtype, PET/CT is not currently recommended (conflicting results/lack of evidence) in the modified IWG criteria to stage, survey, and assess treatment response. Our group recently conducted a retrospective cohort study to examine the prognostic utility of PET/CT imaging (using IHP criteria) in a uniform patient cohort with MCL (53 patients) undergoing dose-intensive chemotherapy (cyclophosphamide, vincristine, doxorubicin and dexamethasone + Rituximab alternating with high-dose methotrexate + cytarabine + R [R-HyperCVAD]) in the front-line setting. With median follow-up of 32 months, we found that interim PET/CT status (positive vs negative) was not associated with PFS (HR, 0.9; confidence interval [CI], 0.3–2.7; P = .8) or OS (HR, 0.6; CI, 0.1–2.9; P = .5). Posttreatment PET/CT status was statistically significantly associated with PFS (HR, 5.2; CI, 2.0–13.6; P = .001) and trended toward significant for OS (HR, 2.8; CI, 0.8–9.6; P = .07). Our data suggest limited value of PET/CT in pretreatment and interim treatment settings. A positive PET/CT result after the completion of therapy identifies a patient subset with an inferior PFS and a trend toward inferior OS.[45]

RECOMMENDATIONS

- The use of PET/CT holds tremendous promise as a means to personalize therapies for patients with lymphoma in the future.
- The current evidence supports the use PET/CT with a narrow focus specifically to prognosticate patients with either DLBCL (posttherapy imaging) or HL (midtreatment and posttherapy imaging) undergoing therapy in the front-line setting.
- However, at present, the current level of evidence (although intriguing) does not support the use of PET/CT imaging in defining response-adaptive treatment algorithms in clinical practice.

- Recently reported and ongoing studies may soon expand the role of PET/CT as a tool for risk stratification and in response-adaptive approaches. The major limitations to the practical application of PET/CT include accuracy (interrater reliability) and validity (clinical relevance), which affect the generalizabilty of clinical research in this area.
- Early steps toward agreement on standardization of PET/CT response criteria and PET/CT imaging protocols may improve the ability to translate results from the research setting to the clinic.
- We strongly support enrollment in clinical trials designed to answer key questions in this area.

REFERENCES

1. Thieblemont C, Briere J, Mounier N, et al. The germinal center/activated B-cell subclassification has a prognostic impact for response to salvage therapy in relapsed/refractory diffuse large B-cell lymphoma: a bio-CORAL study. J Clin Oncol 2011; 29(31):4079–87.
2. Trneny M, Bosly A, Bouabdallah K, et al. Independent predictive value of PET-CT pre transplant in relapsed and refractory patients with CD20 diffuse large B-cell lymphoma (DLBCL) included in the CORAL study. Blood (ASH Annual Meeting Abstracts) 2009; 114(22):881.
3. Gaudio F, Giordano A, Perrone T, et al. High Ki67 index and bulky disease remain significant adverse prognostic factors in patients with diffuse large B cell lymphoma before and after the introduction of rituximab. Acta Haematol 2011;126(1):44–51.
4. Anonymous. A predictive model for aggressive non-Hodgkin's lymphoma. The International Non-Hodgkin's Lymphoma Prognostic Factors Project. N Engl J Med 1993;329(14):987–94.
5. Gutierrez-Garcia G, Cardesa-Salzmann T, Climent F, et al. Gene-expression profiling and not immunophenotypic algorithms predicts prognosis in patients with diffuse large B-cell lymphoma treated with immunochemotherapy. Blood 2011;117(18): 4836–43.
6. Fu K, Weisenburger DD, Choi WW, et al. Addition of rituximab to standard chemotherapy improves the survival of both the germinal center B-cell-like and non-germinal center B-cell-like subtypes of diffuse large B-cell lymphoma. J Clin Oncol 2008;26(28): 4587–94.
7. Kostakoglu L, Goldsmith SJ, Leonard JP, et al. FDG-PET after 1 cycle of therapy predicts outcome in diffuse large cell lymphoma and classic Hodgkin disease. Cancer 2006;107(11):2678–87.

8. Haioun C, Itti E, Rahmouni A, et al. [18F]fluoro-2-deoxy-D-glucose positron emission tomography (FDG-PET) in aggressive lymphoma: an early prognostic tool for predicting patient outcome. Blood 2005;106(4):1376–81.

9. Cheson BD. Role of functional imaging in the management of lymphoma. J Clin Oncol 2011; 29(14):1844–54.

10. Hutchings M, Mikhaeel NG, Fields PA, et al. Prognostic value of interim FDG-PET after two or three cycles of chemotherapy in Hodgkin lymphoma. Ann Oncol 2005;16(7):1160–8.

11. Gallamini A, Rigacci L, Merli F, et al. The predictive value of positron emission tomography scanning performed after two courses of standard therapy on treatment outcome in advanced stage Hodgkin's disease. Haematologica 2006;91(4):475–81.

12. Moskowitz CH, Schoder H, Teruya-Feldstein J, et al. Risk-adapted dose-dense immunochemotherapy determined by interim FDG-PET in advanced-stage diffuse large B-cell lymphoma. J Clin Oncol 2010; 28(11):1896–903.

13. Pregno P, Chiappella A, Bello M, et al. Interim 18-FDG-positron emission tomography/computed tomography (PET) failed to predict different outcome in diffuse large B-cell lymphoma (DLBCL) patients treated with rituximab-CHOP. Blood (ASH Annual Meeting Abstracts) 2009;114(22):99.

14. Juweid ME, Stroobants S, Hoekstra OS, et al. Use of positron emission tomography for response assessment of lymphoma: consensus of the Imaging Subcommittee of International Harmonization Project in Lymphoma. J Clin Oncol 2007;25(5): 571–8.

15. Safar V, Dupuis J, Jardin F, et al. Early 18fluorodeoxyglucose PET scan as a prognostic tool in diffuse large B-cell lymphoma patients treated with an anthracycline-based chemotherapy plus rituximab. Blood (ASH Annual Meeting Abstracts) 2009;114(22):98.

16. Casasnovas RO, Meignan M, Berriolo-Riedinger A, et al. Interim [18F]fluorodeoxyglucose positron emission tomography SUVmax reduction is superior to visual analysis to predict early patient's outcome in diffuse large B-cell lymphoma. Blood (ASH Annual Meeting Abstracts) 2010;116(21):320.

17. Moskowitz C, Hamlin PA Jr, Maragulia J, et al. Sequential dose-dense RCHOP followed by ICE consolidation (MSKCC protocol 01-142) without radiotherapy for patients with primary mediastinal large B cell lymphoma. Blood (ASH Annual Meeting Abstracts) 2010;116(21):420.

18. Horning SJ, Juweid ME, Schoder H, et al. Interim positron emission tomography scans in diffuse large B-cell lymphoma: an independent expert nuclear medicine evaluation of the Eastern Cooperative Oncology Group E3404 study. Blood 2010;115(4): 775–7 [quiz: 918].

19. Huttmann A, Muller S, Jockel KH, et al. Pitfalls of interim positron emission tomography scanning in diffuse large B-cell lymphoma. J Clin Oncol 2010; 28(27):e488–9 [author reply: e490–1].

20. Dorr JR, Buck AK, Stein H, et al. Metabolic targeting in lymphoma therapy. Ann Oncol 2011;22(Suppl 4): iv127.

21. Cashen A, Dehdashti F, Luo J, et al. Poor predictive value of FDG-PET/CT performed after 2 cycles of R-CHOP in patients with diffuse large B-cell lymphoma (DLCL). Blood (ASH Annual Meeting Abstracts) 2008;112(11):371.

22. Gigli F, Nassi L, Negri M, et al. Interim 18f[FDG] positron emission tomography in patients with diffuse large B-cell lymphoma. Blood (ASH Annual Meeting Abstracts) 2008;112(11):3607.

23. Micallef IN, Maurer MJ, Witzig TE, et al. PET scan results of NCCTG N0489: epratuzumab and rituximab in combination with cyclophosphamide, doxorubicin, vincristine and prednisone chemotherapy (ER-CHOP) in patients with previously untreated diffuse large B-cell lymphoma. Blood (ASH Annual Meeting Abstracts) 2009;114(22):137.

24. Sehn LH, Hoskins P, Klasa R, et al. FDG-PET scan guided consolidative radiation therapy optimizes outcome in patients with advanced-stage diffuse large B-cell lymphoma (DLBCL) with residual abnormalities on CT scan following R-CHOP. Blood (ASH Annual Meeting Abstracts) 2010;116(21):854.

25. Cheson BD, Horning SJ, Coiffier B, et al. Report of an international workshop to standardize response criteria for non-Hodgkin's lymphomas. J Clin Oncol 1999;17(4):1244.

26. Cheson BD, Pfistner B, Juweid ME, et al. Revised response criteria for malignant lymphoma. J Clin Oncol 2007;25(5):579–86.

27. Hoppe BS, Moskowitz CH, Zhang Z, et al. The role of FDG-PET imaging and involved field radiotherapy in relapsed or refractory diffuse large B-cell lymphoma. Bone Marrow Transplant 2009;43(12):941–8.

28. Dodero A, Crocchiolo R, Patriarca F, et al. Pretransplantation [18-F]fluorodeoxyglucose positron emission tomography scan predicts outcome in patients with recurrent Hodgkin lymphoma or aggressive non-Hodgkin lymphoma undergoing reduced-intensity conditioning followed by allogeneic stem cell transplantation. Cancer 2010;116(21):5001–11.

29. Zinzani PL, Rigacci L, Stefoni V, et al. Early interim 18F-FDG PET in Hodgkin's lymphoma: evaluation on 304 patients. Blood (ASH Annual Meeting Abstracts) 2010;116(21):3879.

30. Markova J, Kobe C, Skopalova M, et al. FDG-PET for assessment of early treatment response after four cycles of chemotherapy in patients with advanced-stage Hodgkin's lymphoma has a high negative predictive value. Ann Oncol 2009;20(7): 1270–4.

31. Furth C, Steffen IG, Amthauer H, et al. Early and late therapy response assessment with [18F]fluoro-deoxyglucose positron emission tomography in pediatric Hodgkin's lymphoma: analysis of a prospective multicenter trial. J Clin Oncol 2009; 27(26):4385–91.

32. Straus DJ, Johnson JL, LaCasce AS, et al. Doxorubicin, vinblastine, and gemcitabine (CALGB 50203) for stage I/II nonbulky Hodgkin lymphoma: pretreatment prognostic factors and interim PET. Blood 2011;117(20):5314–20.

33. Rigacci L, Zinzani PL, Puccini B, et al. IHP interpretation criteria of interim-PET scan confirms prognostic impact in early stage Hodgkin lymphoma patients without bulky disease. Blood (ASH Annual Meeting Abstracts) 2010;116(21):3890.

34. Avigdor A, Bulvik S, Levi I, et al. Two cycles of escalated BEACOPP followed by four cycles of ABVD utilizing early-interim PET/CT scan is an effective regimen for advanced high-risk Hodgkin's lymphoma. Ann Oncol 2010;21(1):126–32.

35. Meignan M, Gallamini A, Haioun C, et al. Report on the first international workshop on interim-PET-scan in lymphoma. Leuk Lymphoma 2009;50(8):1257–60.

36. Fiore F, Patti K, Viviani S, et al. Effect of early chemotherapy intensification with BEACOPP in high-risk, interim-PET positive, advanced-stage Hodgkin lymphoma on overall treatment outcome of ABVD. ASCO Meeting Abstracts. J Clin Oncol 2010;28(Suppl 15): [abstract 8006].

37. Engert A, Kobe C, Markova J, et al. Assessment of residual bulky tumor using FDG-PET in patients with advanced-stage Hodgkin lymphoma after completion of chemotherapy: final report of the GHSG HD15 trial. Blood (ASH Annual Meeting Abstracts) 2010;116(21):764.

38. Radford J, O'Doherty M, Barrington S, et al. Results of the 2nd planned interim analysis of the RAPID trial (involved field radiotherapy versus no further treatment) in patients with clinical stages 1A and 2A Hodgkin lymphoma and a 'negative' FDG-PET scan after 3 cycles ABVD. Blood (ASH Annual Meeting Abstracts) 2008;112(11):369.

39. Andre MP, Reman O, Federico M, et al. First report on the H10 EORTC/GELA/IIL randomized intergroup trial on early FDG-PET scan guided treatment adaptation versus standard combined modality treatment in patients with supra-diaphragmatic stage I/II Hodgkin's lymphoma, for the Groupe d'Etude Des Lymphomes De l'Adulte (GELA), European Organisation for the Research and Treatment of Cancer (EORTC) Lymphoma Group and the Intergruppo Italiano Linfomi (IIL). Blood (ASH Annual Meeting Abstracts) 2009;114(22):97.

40. Moskowitz AJ, Nimer SD, Zelenetz AD, et al. Pretransplant evaluation with both CT and PET following second-line therapy is essential for predicting outcome in patients with transplant-eligible relapsed and primary refractory Hodgkin lymphoma. Blood (ASH Annual Meeting Abstracts) 2008;112(11):776.

41. Moskowitz CH, Nimer SD, Zelenetz AD, et al. Normalization of FDG-PET pre-ASCT with additional non-cross resistant chemotherapy improves EFS in patients with relapsed and primary refractory Hodgkin lymphoma—Memorial Sloan Kettering Protocol 04-047. Blood (ASH Annual Meeting Abstracts) 2008;112(11):775.

42. Gastinne T, Le Roux PY, Bodet-Milin C, et al. Respective prognostic value of the International Harmonization Project (IHP), Gallamini and London Criteria for interim FDG PET-CT performed after 4 courses of ABVD in Hodgkin's lymphoma. Blood (ASH Annual Meeting Abstracts) 2010; 116(21):3889.

43. Gallamini A, Hutchings M, Rigacci L, et al. Early interim 2-[18F]fluoro-2-deoxy-D-glucose positron emission tomography is prognostically superior to international prognostic score in advanced-stage Hodgkin's lymphoma: a report from a joint Italian-Danish study. J Clin Oncol 2007;25(24): 3746–52.

44. Trotman J, Fournier M, Lamy T, et al. Result of FDG PET-CT imaging after immunochemotherapy induction is a powerful and independent prognostic indicator of outcome for patients with follicular lymphoma: an analysis from the PRIMA study. Blood (ASH Annual Meeting Abstracts) 2010;116(21):855.

45. Mato AR, Zielonka T, Feldman T, et al. Post-treatment (not interim) PET-CT scan status is highly predictive of outcome in mantle cell lymphoma treated with R-HyperCVAD or ASCT. Blood (ASH Annual Meeting Abstracts) 2010;116(21):3131.

The Use of PET in Radiation Therapy for Lymphoma

John P. Plastaras, MD, PhD[a],*, Geoffrey Geiger, MD[a],
Rodolfo Perini, MD[b,c], Eli Glatstein, MD[a]

KEYWORDS

- PET • Radiation therapy • Lymphoma
- 18-Fluorodeoxyglucose

Combined modality treatment has become standard for the cure of many patients with lymphoma in the modern era. Radiation therapy (RT) and chemotherapy complement each other in terms of patterns of relapse. When patients are treated with chemotherapy alone, the most common site of relapse is in previous sites of disease. By contrast, when patients are treated with radiation alone, relapses most often occur outside of the radiated volumes. Because of this complementarity, in most patients the chemotherapy and the radiation can both be truncated in most patients, thereby markedly reducing morbidity resulting from each modality. PET with 18-fluorodeoxyglucose (FDG) had a dramatic impact on the way in which both modalities are used in combination, changing the way clinicians stage patients and how they determine patient response. The way in which to incorporate this information into practical treatment of lymphomas is a developing body of knowledge.

CAN FDG-PET RESPONSE BE USED TO OMIT CONSOLIDATIVE RADIATION?

With the successful cure of many patients with combination chemotherapy regimens, many investigators have attempted to select patients in whom RT can be omitted. Even in favorable-risk, early stage patients with Hodgkin lymphoma (HL), the omission of RT has led to an unacceptable rate of relapse as demonstrated in the EORTC/GELA H9F trial.[1] In curable neoplasms, it is often stated that many patients are "overtreated." The problem is knowing which ones could receive less intensive treatment without increasing the risk of relapses. The so-called "response-adapted strategies" use radiographic responses to chemotherapy to tailor how much additional treatment a given patient needs. Ideally, this would allow individualized less aggressive regimens, without compromising outcomes, decreasing acute and long-term morbidity. Conversely, the minority of patients not responding to therapy on an interim evaluation, presumptively less likely to be cured, can be offered more aggressive treatments. Conventional assessments of response (ie, elimination of nodal mass) are limited in predictive value by virtue that malignant cells in HL only comprise a small fraction of tumor volume.[2] Furthermore, complete response can take time, even in cells that die primarily by apoptosis. Response-adapted decisions need to be made with the proper timing such that the overall "package time" for delivering therapy is not compromised. Metabolic response by FDG-PET offers an opportunity for an interval assessment of response and has been incorporated into the International Workshop Criteria.[3]

Multiple studies have demonstrated that FDG-PET/computed tomography (CT) can differentiate between responders and nonresponders by virtue

a Department of Radiation Oncology, Perelman Center for Advanced Medicine, 3400 Civic Center Boulevard, Philadelphia, PA 19104, USA
b Division of Nuclear Medicine and Molecular Imaging, Department of Radiology, University of Pennsylvania, 3400 Spruce Street, Donner 110-B, Philadelphia, PA 19104, USA
c Division of Hematology and Oncology, Department of Medicine, University of Pennsylvania, 3400 Spruce Street, Donner 110-B, Philadelphia, PA 19104, USA
* Corresponding author.
E-mail address: Plastaras@uphs.upenn.edu

PET Clin 7 (2012) 67–72
doi:10.1016/j.cpet.2011.12.005

of evaluating patients after one to three cycles of chemotherapy and that metabolic response is a reliable surrogate for progression-free survival.[4–7] Preliminary results suggest that about two-thirds of all early stage patients with HL are expected to achieve a metabolic complete response after two cycles of chemotherapy. The concept of treating with two cycles of chemotherapy beyond a complete response has been more accepted in HL than in diffuse large B-cell lymphoma.

Every negative PET in a patient who subsequently relapses should be considered a false-negative. False-positives are harder to define because many patients undergo additional therapy after FDG-PET scanning. There are two fundamental types of errors one can make while using response-adapted strategies: undertreating a false-negative result, or overtreating a false-positive result. For a highly curable disease, the test would need to have a very low rate of false-negatives to avoid undertreatment. The initial studies using postchemotherapy FDG-PET scans to omit radiotherapy in HL are conflicting at this point. Picardi and colleagues[8] randomized 160 patients with bulky HL and negative posttreatment FDG-PET to either RT (32 Gy) to sites of original bulky disease, or observation. With a median follow-up of 40 months, at 1.5 years, 11 patients (14%) in the observation arm relapsed compared with 2 patients (2.5%) in the RT arm. All of the patients who relapsed in the observation arm and one of the two patients in the RT arm developed disease in both the original site of bulky disease and adjacent nodal locations. In contrast, Kobe and colleagues[9] demonstrated a 94% negative predictive value at 12 months of posttreatment FDG-PET/CT for poor risk, limited stage HL patients receiving no RT in an interim analysis of the German HD15 trial. Of note, this analysis included only patients with at least one residual mass of at least 2.5 cm after treatment with six to eight cycles of BEACOPP (311 evaluable patients). This study used a central review panel to determine whether or not there was a complete metabolic response. Patients with residual disease on PET were treated with RT per protocol and 15% of these had relapsed at 12 months. By design, this analysis took place at 12 months as a safety measure, and the authors caution that further follow-up is warranted to confirm this excellent negative predictive value. The differing conclusions from these two studies may be caused by the length of follow-up, the central FDG-PET review panel, or the intensity of the chemotherapy.

For the case of the second type of error (false-positive), Moskowitz and colleagues[10] have recommended repeat biopsy of FDG-avid residua before making major treatment decisions. In a prospective study of patients with high-risk diffuse large B-cell lymphoma treated with four cycles of rituximab, cyclophosphamide, doxorubicin, vincristine, and prednisone, the investigators used the result of the interval evaluation to decide the type of additional treatment; consolidative ifosfamide, carboplatin, and etoposide alone, in patients with a negative interim PET, while ifosfamide, carboplatin, and etoposide plus autologous stem cell transplant in patients with a positive PET and also positive rebiopsy. Of the 38 patients with positive PET who underwent repeat biopsy, 33 were negative ($\approx$87% false-positive rate using biopsy as gold standard) and were treated with the "less aggressive regimen." There is a finite false-negative rate with biopsy, but 26 of the FDG-PET–positive/biopsy-negative 33 patients were still without progression, which was not different than the FDG-PET–negative patients.[10] Although this study was a small, single-institution study, it does make the important point that even though FDG-PET is an excellent tool, it should be viewed with a healthy dose of skepticism. Similarly, in HL, the positive predictive value of postchemotherapy FDG-PET is substantially worse than the negative predictive value.[11–13]

To date, there is not yet prospective randomized evidence that patients benefit from adapted treatment, although there are several ongoing phase III clinical trials. These include H10 EORTC/GELA/IIL randomized intergroup trial,[14] the German HD16 trial,[15] and Christie Hospital NHS Foundation Trust trial.[16] As an example, the HD16 trial randomizes patients with limited stage HL to a standard strategy (two cycles of doxorubicin, bleomycin, vinblastine, and dacarbazine [ABVD] plus 20 Gy IFRT irrespective of FDG-PET results after chemotherapy); or response-adapted strategy (ABVD $\times$ 2 plus 20 Gy IFRT if FDG-PET is positive after chemotherapy; ABVD $\times$ 2 only if FDG-PET is negative after chemotherapy). The H10 EORTC/GELA/IIL study uses three or four cycles of ABVD based on risk grouping and involved node radiotherapy (INRT); accrual on the standard strategy arm completed in June of 2011.[14] If a patient has favorable HL with no negative factors and has achieved a complete response both clinically and radiographically, the authors do not irradiate if the patient is reliable for follow-up. With any negative factors, they recommend consolidative RT.

FDG-PET/CT IN RADIATION TREATMENT PLANNING FOR LYMPHOMA

Over the last three decades, the radiation fields for lymphomas have evolved from large fields based on bony anatomy to much smaller fields in the era of combined modality therapy. Total nodal radiation or subtotal nodal irradiation encompassed all or almost all lymphoid tissue, whereas today's fields are limited to single or contiguous nodal regions. Even the classic "mantle" field has evolved over time, with the frequent and judicious elimination of the axillary components that results in "modified" mantle fields, reducing dose to lung and breast tissue dramatically. The concept of INRT has more recently evolved where the prechemotherapy nodal volume is treated with a small margin of 1 to 2 cm.[17] The appeal of shrinking the fields is the potential reduction in morbidity from large RT fields, but this is balanced by a potential decrement in locoregional control. Imaging methods have been critical in accurately delineating the actual structures that need RT. Lymphangiography and staging laparotomy have been rendered obsolete by CT for staging. CT for treatment planning allows the treating physician to ensure that dose reaches the targets in three-dimensional space, hopefully avoiding many of the treatment failures of the past related to

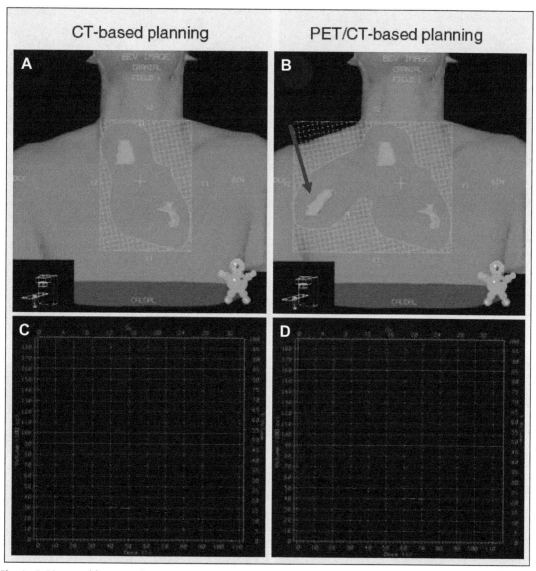

Fig. 1. A 44-year-old man with stage IIA HL who had an FDG-PET–positive focus in the right axilla not identified on the staging CT (red arrow). (A, B) Anterior projections of the different planning treatment volumes. (C, D) Markedly different dose–volume histograms, with body volume on the y-axis and radiation dose on the x-axis. (From Hutchings M, Loft A, Hansen M, et al. Clinical impact of FDG-PET/CT in the planning of radiotherapy for early-stage Hodgkin lymphoma. Eur J Haematol 2007;78:206–12; with permission.)

inadvertent shielding of gross tumor.[18,19] For radiation treatment planning, FDG-PET/CT has brought a whole new level of accuracy to the assessment of nodal involvement. Integrated FDG-PET/CT scanning has further improved imaging accuracy by anatomic correlation and attenuation correction. In addition to avoiding the shielding of important target tissues, CT and FDG-PET/CT have the potential to reduce the volume of normal tissue irradiated by eliminating some of the approximations needed in the two-dimensional era. This concept was prospectively demonstrated in 30 patients with HL where FDG-PET/CT substantially altered the treatment fields in one-third of patients.[20] In seven cases, the volume treated was increased, and in two patients, it was decreased. Furthermore, in one case, RT was safely omitted because of detection of previously undetected advanced disease. FDG-PET information can drastically affect the radiation fields in some cases (**Fig. 1**). The treatment volumes were drastically altered by FDG-PET information when an INRT approach was used.[21] FDG-PET is very helpful in identifying areas of

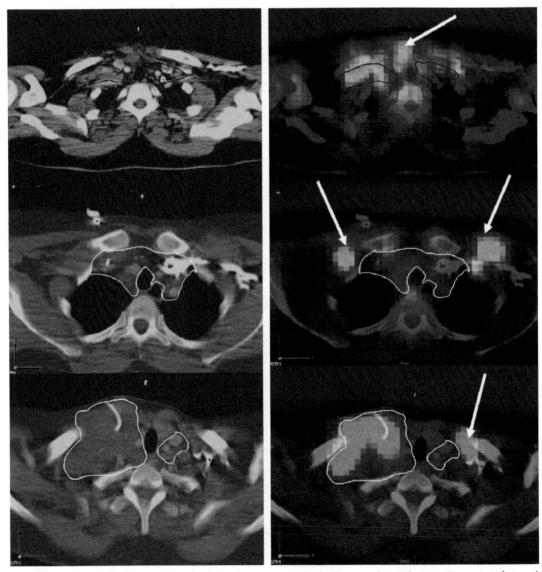

Fig. 2. Examples of FDG-PET–avid lymph nodes that were overlooked on prechemotherapy CT scans. Left panels represent CT scans where target lymph nodes were contoured (*yellow*). Right panels represent the same patients fused with the FDG-PET scans. *Arrows* denote lymph nodes that were overlooked. (*From* Girinsky T, Ghalibafian M, Bonniaud G, et al. Is FDG-PET scan in patients with early stage Hodgkin lymphoma of any value in the implementation of the involved-node radiotherapy concept and dose painting? Radiother Oncol 2007;85:178–86; with permission.)

disease that are not obvious on CT alone. This concept is important in staging, but even more important for RT planning, where the radiation oncologist wants to know where all of the gross disease is located (**Fig. 2**). Interestingly, FDG-PET alone is not sufficient in identifying disease; in early stage HL, only 25% of the lymphomatous volumes contoured on CT were actually FDG avid.[21]

One challenge of incorporating FDG-PET/CT imaging into radiation treatment planning is image fusion with the radiation planning CT scans. The most important set of FDG-PET/CT images are those before chemotherapy. When the patient is ready for consolidative radiation, their anatomy can change because of tumor response and changes in their weight. However, the larger problem is the differing position of the patient from the initial diagnostic FDG-PET or FDG-PET/CT scan to the radiation planning CT scan, performed in a very specific position on a flat treatment table. Deformable fusion algorithms are useful in combining the simulation scan with original pretreatment FDG-PET/CT, but the solutions are far from perfect. It would be ideal to have the radiation oncologist involved from the outset to allow for physical examination and proper initial imaging (eg, flat table at staging FDG-PET/CT). Early involvement of the radiation oncologist is required when using INRT, as delineated by the EORTC/GELA guidelines.[17] Many radiation oncology departments are acquiring PET/CT simulators that allow for streamlined diagnostic and radiation planning imaging to be done in one session.

In addition to using FDG-PET to increase sensitivity compared with CT scanning alone, it is possible to use FDG-uptake differences to guide radiation dosing decisions. Today's doses are 25% to 50% less than 30 years ago if there is no overt disease. Radiation oncologists frequently treat different target volumes to different doses based on their estimation of the burden of disease. The larger volume that is expected to only harbor microscopic amounts of tumor cells can be treated to a lower dose, and a smaller volume of gross tumor can be "boosted" to a higher dose. The rapidity of metabolic changes after two to three cycles of chemotherapy may be used to estimate disease burden and the identification of FDG-avid residua for planning boosts.

DOES RADIATION INTERFERE WITH EARLY INTERVAL FDG-PET SCANNING?

FDG uptake, as an imaging biomarker of glycolysis, is not specific for malignancy and also occurs in inflammatory processes. Appropriate timing of FDG-PET in restaging patients with lymphoma is critical to avoid equivocal interpretations. It is recommended that FDG-PET should be performed at least 3 weeks (preferably 6–8 weeks) after completion of chemotherapy and 8–12 weeks after RT.[3] This is thought to minimize potential RT-induced early inflammatory changes. It is important to remember that these recommendations stem from consensus among different specialists, noting the paucity of human data to support these statements. Small studies by Castellucci and colleagues[22] and Keller and colleagues[23] showed a low rate of postradiation inflammatory changes in patients with lymphoma. As different RT techniques, such as proton therapy, are increasingly applied into routine practice, further studies will be needed to evaluate the optimal time for restaging FDG-PET scans.

SUMMARY

FDG-PET/CT has essentially replaced CT as the primary modality for staging and radiation treatment planning in the last decade. It has been incorporated into the revised response criteria, but response-adapted strategies are still being evaluated. The use of FDG-PET/CT to determine appropriateness of whether to give consolidative radiation, to boost certain volumes, or simply to observe remains unanswered. Ongoing efforts are underway to assess the use of early interim FDG-PET/CT in the selection of good prognosis early stage patients who may be cured by chemotherapy only, without RT. One cannot overemphasize the importance of a multidisciplinary team in the management of patients with lymphoma, as early as in the initial staging, and also in the design of future clinical trials. This will lead to individualized treatment plans, and better outcomes.

REFERENCES

1. Noordijk EM, Thomas J, Fermé C. First results of the EORTC-GELA H9 randomized trials: the H9-F trial (comparing 3 radiation dose levels) and H9-U trial (comparing 3 chemotherapy schemes) in patients with favorable or unfavorable early stage Hodgkin's lymphoma (HL). 2005 ASCO Annual Meeting Proceedings. J Clin Oncol 2005;23(16S, Pt I Suppl):6505.
2. Canellos GP. Residual mass in lymphoma may not be residual disease. J Clin Oncol 1988;6:931–3.
3. Juweid ME, Wiseman GA, Vose JM, et al. Response assessment of aggressive non-Hodgkin's lymphoma by integrated International Workshop Criteria and

fluorine-18-fluorodeoxyglucose positron emission tomography. J Clin Oncol 2005;23:4652–61.

4. Gallamini A, Hutchings M, Rigacci L, et al. Early interim 2-[18F]fluoro-2-deoxy-D-glucose positron emission tomography is prognostically superior to international prognostic score in advanced-stage Hodgkin's lymphoma: a report from a joint Italian-Danish study. J Clin Oncol 2007;25:3746–52.

5. Gallamini A, Rigacci L, Merli F, et al. The predictive value of positron emission tomography scanning performed after two courses of standard therapy on treatment outcome in advanced stage Hodgkin's disease. Haematologica 2006;91:475–81.

6. Hutchings M, Mikhaeel NG, Fields PA, et al. Prognostic value of interim FDG-PET after two or three cycles of chemotherapy in Hodgkin lymphoma. Ann Oncol 2005;16:1160–8.

7. Zinzani PL, Tani M, Fanti S, et al. Early positron emission tomography (PET) restaging: a predictive final response in Hodgkin's disease patients. Ann Oncol 2006;17:1296–300.

8. Picardi M, De Renzo A, Pane F, et al. Randomized comparison of consolidation radiation versus observation in bulky Hodgkin's lymphoma with post-chemotherapy negative positron emission tomography scans. Leuk Lymphoma 2007;48:1721–7.

9. Kobe C, Dietlein M, Franklin J, et al. Positron emission tomography has a high negative predictive value for progression or early relapse for patients with residual disease after first-line chemotherapy in advanced-stage Hodgkin lymphoma. Blood 2008;112:3989–94.

10. Moskowitz CH, Schoder H, Teruya-Feldstein J, et al. Risk-adapted dose-dense immunochemotherapy determined by interim FDG-PET in Advanced-stage diffuse large B-Cell lymphoma. J Clin Oncol 2010; 28:1896–903.

11. de Wit M, Bohuslavizki KH, Buchert R, et al. 18FDG-PET following treatment as valid predictor for disease-free survival in Hodgkin's lymphoma. Ann Oncol 2001;12:29–37.

12. Molnar Z, Simon Z, Borbenyi Z, et al. Prognostic value of FDG-PET in Hodgkin lymphoma for post-treatment evaluation. Long term follow-up results. Neoplasma 2010;57:349–54.

13. Weihrauch MR, Re D, Scheidhauer K, et al. Thoracic positron emission tomography using 18F-fluoro-deoxyglucose for the evaluation of residual mediastinal Hodgkin disease. Blood 2001;98:2930–4.

14. André MP, Reman O, Fédérico M, et al. First report on the H10 EORTC/GELA/IIL randomized intergroup trial on early FDG-PET scan guided treatment adaptation versus standard combined modality treatment in patients with supra-diaphragmatic stage I/II Hodgkin's lymphoma, for the Groupe d'Etude Des Lymphomes De l'Adulte (GELA), European Organisation for the Research and Treatment of Cancer (EORTC) Lymphoma Group and the Intergruppo Italiano Linfomi (IIL) American Society of Hematology. New Orleans, LA, 2009. p. 97.

15. HD16 for early stage Hodgkin lymphoma (HD16 for early stages-treatment optimization trial in the first-line treatment of early stage Hodgkin lymphoma; treatment stratification by means of FDG-PET). Available at: http://clinicaltrials.gov/ct2/show/NCT00736320. Accessed December 27, 2011.

16. PET scan in planning treatment in patients undergoing combination chemotherapy for stage IA or stage IIA Hodgkin lymphoma (a randomised phase III trial to determine the role of FDG-PET imaging in clinical stages IA/IIA Hodgkin's disease). Available at: http://clinicaltrials.gov/ct2/show/NCT00943423. Accessed December 27, 2011.

17. Girinsky T, van der Maazen R, Specht L, et al. Involved-node radiotherapy (INRT) in patients with early Hodgkin lymphoma: concepts and guidelines. Radiother Oncol 2006;79:270–7.

18. Rostock RA, Giangreco A, Wharam MD, et al. CT scan modification in the treatment of mediastinal Hodgkin's disease. Cancer 1982;49:2267–75.

19. Naida JD, Eisbruch A, Schoeppel SL, et al. Analysis of localization errors in the definition of the mantle field using a beam's eye view treatment-planning system. Int J Radiat Oncol Biol Phys 1996;35:377–82.

20. Hutchings M, Loft A, Hansen M, et al. Clinical impact of FDG-PET/CT in the planning of radiotherapy for early-stage Hodgkin lymphoma. Eur J Haematol 2007;78:206–12.

21. Girinsky T, Ghalibafian M, Bonniaud G, et al. Is FDG-PET scan in patients with early stage Hodgkin lymphoma of any value in the implementation of the involved-node radiotherapy concept and dose painting? Radiother Oncol 2007;85:178–86.

22. Castellucci P, Zinzani P, Nanni C, et al. 18F-FDG PET early after radiotherapy in lymphoma patients. Cancer Biother Radiopharm 2004;19:606–12.

23. Keller H, Goda JS, Vines DC, et al. Quantification of local tumor response to fractionated radiation therapy for non-Hodgkin lymphoma using weekly 18F-FDG PET/CT imaging. Int J Radiat Oncol Biol Phys 2010;76:850–8.

Evolving Importance of Diffusion-Weighted Magnetic Resonance Imaging in Lymphoma

Thomas C. Kwee, MD, PhD[a],*,
Sandip Basu, MBBS (Hons), DRM, DNB[b,c],
Drew A. Torigian, MD, MA[c],
Rutger A.J. Nievelstein, MD, PhD[a],
Abass Alavi, MD, PhD (Hon), DSc (Hon)[d]

KEYWORDS

- Diffusion-weighted imaging • Magnetic resonance imaging
- Whole-body imaging • Lymphoma • Hodgkin
- Non-Hodgkin

CURRENT ROLE OF IMAGING IN LYMPHOMA

The lymphomas, Hodgkin lymphoma (HL) and non-Hodgkin lymphoma (NHL), comprise approximately 5% to 6% of all malignancies, and rank fifth in terms of the most frequently occurring type of cancer in the United States. In 2010 in the United States approximately 8490 new cases of HL and 65,540 new cases of NHL were diagnosed, and an estimated 1320 patients with HL and 20,120 patients with NHL died because of their disease.[1] Once the diagnosis of lymphoma has been established histopathologically, it is important to determine the extent of disease (ie, staging). Lymphomas are staged using the Ann Arbor staging system, which comprises 4 stages.[2,3] This system encompasses the number of sites of disease involved, the type of involvement (nodal or extranodal), and the distribution of disease.[2,3] An exception is pediatric NHL, which is staged using the Murphy staging system.[4,5] Accurate staging is important because it determines

treatment planning and predicts prognosis. Furthermore, knowing the sites of involvement at the time of diagnosis makes it possible to accurately restage and assess response at the end of therapy and to document a complete remission.[2,3] Hence, imaging plays a central role in staging of lymphoma from the aforementioned perspectives.[6] Another emerging concept is the use of imaging to provide an early assessment of the response to therapy. Early identification of patients who are likely to show a poor response to therapy would provide the opportunity to adjust individual treatment regimes and to shift to the salvage schedules more rapidly, thus sparing patients unnecessary morbidity and expense of ineffective treatment.

^{18}F-FLUORODEOXYGLUCOSE PET/COMPUTED TOMOGRAPHY

At present, combined ^{18}F-2-fluoro-2-deoxy-D-glucose (FDG) positron emission tomography

[a] Department of Radiology, University Medical Center Utrecht, Heidelberglaan 100, 3584 CX Utrecht, The Netherlands
[b] Radiation Medicine Center (Bhabha Atomic Research Center), Tata Memorial Center Annexe, Jerbai Wadia Road, Parel, Mumbai 400012, Maharashtra, India
[c] Department of Radiology, Hospital of the University of Pennsylvania, 3400 Spruce Street, Philadelphia, PA 19102, USA
[d] Division of Nuclear Medicine, Department of Radiology, Hospital of the University of Pennsylvania, 3400 Spruce Street, Philadelphia, PA 19102, USA
* Corresponding author.
E-mail address: thomaskwee@gmail.com

PET Clin 7 (2012) 73–82
doi:10.1016/j.cpet.2011.11.001
1556-8598/12/$ – see front matter © 2012 Elsevier Inc. All rights reserved.

(PET)/computed tomography (CT) is regarded as the most accurate noninvasive method for the staging of lymphoma.[6,7] In addition, FDG-PET (/CT) may also be performed after a few cycles of chemotherapy to assess early treatment response and predict the final therapeutic outcome.[6–8] Several ongoing trials are expected to provide a definite answer on its utility in this setting in the near future. Well-recognized advantages of FDG-PET are its high lesion-to-background contrast and its ability to visualize and quantify (changes in) tumor glucose metabolism, independent of structural changes. Furthermore, the CT component of an FDG-PET/CT examination allows for the localization of areas with abnormal FDG uptake and the detection of structural (and contrast-enhancement) abnormalities.[6,7] Possible disadvantages of FDG-PET/CT, however, are exposure of the patient to ionizing radiation and its relatively high cost.[9,10]

WHOLE-BODY MAGNETIC RESONANCE IMAGING

Magnetic resonance (MR) imaging is a cross-sectional imaging modality that does not use any ionizing radiation, provides a high soft-tissue contrast, and offers a wide arsenal of anatomic and functional sequences. Furthermore, technological developments have enabled the routine clinical use of whole-body MR imaging.[11] Therefore, whole-body MR imaging may potentially be an alternative to FDG-PET/CT for the evaluation of lymphoma. An alternative view is to consider whole-body MR imaging and FDG-PET as complementary imaging methods, especially given the expected clinical introduction of combined PET/MR imaging systems.[12] Commonly applied sequences for whole-body MR imaging include (contrast-enhanced) T1-weighted and (fat-suppressed) T2-weighted or short inversion-time inversion recovery (STIR) imaging. Several studies have shown that the aforementioned whole-body MR imaging sequences can be used for staging lymphoma.[13–16]

WHOLE-BODY DIFFUSION-WEIGHTED IMAGING

An important MR imaging technique that has recently emerged as a potentially valuable method for whole-body oncological imaging is diffusion-weighted imaging (DWI).[17–20] DWI allows visualization and quantification of (therapy-induced changes in) the random (Brownian) motion of water molecules, without using any contrast agents.[17–20] Because many malignant tumors exhibit an impeded diffusion compared with normal tissues, DWI can provide a high lesion-to-background contrast. For this reason it is a potentially useful technique for the staging of malignancies,[17–20] including lymphomas.[15,21,22] In addition, DWI may be used as an imaging biomarker for the early detection of therapy-induced changes in tumor diffusivity, before structural changes have occurred.[23–26] This article now describes the basics of (whole-body) DWI, and reviews and discusses the evolving importance of whole-body DWI for the staging and therapy response assessment of lymphoma.

BASICS OF (WHOLE-BODY) DWI
Diffusion in Biological Tissue

DWI is sensitive to the random (Brownian) extracellular, intracellular, and transcellular motion of water molecules, driven by their internal thermal energy. The signal intensity in DWI is a function of the Brownian motion of an ensemble of water molecules.[27] For water molecules in the bulk phase, the probability distribution of displacements due to Brownian motion is Gaussian, symmetrically disposed about their original position.[27] In biological tissue, however, the presence of impeding barriers such as cell membranes, fibers, and macromolecules interferes with the free displacement (diffusion) of water molecules. Consequently, the signal intensity at DWI depends on the separation and permeability of these impeding boundaries. Pathologic processes that alter the physical nature of the impeding barriers in biological tissue affect the diffusivity of the water molecules, which can be visualized and quantified using DWI.[17–20,27] The first successful clinical application of DWI was in diagnosing acute ischemic stroke. In acute ischemic stroke, failure of the Na^+,K^+-ATPase pump leads to a net displacement of water from the extracellular to the intracellular compartment, manifest as a precipitous drop in water mobility.[27,28] DWI may also be useful for the evaluation of other diseases, including cancer. Many cancers, including lymphomas, have an increased cellularity compared with normal, healthy tissue. An increase in cellularity may lead to a decrease of the extracellular volume, whereby increased tortuosity of the extracellular space leads to reduced water mobility. On the other hand, (therapy-induced) necrosis and apoptotic processes may lead to a loss of cell membrane integrity and a decrease in cellularity. In turn, this increases the amount of diffusion across the cell membrane and increases the proportion of water molecules in the extracellular space, where water mobility is less impeded. All these processes can be evaluated using DWI, both qualitatively (visually) and quantitatively (by means of so-called apparent diffusion coefficient [ADC] measurements).[17–20,27]

DWI Sequence and Quantification

As introduced by Stejskal and Tanner,[29] the most common approach to render MR imaging sensitive to diffusion is to place two strong symmetric gradient lobes (so-called motion probing gradients [MPGs]) on either side of the 180° refocusing pulse in a (T2-weighted) spin echo sequence (**Fig. 1**). Stationary water molecules within a voxel acquire a phase shift by the first MPG, which is nullified by the second MPG. The resultant signal intensity of that voxel is equal to its signal intensity on an image obtained with the same sequence without the MPGs. However, water molecules within a voxel undergoing diffusion acquire a phase shift by the first MPG, which is not nullified by the second MPG because of a positional difference of the water molecules between the moment of the application of the first MPG and the moment of the application of the second MPG; as a result, the signal is attenuated. The resultant signal intensity (SI) of a voxel containing diffusing water molecules is equal to its intensity on a T2-weighted image, decreased by an amount related to the degree of diffusion:

$$SI = SI_0 \times exp(-b \times ADC), \qquad (1)$$

where SI_0 is the signal intensity on the T2-weighted (or b = 0 s/mm²) image, ADC is the apparent diffusion coefficient, and b is the b-value (which expresses the degree of diffusion weighting), calculated as follows:

$$b = \gamma^2 \times G^2 \times \delta^2(\Delta - \delta/3), \qquad (2)$$

where δ is the duration of one MPG, Δ is the interval between the leading edges of the MPGs, G is the strength of the MPG (see **Fig. 1**), and γ is the gyromagnetic ratio (the ratio of the magnetic moment to the angular momentum of a particle, 42.58 MHz/T for hydrogen).[29,30]

Because the Stejskal-Tanner sequence is based on a T2-weighted spin echo sequence (see **Fig. 1**), the acquired diffusion-weighted image also has T2-weighted contrast, referred to as T2 shine-through. However, unlike T2-weighted imaging, DWI can suppress many unwanted background signals of normal structures that demonstrate perfusion, flow, or a considerable amount of diffusion (eg, signals of gastrointestinal contents, blood vessels, cerebrospinal fluid) while highlighting lesions that exhibit impeded diffusivity. In other words, DWI detects lesions by exploiting both their prolonged T2 value and impeded diffusivity, and provides a high lesion-to-background contrast; in this respect, DWI outperforms conventional MR imaging sequences such as T2-weighted imaging.[17–20]

If one aims to differentiate between potential areas of T2 shine-through and areas with an impeded diffusion, and/or to quantify diffusion, 2 or more images with different b-values should be acquired. The ADC is most frequently calculated using an implicit monoexponential model, as follows:

$$ADC = (1/(b_1 - b_0))ln(S[b_0]/S[b_1]), \qquad (3)$$

where b_1 and b_0 represent 2 different b-values, $S[b_1]$ the signal intensity of the selected region of interest (ROI) on the image acquired with b-value b_1, and $S[b_0]$ the signal intensity of the same ROI on the image acquired with b-value b_0. A pixel by pixel map (so-called ADC map), whose intensity yields quantitative estimation of the regional ADC, can be obtained by postprocessing and applying the equations described above.[27,30] To obtain a perfusion-insensitive ADC, it is recommended to acquire the low b-value DWI dataset with a b-value of 100 s/mm² or greater.[20,23] The high b-value DWI dataset is often acquired using a b-value between 500 and 1000 s/mm². For body imaging, b-values greater than 1000 s/mm² are generally less optimal for ADC calculation because they yield inadequate signal-to-noise ratio.[20,23]

DEVELOPMENT OF WHOLE-BODY DWI

Until recently, the main organ of interest for using DWI was the brain. Extracranial DWI, however, is more challenging. First, because DWI requires

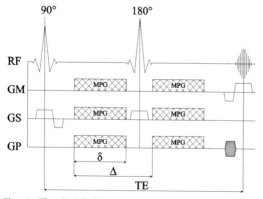

Fig. 1. The Stejskal-Tanner sequence. δ, duration of one MPG; Δ, time interval between the leading edges of the MPGs; GM, readout direction; GP, phase-encoding direction; GS, section-select direction; MPG, motion probing gradient; RF, radiofrequency; TE, echo time.

ultrafast imaging, an echo-planar imaging (EPI) readout is used. EPI is very susceptible to main field inhomogeneities, local susceptibility gradients, and chemical shift, which all may lead to severe image degradation. These artifacts occur in the case of tissue heterogeneity, especially at air-tissue and bone-tissue boundaries.[31,32] Because of the requirement of a larger field of view and the presence of many air-tissue and bone-tissue boundaries in the trunk, extracranial DWI is more prone to EPI-related image distortions. Fortunately, the introduction of parallel imaging, which allows reduction of the echo time, the echo train length, and the k-space filling time, led to substantially fewer image distortions and motion artifacts. As a result, extracranial DWI has become feasible.[17–20] Second, because DWI is sensitive to the motion of water molecules over a few micrometers, bulk tissue motion was initially thought to be a serious impediment when performing DWI of the chest and (upper) abdomen. Therefore, respiratory motion compensation techniques (ie, breath-hold or respiratory gated acquisitions) were thought to be mandatory for DWI of moving organs. However, when using a breath-hold acquisition only thick slices (typically 8–9 mm) can be obtained. The use of thick slices limits lesion detectability, does not allow for the creation of multiplanar reformats and 3-dimensional renderings, and can reduce the reliability of ADC measurements because of partial volume effects. In addition, considerable scan time prolongation under respiratory gating would be a serious impediment for whole-body scanning. This important limitation of DWI in the body has been overcome by the demonstration of the feasibility of DWI under free breathing, also known as the concept of Diffusion-weighted Whole-body Imaging with Background body signal Suppression (DWIBS).[17–20] Details about this concept can be read elsewhere.[19] Advantages of DWI under free breathing over breath-hold and respiratory gated image acquisitions include the possibility to obtain thin slices (typically 4 mm) and its efficient scan time (data can be acquired during the entire respiratory cycle), respectively.[17–20] Of interest, at whole-body DWI (DWIBS concept), many unwanted background structures such as (normal) fat, muscles, flowing blood, and other free fluids are suppressed, while tissues with low water mobility (including many cancerous lesions) are highlighted. The high lesion-to-background contrast is the reason why whole-body diffusion-weighted images and FDG-PET images have striking visual similarities at a first glance. Despite these visual similarities, it is important to always keep in mind that DWI and FDG-PET provide different biological information, which can be regarded as complementary.[20]

GENERAL CHALLENGES ASSOCIATED WITH THE EVALUATION OF WHOLE-BODY DWI

There are several general challenges associated with the interpretation of whole-body diffusion-weighted images. First, an impeded diffusion is not exclusively seen in malignant lesions. Depending on the degree of diffusion weighting (b-value) that is applied, several normal tissues (particularly the brain, spinal cord, peripheral nerves, Waldeyer ring, spleen, lymph nodes, prostate, testis, penis, endometrium, ovaries, and bone marrow) are often visualized as structures of high signal intensity on DWI because of the relatively long T2 value and low water mobility (**Fig. 2**). Furthermore, several nonmalignant lesions (including ischemic and

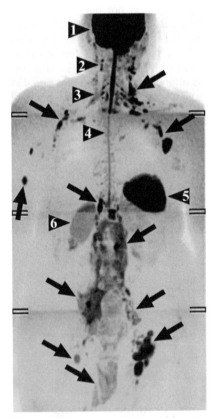

Fig. 2. Whole-body DWI in a 62-year-old woman with stage III follicular lymphoma. Coronal maximum-intensity projection gray-scale inverted whole-body DWI (acquired using a b-value of 1000 s/mm²) shows extensive supradiaphragmatic and infradiaphragmatic lymph node involvement (*arrows*). Also note normal high signal intensity of the brain (*arrowhead 1*), right cervical lymph nodes (*arrowhead 2*), brachial plexus nerves (*arrowhead 3*), spinal cord (*arrowhead 4*), spleen (*arrowhead 5*), and right kidney (*arrowhead 6*).

inflammatory lesions, abscesses, thrombi, and hematoma) can be highlighted on DWI because of the same reasons. The nonspecificity of DWI may occasionally complicate image interpretation in patients with cancer. Second, because of the suppression of many background structures on (high b-value) DWI, there may a lack of an anatomic reference to exactly localize lesions with an impeded diffusion. Third, cardiac motion may lead to signal loss of lesions in the lungs, heart, other mediastinal structures (including esophagus and lymph nodes), and liver (particularly the left hepatic lobe).[33,34] These problems can in part be overcome by using correlative (anatomic) imaging. Studies have shown that the diagnostic performance of DWI with T2-weighted imaging is superior to either DWI or T2-weighted imaging alone.[35–37] A problem that has to be taken into account when performing quantitative diffusion analysis is that cardiac motion may lead to artificially elevated ADCs of nearby lesions.[33,34] Although a cardiac gated acquisition may solve this problem, it considerably prolongs scan time. Furthermore, cardiac gated DWI is technically challenging. Another issue is that the calculation of an ADC requires the acquisition of at least 2 datasets with 2 different b-values.[27,30] Image misregistration between different datasets due to bulk tissue motion (eg, respiratory motion) or EPI-related image distortion may lead to inaccurate ADC measurements. For this reason, it is recommended to check image registration quality between different datasets and to use conservative regions or volumes of interest when performing ADC measurements.

WHOLE-BODY DWI FOR THE STAGING OF LYMPHOMA

Lymphomas are characterized by a relatively long T2 value and a considerably impeded diffusion.[38–46] Therefore, lymphomas exhibit very high signal intensity on native diffusion-weighted images and low signal intensity on ADC maps compared with most normal surrounding tissues. Because of its potentially high lesion-to-background contrast, whole-body DWI may be a valuable technique for the staging of lymphoma (see **Fig. 2**). Furthermore, ADC measurements may potentially be helpful in the evaluation of lymph nodes for lymphomatous involvement (**Fig. 3**).

A study by Kwee and colleagues[15] prospectively compared a combination of conventional whole-body MR imaging (T1-weighted and STIR sequences) and whole-body DWI with CT for the staging of 28 patients with newly diagnosed lymphoma. Lymphomatous lesions were diagnosed at MR imaging based on size criteria and signal abnormalities, without using any ADC maps. Ann Arbor stages of combined conventional whole-body MR imaging and whole-body DWI were equal to those of CT in 75% (21/28), higher in 25% (7/28), and lower in 0% (0/28) of patients, with correct/incorrect overstaging relative to CT in 6 and 1 patient(s), respectively. Of interest, the combination of conventional whole-body MR imaging with whole-body DWI correctly upstaged 4 of 28 patients compared with conventional whole-body MR imaging alone, which well reflects the potential additional diagnostic value of DWI.[15]

Another prospective study by Lin and colleagues[21] compared whole-body DWI with FDG-PET/CT as reference standard for the staging of newly diagnosed diffuse large B-cell lymphoma in 15 patients. Whole-body DWI findings matched FDG-PET/CT findings in 277 regions (94%) ($\kappa = 0.85$, $P<.0001$), yielding sensitivity and specificity for DWI lymph node involvement detection of 90% and 94%. Combining nonquantitative (visual) ADC analysis with size measurement increased the specificity of

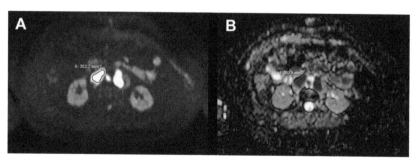

Fig. 3. Example of an ADC measurement of a lymphomatous para-aortic lymph node in a 72-year-old woman with nodal marginal zone lymphoma. Axial diffusion-weighted image (acquired using a b-value of 1000 s/mm^2) (*A*) and corresponding ADC map (created using b-values of 0 and 1000 s/mm^2) (*B*) with region of interest in a pathologically enlarged para-aortic lymph node revealed a relatively low ADC of 0.51×10^{-3} mm^2/s, suggestive of lymphoma. (*From* Kwee TC, Ludwig I, Uiterwaal CS, et al. ADC measurements in the evaluation of lymph nodes in patients with non-Hodgkin lymphoma: feasibility study. MAGMA 2011;24(1):5; with permission.)

whole-body DWI to 100%, with 81% sensitivity. For organ involvement, the two techniques agreed in all 20 recorded organs (100%). Ann Arbor stages agreed in 14 (93%) of the 15 patients. The investigators concluded that whole-body DWI with visual ADC analysis can potentially be used for lesion detection and staging in patients with diffuse large B-cell lymphoma.[21]

In yet another study by Van Ufford and colleagues,[22] the combination of conventional whole-body MR imaging (T1-weighted and STIR sequences) and whole-body DWI was prospectively compared with FDG-PET/CT for the staging of 22 patients with newly diagnosed lymphoma. Lymphomatous lesions were diagnosed at MR imaging based on size criteria and signal abnormalities, without using any ADC maps. Whole-body MR imaging combined with DWI (MRI-DWI) was independently evaluated by two blinded observers. Interobserver agreement was assessed and whole-body MRI-DWI was compared with FDG-PET/CT. K values for interobserver agreement at whole-body MRI-DWI for all nodal regions together and for all extranodal regions together were 0.676 and 0.452, respectively. K values for agreement between whole-body MRI-DWI and FDG-PET/CT for all nodal regions together and for all extranodal regions together were 0.597 and 0.507, respectively. Ann Arbor stage according to whole-body MRI-DWI was concordant with that of FDG-PET/CT in 77% (17/22) of patients, whereas understaging and overstaging relative to FDG-PET/CT occurred in 0% (0/22) and 23% (5/22) of patients, respectively. In 9% (2/22) of patients, whole-body MRI-DWI overstaging relative to FDG-PET/CT would have had therapeutic consequences. Van Ufford and colleagues[22] concluded that overall interobserver agreement at whole-body MRI-DWI is moderate to good. Overall agreement between whole-body MRI-DWI and FDG-PET/CT is moderate. Furthermore, whole-body MRI-DWI does not understage relative to FDG-PET/CT in patients with newly diagnosed lymphoma. In a minority of patients, whole-body MRI-DWI leads to clinically important overstaging relative to FDG-PET/CT. Van Ufford and colleagues[22] emphasized that FDG-PET/CT remains the gold standard for the staging of lymphoma until future, larger studies have shown that whole-body MRI-DWI provides correct upstaging in such cases.

In the studies by Kwee and colleagues,[15] Lin and colleagues,[21] and Van Ufford and colleagues,[22] whole-body diffusion-weighted images (without or with the use of ADC maps) were only qualitatively (visually) assessed. To investigate whether quantitative diffusion (ADC) measurements can be used to discriminate normal lymph nodes from lymphomatous lymph nodes, and indolent lymphomas from aggressive lymphomas in patients with NHL, Kwee and colleagues[46] prospectively performed DWI in 18 healthy volunteers and 32 patients with newly diagnosed NHL (indolent: n = 16; aggressive: n = 16). ADCs of normal lymph nodes were compared with those of lymphomatous lymph nodes, and ADCs of indolent lymphomas were compared with those of aggressive lymphomas. ADCs (in 10^{-3} mm^2/s) of lymphomatous lymph nodes (0.70 ± 0.22) were significantly lower ($P<.0001$) than those of normal lymph nodes (1.00 ± 0.15). Area under the receiver-operating characteristic curve was 0.865. On the other hand, ADCs of indolent lymphomas (0.67 ± 0.21) were not significantly different ($P = .2997$) from those of aggressive lymphomas (0.74 ± 0.23). The investigators concluded that ADC measurements show promise as a highly specific tool for the discrimination of normal lymph nodes from lymphomatous lymph nodes, but appear to be of no utility in differentiating indolent from aggressive lymphomas.[46]

The evidence accumulated so far[15,21,22,46] shows that whole-body DWI is a feasible and promising method for the staging of lymphoma. However, further research in larger patient samples is needed to show the (additional) diagnostic value of whole-body DWI compared with conventional (T1-weighted, T2-weighted, or STIR) whole-body MR imaging alone, and to assess whether it can be an alternative to FDG-PET/CT. In addition, larger studies should prospectively establish the value of ADC measurements in the staging workup of patients with lymphoma.

WHOLE-BODY DWI FOR THERAPY RESPONSE ASSESSMENT IN LYMPHOMA

Another promising application of DWI is its use as an imaging biomarker for the (early) assessment of response to anticancer therapy (**Fig. 4**). First, pretreatment ADCs in responding lesions have been reported to be significantly lower (ie, lower water mobility) than those of nonresponding lesions in several other cancers.[47–49] The biological basis for this finding remains unclear, but it can be speculated that a higher pretreatment ADC (ie, higher water mobility) is observed in necrotic tissue and in tissue with loss of cell membrane integrity, which may correspond to a more aggressive phenotype. Second, it has also been reported that, after initiation of therapy, responding lesions show a significantly higher increase in ADC early after initiation of therapy (ie, higher increase in water mobility) than nonresponding lesions,[47–50] which can be attributed to

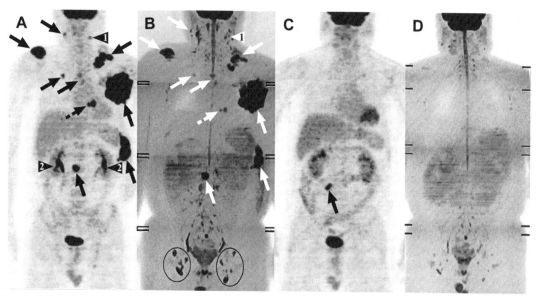

Fig. 4. Comparison of prechemotherapy and postchemotherapy FDG-PET and whole-body DWI in a 44-year-old man with stage III diffuse large B-cell lymphoma. (*A*) Coronal maximum-intensity projection FDG-PET and (*B*) coronal maximum-intensity projection gray-scale inverted whole-body DWI (acquired using a b-value of 1000 s/mm^2) before initiation of chemotherapy. Both images show cervical, bilateral supra/infraclavicular, mediastinal, left axillary, para-aortic lymph node, splenic involvement (*continuous arrows*), and cardiac involvement (*dashed arrow*). FDG-PET (*C*) and DWI (*D*) at the end of treatment show resolution of all preexisting lesions. A limitation of DWI is that the discrimination between normal and metastatic lymph nodes is still based on size criteria because of the lack of prospectively validated ADC criteria for malignancy; the FDG-PET positive left cervical lymph node (*A, arrowhead 1*) cannot conclusively be identified as malignant at DWI (*B, arrowhead 1*). DWI also shows prominent bilateral inguinal lymph nodes (*encircled*), which are normal according to FDG-PET. On the other hand, thanks to its higher spatial resolution, DWI visualizes two separate cardiac lesions (*dashed arrow*), whereas FDG-PET shows only one large cardiac lesion (*dashed arrow*). DWI also allows better evaluation of the urinary tract than FDG-PET, whereby potential lesions can be obscured because of FDG accumulation (*arrowheads 2*). Note the physiologic FDG uptake in the large intestine (*C, arrow*), which should not be confused with persistent malignant lymphoma. (*From* Kwee TC, Takahara T, Ochiai R, et al. Diffusion-weighted whole-body imaging with background body signal suppression (DWIBS): features and potential applications in oncology. Eur Radiol 2008;18(9):1947; with permission.)

changes in cell density resulting from therapy-induced necrosis and/or apoptotic processes. Because these changes in diffusion occur well before changes in tumor size,[47–50] DWI has potential as an imaging biomarker for the early assessment of response to anticancer therapy.

A recent study by Huang and colleagues[25] investigated the feasibility of T2-weighted imaging and DWI for in vivo detection of response to chemotherapy of human diffuse large B-cell lymphoma (DLBCL) xenografts in severe combined immunodeficient mice. Each cycle of combination chemotherapy with cyclophosphamide, hydroxy-doxorubicin, Oncovin, prednisone, and bryostatin 1 (CHOPB) was administered to tumor-carrying mice weekly for up to 4 cycles. T2-weighted imaging and DWI were performed before the initiation of CHOPB and after each cycle of CHOPB. To corroborate the MR imaging results, histologic analyses were performed on control tumors and treated tumors after completion of all MR imaging studies. DWI revealed a significant (*P*<.03) increase in the mean ADC in CHOPB-treated tumors as early as 1 week after initiation of CHOPB. However, a significant (*P*<.03) decrease in mean T2 value was observed only after 2 cycles of CHOPB. Both MR imaging methods produced high-resolution (0.1 × 0.1 × 1.0 mm^3) maps of regional therapeutic response in the treated tumors based on local ADC and T2 value. Of interest, due to an unknown reason, only a specific region of the tumors (in 3 of the 5 tumors) corresponding to about one-third of the tumor volume exhibited a response-associate increase in ADC and decrease in T2 value. An adjacent region exhibited an increase in T2 value and no change in ADC. The rest of the tumor was indistinguishable from sham-treated controls by MR imaging criteria. The therapeutic response of the treated tumors detected by MR imaging was accompanied by changes in tumor cell density, proliferation, and apoptosis revealed by histologic studies performed on completion of the longitudinal study. Huang and colleagues[25] concluded that DWI and T2-weighted imaging can detect the therapeutic response of treated tumors after 1 or 2 cycles of CHOPB, respectively. In addition, DWI and T2-weighted imaging delineate the spatial distribution of changes in ADC and T2 value, respectively, within the tumors, thereby detecting the heterogeneity of tumor therapeutic response which, in turn, may be used to guide multimodal therapeutic approaches. The same investigators[25] also concluded that DWI has higher sensitivity than T2-weighted imaging in detecting early therapeutic response of NHL tumors.

Lin and colleagues[26] prospectively evaluated both whole-body DWI and FDG-PET/CT as reference standard in 15 patients with DLBCL before initiation and after 4 cycles of chemotherapy. ADC of residual masses (lymph node and organ lesions) was assessed both visually and quantitatively, including measurement of mean ADC. After chemotherapy, among 85 examined lymph node regions residual nodes were present in 62 (73%) regions at DWI. Of these 62 regions, 26 had persistent lymph nodes with longest transverse diameter greater than 10 mm (ie, positive based on DWI size criteria). The mean ADC (in 10^{-3} mm^2/s) of these 26 regions significantly ($P<.0001$) increased from 0.658 ± 0.153 at baseline to 1.501 ± 0.307. Only 6 of these 26 regions were considered positive at FDG-PET/CT. Combining visual ADC analysis with size criteria reduced the number of false-positive results of DWI from 20 to 2 regions. For organ involvement, ADCs also increased compared with the baseline values (1.558 ± 0.424 vs 0.675 ± 0.135, respectively; $P = .0009$). Lin and colleagues[26] concluded that whole-body DWI with ADC mapping can show a significant increase in ADC values of residual masses persisting after treatment, and may help to assess the treatment response in patients with DLBCL.

It is clear that more studies with larger sample sizes are required to establish the utility of DWI as an imaging biomarker for the (early) prediction of therapeutic effectiveness in patients with lymphoma. Such studies should also compare DWI metrics with patient outcome in terms of progression-free survival or overall survival. Other issues that require further investigation are the optimal timing of DWI acquisition during therapy and the assessment of repeatability and reproducibility (interobserver and intraobserver variability) of ADC measurements. Such information is critical in ascribing ADC changes to drug effects, rather than to measurement errors and technical or biological variations.

SUMMARY

DWI is a noninvasive MR imaging technique that is sensitive to the random (Brownian) motion of water molecules. Major advantages of this technique are the high lesion-to-background contrast that can be achieved, and the opportunity to visualize and quantify (therapy-induced) changes in tissue diffusivity. Thanks to technical developments, it has become possible to perform DWI in the entire body. Early studies show that whole-body DWI is a feasible and promising method for staging lymphoma, and that it may be used as an imaging biomarker for the (early) assessment of therapeutic effectiveness. Further research is warranted to establish the clinical role of whole-body DWI in the evaluation of lymphoma in terms of staging performance, prognostic capabilities, and cost effectiveness.

REFERENCES

1. Jemal A, Siegel R, Xu J, et al. Cancer statistics, 2010. CA Cancer J Clin 2010;60(5):277–300.
2. Armitage JO. Staging non-Hodgkin lymphoma. CA Cancer J Clin 2005;55(6):368–76.
3. Connors JM. State-of-the-art therapeutics: Hodgkin's lymphoma. J Clin Oncol 2005;23(26):6400–8.
4. Murphy SB. Classification, staging and end results of treatment of childhood non-Hodgkin's lymphomas: dissimilarities from lymphomas in adults. Semin Oncol 1980;7(3):332–9.
5. Murphy SB, Fairclough DL, Hutchison RE, et al. Non-Hodgkin's lymphomas of childhood: an analysis of the histology, staging, and response to treatment of 338 cases at a single institution. J Clin Oncol 1989;7(2):186–93.
6. Kwee TC, Kwee RM, Nievelstein RA. Imaging in staging of malignant lymphoma: a systematic review. Blood 2008;111(2):504–16.
7. Delbeke D, Stroobants S, de Kerviler E, et al. Expert opinions on positron emission tomography and computed tomography imaging in lymphoma. Oncologist 2009;14(Suppl 2):30–40.
8. Terasawa T, Lau J, Bardet S, et al. Fluorine-18-fluorodeoxyglucose positron emission tomography for interim response assessment of advanced-stage Hodgkin's lymphoma and diffuse large B-cell lymphoma: a systematic review. J Clin Oncol 2009; 27(11):1906–14.
9. Huang B, Law MW, Khong PL. Whole-body PET-CT scanning: estimation of radiation dose and cancer risk. Radiology 2009;251(1):166–74.
10. Plathow C, Walz M, Lichy MP, et al. Cost considerations for whole-body MRI and PET/CT as part of oncologic staging. Radiologe 2008;48(4):384–96 [in German].

11. Lauenstein TC, Semelka RC. Whole-body magnetic resonance imaging. Top Magn Reson Imaging 2005;16(1):15–20.

12. Antoch G, Bockisch A. Combined PET/MRI: a new dimension in whole-body oncology imaging? Eur J Nucl Med Mol Imaging 2009;36(Suppl 1):113–20.

13. Brennan DD, Gleeson T, Coate LE, et al. A comparison of whole-body MRI and CT for the staging of lymphoma. AJR Am J Roentgenol 2005; 185(3):711–6.

14. Kellenberger CJ, Miller SF, Khan M, et al. Initial experience with FSE STIR whole-body MR imaging for staging lymphoma in children. Eur Radiol 2004; 14(10):1829–41.

15. Kwee TC, Quarles van Ufford HM, Beek FJ, et al. Whole-body MRI, including diffusion-weighted imaging, for the initial staging of malignant lymphoma: comparison to computed tomography. Invest Radiol 2009;44(10):683–90.

16. Punwani S, Taylor SA, Bainbridge A, et al. Pediatric and adolescent lymphoma: comparison of whole-body STIR half-Fourier RARE MR imaging with an enhanced PET/CT reference for initial staging. Radiology 2010;255(1):182–90.

17. Takahara T, Imai Y, Yamashita T, et al. Diffusion weighted whole body imaging with background body signal suppression (DWIBS): technical improvement using free breathing, STIR and high resolution 3D display. Radiat Med 2004;22(4):275–82.

18. Koh DM, Collins DJ. Diffusion-weighted MRI in the body: applications and challenges in oncology. AJR Am J Roentgenol 2007;188(6):1622–35.

19. Kwee TC, Takahara T, Ochiai R, et al. Diffusion-weighted whole-body imaging with background body signal suppression (DWIBS): features and potential applications in oncology. Eur Radiol 2008;18(9):1937–52.

20. Kwee TC, Takahara T, Ochiai R, et al. Complementary roles of whole-body diffusion-weighted MRI and ^{18}F-FDG PET: the state of the art and potential applications. J Nucl Med 2010;51(10):1549–58.

21. Lin C, Luciani A, Itti E, et al. Whole-body diffusion-weighted magnetic resonance imaging with apparent diffusion coefficient mapping for staging patients with diffuse large B-cell lymphoma. Eur Radiol 2010;20(8):2027–38.

22. Van Ufford HM, Kwee TC, Beek FJ, et al. Newly diagnosed lymphoma: initial results with whole-body T1-weighted, STIR, and diffusion-weighted MRI compared With ^{18}F-FDG PET/CT. AJR Am J Roentgenol 2011;196(3):662–9.

23. Padhani AR, Liu G, Koh DM, et al. Diffusion-weighted magnetic resonance imaging as a cancer biomarker: consensus and recommendations. Neoplasia 2009; 11(2):102–25.

24. De Bazelaire C, de Kerviler E. From multislice CT to whole-body biomarker imaging in lymphoma patients. Eur Radiol 2011;21(3):555–8.

25. Huang MQ, Pickup S, Nelson DS, et al. Monitoring response to chemotherapy of non-Hodgkin's lymphoma xenografts by T(2)-weighted and diffusion-weighted MRI. NMR Biomed 2008;21(10):1021–9.

26. Lin C, Itti E, Luciani A, et al. Whole-body diffusion-weighted imaging with apparent diffusion coefficient mapping for treatment response assessment in patients with diffuse large B-cell lymphoma: pilot study. Invest Radiol 2011;46(5):341–9. DOI:10.1097/RLI.0b013e3182087b03.

27. Sotak CH. Nuclear magnetic resonance (NMR) measurement of the apparent diffusion coefficient (ADC) of tissue water and its relationship to cell volume changes in pathological states. Neurochem Int 2004;45(4):569–82.

28. Schaefer PW, Grant PE, Gonzalez RG. Diffusion-weighted MR imaging of the brain. Radiology 2000;217(2):331–45.

29. Stejskal EO, Tanner JE. Spin diffusion measurements: spin echoes in the presence of a time-dependent field gradient. J Chem Phys 1965; 42(1):288–92.

30. Bammer R. Basic principles of diffusion-weighted imaging. Eur J Radiol 2003;45(3):169–84.

31. Poustchi-Amin M, Mirowitz SA, Brown JJ, et al. Principles and applications of echo-planar imaging: a review for the general radiologist. Radiographics 2001;21(3):767–79.

32. Liu G, Ogawa S. EPI image reconstruction with correction of distortion and signal losses. J Magn Reson Imaging 2006;24(3):683–9.

33. Nasu K, Kuroki Y, Sekiguchi R, et al. Measurement of the apparent diffusion coefficient in the liver: is it a reliable index for hepatic disease diagnosis? Radiat Med 2006;24(6):438–44.

34. Kwee TC, Takahara T, Niwa T, et al. Influence of cardiac motion on diffusion-weighted magnetic resonance imaging of the liver. MAGMA 2009;22(5): 319–25.

35. Tsushima Y, Takano A, Taketomi-Takahashi A, et al. Body diffusion-weighted MR imaging using high b-value for malignant tumor screening: usefulness and necessity of referring to T2-weighted images and creating fusion images. Acad Radiol 2007; 14(6):643–50.

36. Fischer MA, Nanz D, Hany T, et al. Diagnostic accuracy of whole-body MRI/DWI image fusion for detection of malignant tumours: a comparison with PET/CT. Eur Radiol 2011;21(2):246–55.

37. Koyama H, Ohno Y, Aoyama N, et al. Comparison of STIR turbo SE imaging and diffusion-weighted imaging of the lung: capability for detection and subtype classification of pulmonary adenocarcinomas. Eur Radiol 2010;20(4):790–800.

38. Sumi M, Sakihama N, Sumi T, et al. Discrimination of metastatic cervical lymph nodes with diffusion-weighted MR imaging in patients with head

and neck cancer. AJNR Am J Neuroradiol 2003;24: 1627–34.

39. Sumi M, Van Cauteren M, Nakamura T. MR microimaging of benign and malignant nodes in the neck. AJR Am J Roentgenol 2006;186(3):749–57.

40. Abdel Razek AA, Soliman NY, Elkhamary S, et al. Role of diffusion-weighted MR imaging in cervical lymphadenopathy. Eur Radiol 2006;16(7):1468–77.

41. King AD, Ahuja AT, Yeung DK, et al. Malignant cervical lymphadenopathy: diagnostic accuracy of diffusion-weighted MR imaging. Radiology 2007; 245(3):806–13.

42. Holzapfel K, Duetsch S, Fauser C, et al. Value of diffusion-weighted MR imaging in the differentiation between benign and malignant cervical lymph nodes. Eur J Radiol 2009;72(3):381–7.

43. Sumi M, Nakamura T. Diagnostic importance of focal defects in the apparent diffusion coefficient-based differentiation between lymphoma and squamous cell carcinoma nodes in the neck. Eur Radiol 2009; 19(4):975–81.

44. Koşucu P, Tekinbaş C, Erol M, et al. Mediastinal lymph nodes: assessment with diffusion-weighted MR imaging. J Magn Reson Imaging 2009;30(2):292–7.

45. Perrone A, Guerrisi P, Izzo L, et al. Diffusion-weighted MRI in cervical lymph nodes: differentiation between benign and malignant lesions. Eur J Radiol 2011;77(2):281–6.

46. Kwee TC, Ludwig I, Uiterwaal CS, et al. ADC measurements in the evaluation of lymph nodes in patients with non-Hodgkin lymphoma: feasibility study. MAGMA 2011;24(1):1–8.

47. Kim S, Loevner L, Quon H, et al. Diffusion-weighted magnetic resonance imaging for predicting and detecting early response to chemoradiation therapy of squamous cell carcinomas of the head and neck. Clin Cancer Res 2009; 15(3):986–94.

48. Cui Y, Zhang XP, Sun YS, et al. Apparent diffusion coefficient: potential imaging biomarker for prediction and early detection of response to chemotherapy in hepatic metastases. Radiology 2008; 248(3):894–900.

49. Liu Y, Bai R, Sun H, et al. Diffusion-weighted imaging in predicting and monitoring the response of uterine cervical cancer to combined chemoradiation. Clin Radiol 2009;64(11):1067–74.

50. Hamstra DA, Galbán CJ, Meyer CR, et al. Functional diffusion map as an early imaging biomarker for high-grade glioma: correlation with conventional radiologic response and overall survival. J Clin Oncol 2008;26(20):3387–94.

Novel PET Radiotracers for Potential Use in Management of Lymphoma

Lale Kostakoglu, MD, MPH

KEYWORDS

- PET • Radiotracer • Imaging • Lymphoma

The advent of integrated PET and computed tomography (CT) imaging using [^{18}F]fluorodeoxyglucose (FDG) PET/CT has changed the diagnostic algorithm-+ in lymphoma, culminating in management imuyhfgds plications. Metabolic imaging using PET technology provides a sensitive means to accurately determine the extent of disease involvement for a better management strategy at staging. It also offers valuable information to evaluate therapy response and to identify sites of recurrent disease. Although PET using ^{18}F-FDG has proved useful for diagnosis and therapy monitoring in patients with lymphoma, the specificity of FDG uptake has been critically questioned because of its dependence on glucose metabolism, which may indiscriminately increase in benign conditions such as inflammatory or infectious processes.[1–4]

There are 6 well-defined hallmarks of cancer, including sustenance of proliferative signals, angiogenesis, replicative immortality, invasion and metastases, resistance to cell death, and evasion of growth suppressors (**Fig. 1**). All of these features serve as specific references against which targeted imaging and therapy agents are developed to better outline and counteract these mechanisms,[5] respectively. In this context, recently introduced effective therapy agents targeting specific molecular pathways have stimulated the development of various labeled molecules defining tumor biology (**Table 1**). There is a plethora of ongoing preclinical and clinical trials using these specific imaging

probes with a common prospect of improving diagnostic and prognostic accuracy. In particular, the disease progress of patients with aggressive chemorefractory lymphoma would benefit greatly from novel therapies arising from investigation of dysregulated oncogenic processes that occur during lymphomagenesis. Several promising therapies against non-Hodgkin lymphoma (NHL) are in development that target apoptosis, neoangiogenesis, mammalian target of rapamycin (mTOR) complex, proteasome, and immune kinases of the B-cell receptor signaling pathway. Imaging procedures may be used to characterize the biologic features of lymphomas with respect to the oncogenic pathways mentioned earlier. The information obtained with these techniques is expected to individualize treatment, and makes imaging-based methods promising tools for tumor detection, therapy planning, and therapy monitoring. The unmet need in noninvasive imaging for better management of lymphoma is summarized in **Box 1**.

This article discusses the potential role of emerging novel PET imaging markers in the management of lymphoma, although there are few data supporting the role of these novel radiotracers in this realm.

IMAGING TUMOR PROLIFERATION

An important hallmark of cancer is propagated tumor growth and dissemination through proliferative signaling capacity. The mitogenic signals in

Division of Nuclear Medicine, Department of Radiology, Mount Sinai School of Medicine, New York, NY 10029, USA
E-mail address: lale.kostakoglu@mountsinai.org

PET Clin 7 (2012) 83–117
doi:10.1016/j.cpet.2011.12.002
1556-8598/12/$ – see front matter © 2012 Elsevier Inc. All rights reserved

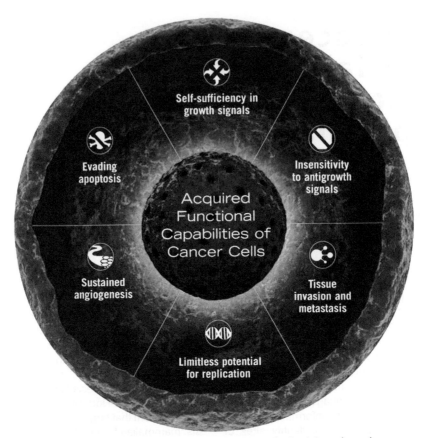

Fig. 1. Hallmarks of cancer. Six well established alterations in cell physiology have been suggested as the promoter of malignant growth: self-sufficiency in growth signals, insensitivity to growth-inhibitory (antigrowth) signals, evasion of programmed cell death (apoptosis), limitless replicative potential, sustained angiogenesis, and tissue invasion and metastasis. Each of these changes that occur during oncogenic transformation represents a potential target against which anti-cancer treatments can be developed. (*From* Hanahan D, Weinberg RA. The hallmarks of cancer. Cell 2000;100:57–70. Available at: http://www.biooncology.com/molecular-causes-of-cancer/index.html. Accessed December 4, 2011; with permission.)

normal tissues are highly regulated to ensure a homeostasis of cell number and function, whereas cancer cells become autonomous under the influence of growth factors that promote cell growth through a cascade of downstream signaling pathways.[6,7]

The noninvasive assessment of tumor proliferative activity by a functional imaging modality may provide a selection tool for individualized treatment. The probe 3'-deoxy-3'-^{18}F-fluorothymidine (FLT) was first introduced by Shields and colleagues[8] and subsequently became the most extensively investigated probe for noninvasive measurement of cancer cell proliferative capacity.[9,10]

Relevance in Lymphoma

A positive correlation was found between the proliferation and aggressiveness of the B-cell

NHLs as measured with Ki-67 expression reflecting increased cellular proliferation.[11] In this regard, FLT PET can be used to determine tumor grade and early transformation to a higher grade subtype in patients with indolent forms of lymphoma. Another useful application entails the evaluation of proliferative activity as a prognostic marker. Newly recognized correlations between specific biomarkers and the International Prognostic Index (IPI) highlight the importance of biologic factors in prognostic models. Emerging data from tissue microarrays show that, using BCL2, Ki-67, and IPI, improved discrimination of low-risk patients with diffuse large B-cell lymphoma (DLBCL) treated with rituximab and chemotherapy.[12] In another study of de novo DLBCL (n = 111), a high Ki-67 index of greater than 80% and bulky disease were found to be significant adverse prognostic factors for overall survival and progression-free survival before and after the introduction of

Table 1
PET radiotracers for imaging cancer biology

Radiopharmaceutical	Measured Activity
FDG	Glucose use
FLT	Cellular proliferation
[18]F-Fluoromisonidazole[a]	Tissue hypoxia
[64]Cu-ATSM	Tissue hypoxia
^{18}F-FAZA	Tissue hypoxia
[18]F-Fluoroannexin	Apoptosis
^{18}F-ML-10	Apoptosis
[18]F-Galacto-RGD	Angiogenesis
^{18}F-AH111585 (fluciclatide/GE 135)	Angiogenesis
[11]C-Methionine	Amino acid
[11]C-Thyrosine	Amino acid
[11]C-Acetate	Tricarboxylic acid cycle
[11]C-Choline or ^{18}F-choline	Phosphatidylcholine

rituximab.[13] FLT PET imaging as a surrogate of histopathologic proliferative activity could be used to identify high-risk subgroups in DLBCL. This consideration is particularly important in light of inherent tumor heterogeneity and resultant sampling errors.

In the posttherapy setting, the nonspecific FDG accumulation in glucose-consuming tumor

Box 1
Unmet need for management in cancer imaging

Before therapy

Characterize in vivo tumor biology for prognostication and prognosis

Predict response to conventional anticancer therapy agents for risk stratification

Identify specific targets for selection of patients for targeted drugs

Predict response to targeted/biologic drugs

Predict response to radiotherapy

Determine chemoresistance

During therapy

Measure early tumor response to therapy with high specificity

Measure response to radiation therapy

Measure response to targeted/biologic therapy

Predict survival (overall and progression free)

stromal cells including activated macrophages, fibroblasts, and granulation tissue[14,15] can potentially lead to overtreatment. FLT as a promising specific probe for proliferating tumor tissue can be used to determine therapy response with the expectation of a lower false-positive rate. Moreover, some indolent lymphoma histologies, including marginal zone lymphoma and chronic lymphocytic leukemia (CLL)/small lymphocytic lymphoma (SLL), may accumulate FDG at low levels, precluding a role for FDG PET imaging in their management.[16,17] In mantle cell lymphoma (MCL), although its sensitivity is high, no proven benefit has been validated for FDG PET either for response assessment or posttreatment surveillance.[18] Hence, there is a justified need for selective targeting of tumor-specific cellular processes in which FLT PET can serve a niche clinical need.

Mechanism of Uptake

FLT is a pyrimidine analogue and reflects the activity of a thymidine kinase-1 during the S phase of DNA synthesis.[19] Similar to thymidine, FLT enters the cell via the equilibrative nucleoside transporter (ENT1)–mediated facilitated transport and subsequently is phosphorylated by thymidine kinase-1 (TK1) to thymidine monophosphate (TMP) (**Fig. 2**). Because the number of cells in the S phase of the cell cycle is higher in tumors compared with normal tissue, the requirement for nucleotides increases for DNA synthesis. Among the 4 nucleotides required for DNA synthesis, thymidine is the only one incorporated exclusively into DNA and not RNA. However, the incorporation of FLT into DNA is less than 1%, which makes toxicity concerns irrelevant. During DNA synthesis, TK_1 activity increases almost tenfold reflecting cellular proliferation, although indirectly,[20] as measured by increases in FLT uptake. Because of its impermeable constitution and resistance to degradation, phosphorylated FLT is metabolically trapped inside the cells in competition with catabolic dephosphorylation mediated by dNT1 and FLT efflux.[21] FLT uptake and PET quantitative parameters (standard uptake value [SUV] and FLT flux) have been shown to correlate with tissue proliferation measurements, including the Ki-67 score in human cancers.[22] FLT PET might, therefore, be a useful tool for assessing tumor aggressiveness, predicting outcome, and monitoring response to treatment.

Among additional radiolabeled thymidine analogues, the pyrimidine analogue, 1-(2′-deoxy-2′-fluoro-β-ᴅ-arabinofuranosyl)thymine (FMAU), labeled with ^{11}C or ^{18}F, has shown encouraging results.[23,24] In vitro studies have shown that the

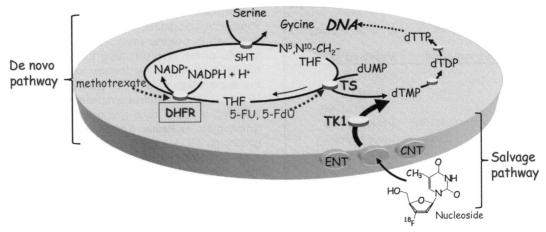

Fig. 2. De novo pathway of thymidylate synthesis (thymidine monophosphate, TMP): monophosphorylation of dUMP by thymidylate synthase (TS) and salvage pathway of TMP synthesis (phosphorylation of exogenous thymidine by thymidine kinase 1, TK1). The de novo pathway can be blocked by drug treatment (5-fluorouracil, methotrexate) potentially causing an upregulation of the salvage pathway and subsequent increase of the uptake and retention of nucleosides such as [^{18}F]FLT. The key process for the metabolic trapping of [^{18}F]FLT is an intracellular transport via nucleoside transporters which are located in the cellular membrane (equilibrative and concentrative nucleoside transporters ENT, CNT) and subsequent phosphorylation by TK1. CNT, concentrative nucleoside transporter; DHFR, dihydrofolate reductase; dTMP, deoxythymidine monophosphate; dUMP, deoxyuridine monophosphate; ENT, equilibrative nucleoside transporter; 5-FdU, 5-fluoro-2'-deoxyuridine; 5-FU, 5-fluorouracil; SHT, serine hydroxymethyl transferase; THF, tretrahydrofolate; TK1, thymidine kinase; TS, thymidylate synthase. (*From* Buck AK. Molecular imaging of proliferation in vivo: positron emission tomography with [^{18}F]fluorothymidine. Methods 2009;48:206; with permission.)

amount of FMAU incorporated into DNA is proportional to the level of DNA synthesis and the rate of proliferation.[24] However, there are no data available comparing the diagnostic efficacy and toxicity of FMAU with FLT.

Biodistribution

The highest physiologic FLT accumulation occurs in bones with hematopoietic marrow (**Fig. 3**). FLT undergoes glucuronidation resulting in significant liver uptake. FLT is excreted through the kidneys and there is also a moderate degree of uptake in the spleen. The low background activity in the neck and chest, and no uptake in the brain, muscles, and myocardium, provide an advantage compared with FDG imaging in these anatomic locations.[25]

Timing

Although the widely adopted period between injection and imaging is 60 minutes, variable times have also been used in the literature with the premise that longer waiting periods may increase the sensitivity of FLT PET imaging (see later discussion). The administered dose is 0.07 mCi/kg with a maximum of 5 mCi (18.5 mBq). A dose of 5mCi FLT results in an effective total body dose equivalent of 3.0 to 4.0 mSv.

Reproducibility

The reproducibility of imaging parameters is a prerequisite for comparison of interpatient and intrapatient data, particularly when sequential imaging is involved to determine therapy response. Several studies have shown that serial FLT PET imaging can be performed with high reproducibility when reproducibility or measured error is defined as the percent difference between the 2 scans.[26–28] Compared with FDG, SUVmax reproducibility levels were similar, with a mean percentage difference of 2% to 17% and 1% to 15% for the FDG and FLT lesions, respectively. The worst-case SUVmean error was 21%.[28] Compartmental and graphical kinetic analyses were also reproducible ($r^2 = .59$; $P = .015$).[26] When monitoring response in individual patients, changes of more than 20% to 25% in SUVmax and Patlak-derived Ki, are likely to represent treatment effects.[27]

The Factors Influencing FLT Uptake

Certain factors should be considered while interpreting FLT PET studies. Some of the factors that have an impact on FLT uptake may also be manipulated to enhance its uptake profile and thereby increase its sensitivity.

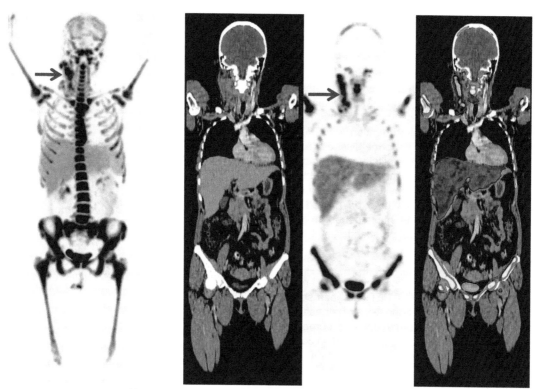

Fig. 3. Biodistribution of [^{18}F]FLT in a patient with DLBCL. (*Courtesy of* Dr Andreas Buck, Universitätsklinikum Würzburg.)

Activation of the salvage pathway and flare phenomenon

Despite reduced cellular proliferation rate, increased FLT retention could be observed because of inhibition of thymidylate synthase (TS) and subsequent increase in TK_1 activity (see **Fig. 2**). This observation is considered to be a result of activation of a salvage pathway after drug-related inhibition of de novo synthesis of thymidine monophosphate (TMP) by some cytotoxic drugs including 5-fluorouracil (5-FU), cisplatin, or methotrexate (MTX). De novo thymidine synthesis could be a limitation and confounding factor for qualitative and quantitative evaluation of tumor proliferation using FLT PET imaging. Thus, this phenomenon should be recognized for accurate interpretation of FLT PET studies, particularly early in the course of therapy with the relevant cytotoxic drugs.[29] The altered pharmacokinetics of FLT were investigated using this mechanism following various pharmaceutical interventions at nontoxic concentrations to overcome the inferior sensitivity of FLT.[30] This caveat can also be exploited to promote FLT uptake by the proliferating tumor cells. The incubation of tumor cells with 5-FU or methotrexate (MTX), both of which are known to block the de novo pathway through inhibiting TS, caused a sevenfold to tenfold increase in respective FLT uptake.[30] Similarly, in

mice xenografts, 5-fluoro-2′-deoxyuridine (FdUrd) increased FLT uptake by a factor of 3.0 to 8.0 compared with controls.[31] In patients with breast cancer, capecitabine, another inhibitor of TS, increased tumor FLT retention and the rate constant for the net irreversible transfer of radiotracer from plasma to tumor (Ki) by approximately 30% and 70%, respectively.[32]

Although the results of these investigational studies may be clinically relevant for future diagnostic applications designed to increase the sensitivity of FLT PET imaging, cytostatic action of these interventional drugs on RNA synthesis could limit their clinical usefulness.[30] Hence, further studies in humans are warranted to confirm an effective and a reliable increase of FLT uptake in different tumors with no adverse effects.

Competition from the endogenous thymidine pool

Endogenous thymidine competes with the cellular uptake of exogenous FLT, further limiting FLT uptake in target cells. The variability in efficacy of TS among individuals and the availability of thymidine because of its nutritional status may lead to variable FLT tumor uptake even in tumors of similar proliferation activity. Hence, previously discussed pharmacologic interventions could improve the consistency of FLT tumor uptake by rendering a more homogeneous medium.

Longer time interval after FLT injection

In lymphoma xenografts, tumor uptake of FLT was not significantly different between retention periods of 1 hour and 3 hours after injection.[31] Nonetheless, because of greater washout from normal tissues, high tumor retention of FLT led to markedly improved tumor/normal tissue ratios at 3 hours. Although these results suggest that delayed FLT PET imaging may be preferable to obtain better detection sensitivity, the superiority of 90-minute imaging is yet to be proved and currently a 60-minute retention period may be preferable from a practical perspective.[33]

Sensitivity

In both preclinical and clinical settings, in a multitude of tumor models, FLT PET has been shown to be a less sensitive diagnostic probe based on its lower tumor-to-nontumor contrast compared with FDG.[34–37] As previously mentioned, in certain anatomic locations, including the neck, brain, and the abdominal cavity, the sensitivity of FLT PET can be favorable because of better delineation of tumor outlines because of lower background activity. In contrast, high physiologic bone marrow and liver uptake is deemed to interfere with detection of malignant processes. FDG PET is probably superior to FLT in the detection of hepatic metastases, although there are no comparative data proving this hypothesis.

Several groups validated FLT PET imaging for lung, head and neck, gastrointestinal, and breast cancers with varying sensitivities and specificities (**Table 2**).[34–48]

In lymphoma, at staging, FLT PET was reported to produce images of high contrast; however, the mean FLT uptake was lower compared with respective FDG uptake (SUVmax 4.6 vs 5.1).[48] Compared with routine staging procedures, a larger number of lesions were detected on FLT PET, yielding a sensitivity of 98%; nonetheless, FLT PET did not change the clinical stage determined by the standard staging procedures. Although the existing data are preliminary, the FLT uptake is low in Hodgkin lymphoma (HL), showing a maximum average SUV of 2.7, which was about 30% lower than that of FDG.[48]

In summary, these preliminary results suggest a lower sensitivity for FLT compared with FDG, which makes it unlikely that FLT applications will supplant those of FDG for staging purposes. However, the higher specificity and superior positive predictive values associated with FLT PET should be exploited as a major advantage for tumor grading. FLT PET is also promising for improving the accuracy of therapy response evaluation and thereby patient selection for potential treatment modifications during the early course of ongoing treatment.

Specificity

The specificity of a radiotracer relates to both the specificity of the probe for malignant tissues and the specificity of the tracer with respect to its representation of its biologic counterpart with high fidelity.

Inflammation versus Selective Tumor Uptake

In contrast with the FDG uptake mechanism, FLT is deemed to reflect increased cell proliferation, which is one of the key features of oncogenic transformation. FLT showed higher selectivity indices than FDG as measured by tumor/inflammation ratios and selective localization in tumors, confirming the hypothesis that FLT has a higher tumor specificity (**Fig. 4**).[49,50] In humans, FLT PET/CT was found more helpful than FDG PET/CT in differentiating inflammation from tumor during therapy in esophageal cancer. Those patients who underwent scans after completing the radiotherapy course showed no tumor uptake on FLT PET/CT but there was high uptake on FDG PET/CT at sites where pathologic examination revealed inflammatory infiltrates but no residual tumor.[51] However, there are contrasting results that are addressed later.

Reactive Lymphoid Hyperplasia

In a previous study, it was concluded that FDG-avid follicular dendritic cells might be the cause of FDG uptake in reactive cervical lymph nodes, resulting in false-positive results.[52] The research question of whether or not this limitation could be solved with FLT as a more specific PET tracer was addressed in a preliminary study in patients with head and neck cancers.[53] On correlation with immunohistochemical assessment of the cell proliferation markers Ki-67 and iododeoxyuridine, the sensitivity and specificity of FLT PET for the detection of metastatic nodes were 100% and 40%, respectively. Labeling indices for Ki-67 and iododeoxyuridine were higher in the germinal centers harboring B-lymphocytes than in the metastatic deposits. Furthermore, the median numbers of germinal centers per lymph node and the absolute area occupied by germinal centers were significantly higher in the nonmetastatic (reactive) lymph nodes than in the negative lymph nodes. Although preliminary data suggest that the active proliferation of B-lymphocytes could lead to

Table 2
Sensitivity of FLT PET in various tumors in chronological order

Author	References	Year	Malignancy	Patient#	FLT Sensitivity (%)	Correlation, proliferation marker[a]
Vesselle et al (2002)	54	2002	Lung cancer	10	100	$r = 0.84$; $P<.001$
Francis et al (2003)	34	2003	Colorectal cancer	10	100	$r = 0.8$; $P<.01$
Wagner et al (2003)	56	2003	Lymphoma	9	100	$r = 0.95$; $P<.005$
Cobben et al (2004)	37	2004	Laryngeal cancer	21	88	N/A
Smyczek-Gargya et al (2004)	46	2004	Breast cancer	12	92	$r^2 = 0.01$; $P>.05$
Cobben et al (2004)	241	2004	Bone/soft tissue sarc	19	100	$r = 0.55$-0.75; $P<.05$
Buck et al (2005)	39	2005	Lung cancer	47	90	N/A
Yap et al (2006)	36	2006	Lung cancer	11	79	$r = 0.6$; $P = .02$
Buck et al (2006)	48	2006	Lymphoma	34	92	$r = 0.84$; $P<.0001$
Kenny et al (2005)	57	2005	Breastt caner	15	100	$r = 0.92$, $P<.0001$
Yamamoto et al (2007)	35	2007	Lung cancer	18	72	$r = 0.77$; $P<.0002$
Troost et al (2007)	53	2007	HNSCC	10	N/A	$r^2 = 0.55$, $P = .0004$
Herrmann et al (2007)	84	2007	Aggressive NHL	22	100	N/A
Herrmann et al (2008)	40	2007	Pancreatic cancer	31	71.4	N/A
Buck et al (2008)	242	2008	Bone/soft tissue sarc	22	100	$r = 0.71$; $P<.0001$
Linecker et al (2008)	44	2008	HNSCC	20	95	$P>.05$
Been et al (2009)	45	2009	HNSCC	14	86	N/A
Yamamoto (2009)	41	2009	Colorectal cancer	26	100	$P>.05$
Troost et al (2010)	43	2010	HNSCC	17	100	$P = .44$
Yue et al (2010)	51	2010	Esophageal cancer	21	91	N/A
Yang W et al (2010)	38	2010	Lung cancer	31	74	$r = 0.644$; $P<.01$
Hoshikawa et al (2011)	42	2011	HNSCC	43	100	$r = -0.103$; $P = .58$
Herrmann et al (2011)	85	2011	Aggressive NHL	66	100	$P = .18$
Ott et al (2011)	64	2011	Gastric cancer	45	100	$r = 0.017$; $P = .921$
Zander et al (2011)	74	2011	Lung cancer	34	100	N/A

Abbreviation: N/A, Not Applicable.
[a] Ki67 or IdUrd = iododeoxyuridine labeling index or cyclin D1 labeling.

false-positive FLT PET results, larger samples should be investigated to confirm the role of FLT in discerning inflammation from malignant processes.

Correlation Between TK-1, Proliferative Index, and FLT

In most of the published data, a strong correlation has been shown between FLT uptake and the tumor histologic grades as well as cellular proliferation rates as measured by Ki-67 immuno-staining,[35,36,38,54,55] whereas FDG uptake did not show any correlation (see **Table 2**). In a pilot study of 11 patients with indolent or aggressive lymphoma, FLT PET findings were comparable with those of FDG PET in the ability to detect malignant lesions by PET scan (**Fig. 5**).[56] After incubation with FLT for 240 minutes, 12.5% ($\pm$ 1.0%) of radioactivity applied to the medium was intracellularly trapped. Furthermore, close correlation was found ($r = 0.95$, $P<.005$) between FLT uptake and the Ki-67–labeling index of tissue biopsies in these patients.

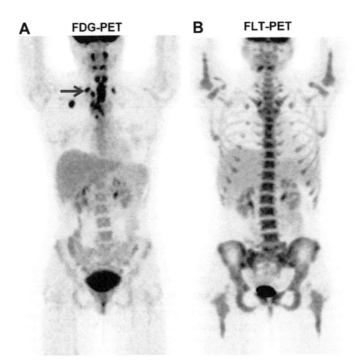

Fig. 4. No significant uptake in inflammatory or infectious processes with FLT versus FDG. Coronal images of FDG PET (*A*) and FLT PET (*B*) in a patient with a diagnosis of laryngotracheitis. (*A*) FDG-PET coronal image demonstrates increased radiotracer uptake corresponding to the larynx and trachea (*arrow*) as well as in multiple lymph nodes demonstrating increased FLT uptake, representing an inflammatory/infectious process and associated reactive changes in the locoregional lymph nodes, respectively. (*B*) FLT PET coronal image demonstrates normal distribution of radiotracer with no increased uptake in the region of the trachea or larynx and regional lymph nodes as seen on the FDG PET image. This finding suggests the lack of non-specific FLT accumulation in infectious processes and a more specific uptake pattern compared to FDG in malignant processes. (*Courtesy of* Dr Andreas Buck, Universitätsklinikum Würzburg.)

In breast cancer, similar results were found using the Ki-67 labeling index; however, the correlation coefficient for Ki, the net irreversible transfer of radiotracer from plasma to tumor tissue, was higher than that of SUVmax (0.92 vs 0.79).[57] The more clinically applicable method, SUV, should be interpreted with the knowledge that they can be influenced by some factors including changes in radiotracer delivery, dephosphorylation within the tumor, and changes in systemic clearance after treatment. There are also conflicting data in head and neck cancer and colon cancer, which showed no consistent correlation between FLT SUVs and tumor proliferative indices.[42,43] In most tumors, TK-1 staining of varying intensity was present but correlated with neither iododeoxyuridine binding nor FLT uptake.[43] This weak correlation may, in part, be explained by differences in biomarker characteristics, resolution, and quantification methods. Furthermore, the temporal difference between surgery and PET imaging may yield negative results based on ongoing therapy effects until the time of tissue sampling leading to further decreases in tumor proliferation rates.

Further phase II to III studies will determine whether FLT PET/CT is specific enough to distinguish between malignant and nonmalignant cells with respect to tumor proliferative capacity.

Evaluation of Therapy Response

Although FDG PET is currently the mainstay for evaluation of metabolic changes during or after completion of conventional therapy, FLT PET is envisioned as a more specific tool for monitoring anticancer treatment as a surrogate marker of cellular proliferation. Therefore, it is likely to provide early evidence of response with more definitive results than merely relying on changes in glucose metabolism. In addition to preclinical animal PET studies used in the development of novel therapeutic strategies,[58-63] preliminary clinical reports also support the role of FLT as a promising response surrogate, particularly in breast cancer, lung cancer, lymphoma, and colorectal cancer. In breast cancer, Kenny and colleagues[55] reported that FLT PET can detect changes in tumor proliferation early during cytotoxic therapy.

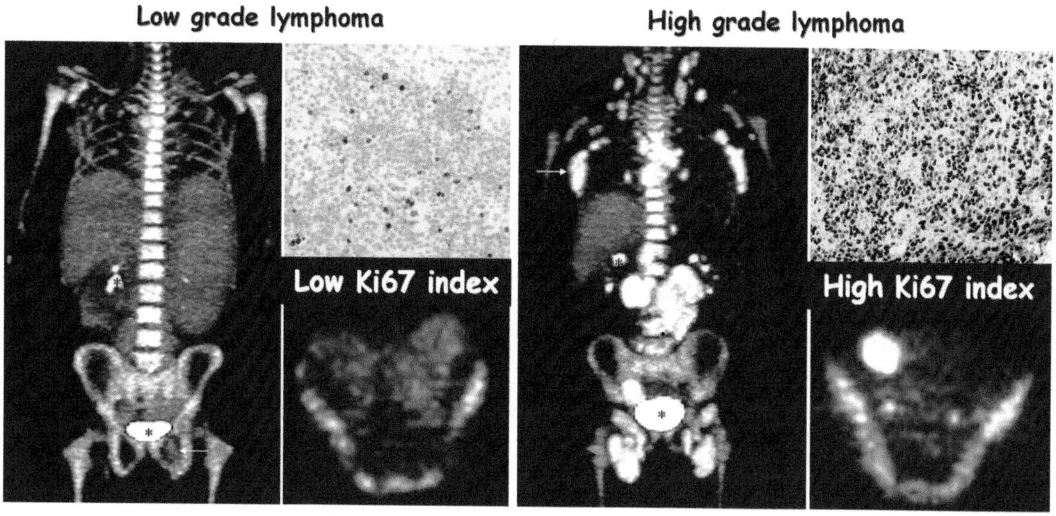

Low grade lymphoma

High grade lymphoma

Low Ki67 index

High Ki67 index

Fig. 5. FLT may be superior to FDG to diagnose the transformation from low-grade lymphoma to high-grade lymphoma. Follicular lymphoma grade-I versus Large cell anaplastic lymphoma. Exploting this feature pre therapy grading of tumors particularly relevant in lymphoma, can be done. The management dramatically changes once the lymphoma transforms to a higher grade and detected earlier survival benefits can be obtained. (*From* Buck AK, Bommer M, Stilgenbauer S, et al. Molecular imaging of proliferation in malignant lymphoma. Cancer Res 2006;66:11058, with permission; and Tatum JL, Kelloff GJ. Hypoxia: importance in tumor biology, noninvasive measurement by imaging, and value of its measurement in the management of cancer therapy. Int J Radiat Biol 2006;82(10):699–757; with permission.)

Decreases in Ki and SUVmax at 1 week discriminated between clinical response and stable disease ($P = .022$ for both parameters). In all tumors with partial or complete responses, a significant reduction in tracer uptake (approximately 41%) has been observed, whereas, in patients without response, there was an increase in FLT uptake. In patients with gastric cancers, although there was no significant association between clinical or histopathologic response and FLT or FDG parameters, FLT uptake 2 weeks after initiation of therapy was found to be the only imaging parameter with significant prognostic impact.[64] However, there were no significant differences in the magnitude of FLT decrease between responders and nonresponders in patients with metastatic germ cell tumors (GCT), after 1 cycle of chemotherapy.[65]

Data from various tumor models should be reviewed in the context of individual tumor biology and primary therapy objectives. Response in a patient with an incurable tumor such as locally advanced solid tumors is biologically different from response in a patient with a potentially curable tumor such as lymphoma or GCT. In locally advanced cancers, the goal of neoadjuvant chemotherapy is to downstage an inoperable tumor to increase tumor resectability and the chance of achieving long-term tumor control by eliminating microscopic disease.[66] The goal of curative therapy is to eradicate disease, as in patients with HL and DLBCL, and attaining a durable complete response requires a risk-adapted therapy approach that probably includes imaging to optimize therapy, aiming at a treatment strategy that operates at the maximum tolerable dose level. For neoadjuvant therapy, robust end points include cellular response surrogates (eg, histopathologic response, chemical response) or imaging response to identify those patients who would benefit from alternative strategies if response is not optimal. One should therefore be careful when applying these criteria to treatment strategies of curative intent. Similar to FDG, FLT may have a niche as a surrogate marker in the determination of optimal management to improve outcome by optimizing individualized therapy with both intents.

The potential role of FLT PET imaging in patient management cannot be emphasized enough in light of emerging targeted cytostatic anticancer agents whose mode of operation is through inhibition of signal transduction pathways of cell proliferation. These forms of therapies exert their anticancer effect by rapid interruption of cell division that is not always associated with decrease in size or tumor glucose metabolism. FLT is a suitable probe for early evaluation of efficacy of biologic anticancer agents.[67,68] A rapid decline in FLT uptake is described after biologic anticancer treatment in various solid tumors, proving superior to conventional response parameters including morphologic alterations defined by CT or magnetic resonance (MR) imaging.[69–76]

Targeting the mTOR pathway is a potential means of overcoming cisplatin resistance, which is in various stages of clinical development and investigation in human patients with lymphoma.[77,78] Reduction in FLT uptake has shown a good correlation with the level of mTOR inhibition by the anticancer agent everolimus. The reduction of FLT uptake observed at day 2 in the everolimus group preceded changes in tumor volume.[62]

These investigational data support FLT PET imaging as a potential modality to identify patients likely to benefit from targeted therapies early in their treatment course.

Response to radiation therapy

The assessment of radiotherapy response is challenged by radiation-induced fibrosis, infiltration with inflammatory cells, and desmoplastic reaction as a result of vascular proliferation, all of which contribute to false-positive findings obtained with FDG PET imaging as well as with anatomic modalities. A potential role for FLT PET in monitoring radiotherapy is supported by animal studies that have shown a rapid reduction in FLT uptake following therapy.[79,80] Most human studies evaluating radiotherapy response, although preliminary, were performed in patients with head and neck cancer. A proof-of-concept study showed that even a dose of only 2 Gy of radiation could induce a marked reduction of FLT uptake in the irradiated bone marrow, accompanied by decreases in the fraction of proliferating bone marrow. Hence, FLT uptake can monitor the distinctive biologic responses of epithelial cancers and highly radiosensitive normal tissue changes during chemotherapy-radiotherapy.[81] Through kinetic analysis, a decrease in FLT uptake in irradiated marrow was shown to represent a decrease in the net phosphorylation rate of FLT.[82] Early after initiation of chemoradiation therapy in patients with head and neck squamous cell carcinoma (HNSCC), there was a 76% decrease in SUVmax (at 10 Gy) that showed excellent correlation with influx parameters from compartmental and Patlak analyses.[33] In a limited group of patients with laryngeal cancer, after radiotherapy, FLT biodistribution was affected to a lesser extent by radiotherapy than was FDG uptake.[45] However, during radiotherapy, it became increasingly difficulty to perform segmentation of the tumor subvolume from the background and the proliferative activity in the nearby nontumor tissues. These findings raise questions as to the technical feasibility of future dose escalations to these regions based on the concerns of the impacts on nearby tissues.[43]

In rectal cancer (n = 10), the degree of reduction in FLT uptake early in the course of neoadjuvant chemoradiotherapy did not correlate with histopathologic tumor regression. These results suggest therapy-induced growth arrest of tumor cells that may be attributable to sublethal toxicity of chemoradiotherapy.[83] One more concept that may be applicable to false-negative findings is the possibility of a stunning effect on FLT transport through the cell membranes or on phosphorylation process required for intracellular trapping following chemoradiotherapy that would preclude a positive. However, definitive conclusions should not be extrapolated from these early data because of small sample sizes and/or short follow-up periods. Further FLT PET/CT studies are warranted to determine the role of this imaging modality in response-adapted radiotherapy strategies.

FLT Imaging in Lymphoma

Imaging at staging

Based on the biodistribution characteristics of FLT, lymphoma manifestations in the neck and around the heart can be detected without challenges, unlike those involved with FDG PET imaging. However, evaluation of lymphoma involvement in the bone marrow and the liver is limited by significant physiologic uptake. In a prior study, in a mixed group of patients with lymphoma (21 dL BCL, 11 indolent NHL), FLT PET detected 15% more lesions compared with routine staging procedures not including FDG PET; however, the Ann Arbor staging classification remained unchanged.[48] The sensitivity of FLT PET was 98% versus 100% for FDG PET imaging (n = 21). FLT PET missed known bone or bone marrow lesions. In a study of patients with high-grade NHL (n = 22), FLT PET produced images of high contrast with a mean FLT SUVmax of 8.1 (median, 7.4; standard deviation [SD], 3.9; range, 2.6–19.4).[84]

Differentiation between high-grade and low-grade lymphoma

Aggressive NHL, mainly DLBCL, had approximately a 2.5 times higher FLT uptake (mean 5.9 vs 2.3) compared with indolent lymphoma ($P<.0001$). Using a cutoff for FLT SUVmax of 3.0, aggressive lymphoma could be differentiated from an indolent histology with higher accuracy than FDG PET (area under the curve, 0.98 vs 0.78).[48] These findings were consistent with the significant correlation found between the proliferation fraction of the biopsied tumors and corresponding FLT uptake ($r = 0.84$, $P<.0001$). Hence,

FLT could potentially be the future imaging modality of choice for noninvasive determination of tumor grading (see **Fig. 5**).

More recently, in a prospective study in 66 patients with aggressive NHL, all lymphoma lesions showed focally increased FLT uptake (mean SUV, 7.3). In addition, a significant correlation was found between the IPI score and initial FLT uptake. These data are promising for risk stratifying patients before therapy, especially with the increasing demand for a more specific prognostic tool. However, FLT PET will not be ready to take a leading role in implementing risk-adapted treatments until it is proved to be superior to existing risk stratification systems.[85]

Evaluation of response to therapy

The clinical usefulness of FLT as an early response surrogate has been shown by several investigators in both preclinical and clinical studies.[86–90] In follicular lymphoma mice xenografts, reduction of tumor FLT uptake was observed as early as 48 hours after cyclophosphamide treatment.[86] In treated and untreated tumors, linear regression analysis showed a significant correlation of Ki-67 index and FLT uptake ($P = .0002$, $r = 0.56$). Cytotoxic chemotherapy caused a significantly greater decrease in proliferation fraction (50%) compared with immunotherapy or radioimmunotherapy (7%). Tumor FLT uptake decreased by 72% and 28% after chemotherapy and immunotherapy, respectively. These findings provide grounds for consideration of use of FLT PET only for early evaluation of cytotoxic treatment response.

Because FLT uptake is not expected to be influenced by the temporary increase in inflammatory cells, it is presumed that it reflects tumor response more accurately than FDG. In mice xenografts of human MCL, FDG and FLT uptake decreased at day 2 of cyclophosphamide or mTOR inhibition. After cyclophosphamide treatment, although FDG uptake started increasing between day 4 and day 7, FLT uptake remained stable. Histologic evaluation confirmed an increase in apoptotic or necrotic tumor fraction, followed by an influx of inflammatory cells. Cyclin D1 expression decreased from D1 until D4 and returned to baseline at D7. However, a temporary increase in FLT uptake was noted a week after the administration of mTOR inhibition, which suggests that drug-specific responses should be considered when using PET for early treatment monitoring.[87] In high-grade lymphoma xenotransplants, the decrease in FLT uptake at 24 hours of therapy correlated with reduced proliferation and induction of apoptosis. In light of these animal models, a strong argument can be made in favor of using FLT as an early response surrogate in lymphoma.[88] However, the limited applicability of in vitro and animal studies to humans must be considered, because there are vast differences in pharmacokinetics and pharmacodynamics between animals and humans.

A multitude of pilot human studies have shown a potential benefit for early prediction of response based on FLT PET studies (**Fig. 6**).[55,76,84,89] Within 1 and 6 weeks after initiation of therapy, a significant tumor SUV decline of 77% and 85% was

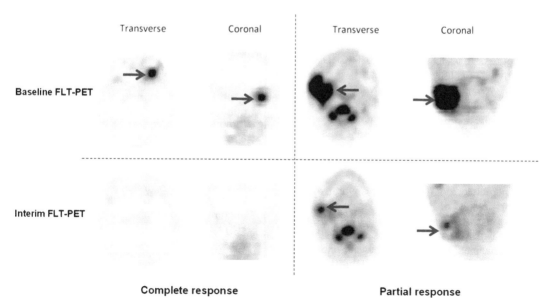

Complete response   Partial response

Fig. 6. FLT PET in evaluation of response to therapy in DLBCL. (*Courtesy of* Dr Andreas Buck, Universitätsklinikum Würzburg.)

noted, respectively. Two days after administration of the monoclonal antibody rituximab (anti-CD20 mAb), no meaningful FLT decrease was observed, mirroring findings in animal experiments suggesting that rituximab does not induce short-term antiproliferative effects.[84] However, in patients treated with dexamethasone before rituximab administration, as early as 2 days after therapy, FLT uptake was significantly lower compared with that of the baseline. Overall response to chemotherapy correlated well with reduction of tumor FLT uptake after administration of R-CHOP. There was no statistically significant difference between initial FLT uptake in patients achieving a partial remission (PR) or complete remission (CR) based on CT criteria ($P = .09$). After the first cycle (2–7 days after completion of R-CHOP), a marked difference was noted in tumor FLT retention between patients reaching PR versus those achieving a CR at the end of therapy. After a median follow-up of 12.6 months, only 2 patients developed relapse after initial response. In another study, in 48 patients with HL (n = 15) or NHL (n = 33) with residual masses of greater than 2.0 cm, the overall survival for patients with a negative FDG PET or FLT PET result was significantly higher than for those with a positive PET, irrespective of the tracer used. FLT alone was able to discriminate between patients with long or short overall survival. However, these data did not suggest any advantage for combining FDG and FLT PET studies rather than FDG PET alone with respect to prediction of survival. Although FDG detected only 10% more lesions than FLT, the additional characterization of tumor tissue with respect to proliferation might be useful for the better identification of patients with recurrence.[90] More recently, in a prospective study in 66 patients with aggressive NHL treated with R-CHOP, the initial mean SUV was significantly higher in patients who showed progressive disease and partial response than in patients who achieved CR ($P = .049$). In addition, a significant correlation between IPI score and initial FLT uptake was found to support a role for FLT as a prognostic indicator. Thus, FLT PET may play a role in risk-adapted treatment.[85]

As a hematologic malignancy, it is worthwhile to review the results of a study assessing treatment response in acute myeloid leukemia (AML), a proliferative malignancy of the hematopoietic system. In 8 adult patients with AML receiving induction chemotherapy, those who entered CR had threefold lower FLT uptake in the bone marrow than those patients with resistant disease (SUVmax 3.6 vs 11.4, $P<.001$).[91] FLT PET results for patients in CR were independent of assessment time point

between days 2 and 6 of therapy, suggesting that FLT PET scans acquired as early as 2 days after chemotherapy initiation may predict clinical response. This pilot study suggests that FLT PET imaging during induction chemotherapy may serve as an early biomarker of treatment response in AML. Given that many patients with a negative postinduction bone marrow biopsy fail to achieve a complete remission, FLT PET imaging may provide a more accurate tool for early assessment of treatment response in AML and deserves further study.

Whether or not imaging of proliferation provides superior information compared with established response parameters is yet to be proved. In this regard, FLT PET has not been sufficiently evaluated to claim a definitive prognostic role among other indicators. Based on the promising pilot studies summarized earlier, its potential in guiding individualized management should be further explored in a multicentral setting.

SUMMARY

There are multiple potential applications for FLT PET in lymphoma (**Box 2**). The role for FLT PET in determination of the extent of disease involvement does not seem justified in the absence of

---

Box 2
Potential clinical applications of noninvasive imaging of proliferation

- Differential diagnosis of benign from malignant tumor lymphoproliferative disorders
- Staging of HL and high-grade NHL lymphoma
- Detection of disease extent in organs with high metabolic activity (eg, brain lesions, Waldeyer ring)
- Lymphoma grading and assessment of tumor aggressiveness by identification of lesions with low and high proliferative activity; guiding biopsy in patients with low-grade tumors to determine transformation to a more aggressive condition
- Early detection of response to therapy, particularly in aggressive NHL
- Differentiation of inflammation from viable residual disease in HL (may be a niche imaging for patients with positive interim FDG PET results)
- Assessment of response to targeted drugs that are more cytostatic than cytotoxic
- Monitor response to radiation therapy
- Assessment of prognosis (disease-free survival, overall survival)

supporting comparative data with FDG PET. FDG whose tumor uptake is at least twice as much as FLT will probably hold its place as initial staging for lymphoma. Moreover, the overall lower uptake in tumors and higher background activity in the liver and bone marrow further dampens the enthusiasm to use this tracer as a staging tool. Nonetheless, FLT PET seems to be a useful diagnostic tool to differentiate indolent from transformed lymphoma, with a substantial potential to alter management in this population. This use will probably only be justified in those patients with clinical suspicion of transformation rather than as a screening method to determine transformation.

In the posttherapy setting, FLT seems to have a niche based on convincing preliminary data for specifically evaluating proliferative activity. This application could bring new implications in treatment selection or monitoring in patients undergoing induction or curative therapy as well as in those patients presenting with suspected recurrent cancer. Furthermore, FLT imaging as a proliferative marker can provide biologic information regarding repopulation of clonogenic tumor cells for radiotherapy planning with an intention to escalate the dose to regions with rapid cell repopulation. However, larger prospective multicenter studies are warranted to establish the role of FLT PET in management of patients who have cancer.

IMAGING TUMOR HYPOXIA

Hypoxia is a common milieu in many human cancers that contributes to tumor progression and resistance to both chemotherapy and radiotherapy (**Table 3**). The major factors that propagate tumor cell hypoxia include inadequate blood flow as a consequence of deficient tumor neovasculature, reduced tissue oxygenation caused by fast tumor growth, and anemia.[92] A large body of clinical evidence suggests that the aggressive behavior of cancer cells and broad resistance to therapy is orchestrated by hypoxia-inducible factor-1 α (HIF-1α).[93,94] Other factors, including genetically driven events such as the loss of function of the Von Hippel-Lindau (VHL) tumor suppressor protein, contribute to activation of HIF-1α. Because of the central role of HIF-1α in cancer biologic behavior, it has become a major target for the development of anticancer drugs.[95] The difficulties associated with earlier hypoxia evaluation methods, such as invasive oxygen electrodes, can be largely overcome by molecular imaging methods to identify, localize, and quantify a tumor's oxygenation status. Conceivably, the decrease in tumor hypoxic fraction can be monitored by imaging during hypoxia-directed therapy.

Relevance in Lymphoma

In evaluating different hypoxia tracers, the intent is not determination of extent of tumor but rather the measurement of hypoxic subvolumes. The potential applications of tumor hypoxia imaging in lymphoma probably mirror those in solid tumors. The negative correlation of hypoxia with treatment response and ultimate outcome strongly suggests a clinical role for noninvasive evaluation of tumor hypoxic fraction to direct treatments to overcome inherent radioresistance. Pretherapy information on the oxygenation status

Table 3
Hypoxia-induced mechanisms of resistance to anticancer therapy

Effect of Hypoxia	Mechanism	Affected Therapy
DNA free radicals	Failure to induce DNA breaks	Radiotherapy
Cell cycle arrest in G1 or G2 phase	Repair before progression to S or M phase	Cycle-selective chemotherapy agents
Distance from vessels	Compromised drug delivery	Drugs bound in tumor cells
Extracellular acidification	Decreased delivery/uptake	Basic drugs
Resistance to apoptosis	Genetic selection of TP53 mutations	Various drugs
Genomic instability	Induction of mutations	Various drugs
DNA repair suppression	Suppression of multidrug resistance protein	DNA methylating agents
HIF1 stabilization	Expression of ABC transporters	ABC transporter substrates

Abbreviation: ABC, ATP-binding cassette.
Data from Wilson WR, Hay MP. Targeting hypoxia in cancer therapy. Nat Rev Cancer 2011;11:393–410.

of a tumor microenvironment could bring implications for alternative treatment selection and to monitor the effects of treatment. Recent advances in conformal radiotherapy and using PET technology as a tool for therapy planning have made it possible to perform hypoxia-directed intensity-modulated radiotherapy.[96,97]

Tissue microarray analyses performed in molecular classification of DLBCL recently showed higher levels of HIF expression compared with follicular lymphoma (FL) (44% vs 11%, $P = .002$), probably consistent with the more aggressive clinical course of DLBCL compared with FL. Analysis of both DLBCL and FL also confirmed inferior survival trends with high HIF expression; 2-year EFS 44% versus 67% for DLBCL and 71% versus 90% for FL (not significant).[98] The implications of these results can further be considered for applications in prognostication of lymphoma. The commonly used clinicopathologic parameters for evaluation of prognostic risk factors, including international prognostic score (IPS) and IPI, for HL and NHL, respectively, are limited, with considerable overlaps among different risk categories.[99,100] Hypoxia, as a promoter of tumor aggressive behavior and a predictor of resistance to anticancer therapy, can be used as an adverse prognostic marker in lymphoma. Further studies are necessary to determine whether hypoxia or HIF-1α is an independent, or at least complementary, prognostic factor for lymphoma.

Mechanism of Uptake

Most prior investigations have been focused on radiolabeled 2-nitroimidazole–based radiosensitizers whose retention within the cell depends on tissue oxygenation.[92,101] These molecules are lipophilic, freely diffusible through cell membranes, and they bind covalently to intracellular molecules at levels that are inversely proportional to intracellular oxygen concentration. As soon they enter the cell, nitroimidazols are reduced to free radical anions, regardless of the intracellular oxygen concentration. This process is reversible in the presence of oxygen; however, under hypoxic conditions (O_2 <10–20 mm Hg), this free anion undergoes further reductions to produce more chemically reactive species that lead to selective trapping of the tracer within hypoxic cells.[102] [^{18}F]Fluoromisonidazole ([^{18}F]FMISO), one of the earliest radiosensitizers used in radiation therapy, is the most widely used PET radiotracer for mapping out hypoxic tumor subvolumes.[103–106]

The ^{64}Cu-labeled acetyl derivative of pyruvaldehyde bis [N^4-methylthiosemicarbazonato] copper(II) complex, Cu-ATSM, is another class of radiopharmaceuticals developed for imaging hypoxia. It is freely diffusible and has the advantage of having a longer $T_{1/2}$ of ^{64}Cu (12.8 hours vs 110 minutes for ^{18}F) for practical clinical use, although the mechanism of retention is not well established. The reduction of Cu(II)-ATSM takes place in both normoxic and hypoxic cells, resulting in formation of unstable Cu(I)-ATSM. These unstable species are completely dissociated in hypoxic cells, becoming irreversibly trapped. Similar to FMISO, this radiopharmaceutical has rapid washout from normoxic regions. Nonetheless, the concentration of NADH, a reducing agent for copper, is increased under extended hypoxic conditions, thus limiting the role of Cu-ATSM in measuring prompt reoxygenation response.[107]

Another alternative investigational nitroimidazole derivative is ^{18}F-labeled fluoroazomycin-arabinoside ([(^{18})F]FAZA or FAZA), which has proved useful to identify tumor hypoxia in several human cancers with suitable tumor/background ratios.[108,109]

FMISO versus Cu-ATSM

The main shortcoming of ^{18}F-FMISO is its low contrast ratio between hypoxic and normoxic tissues and its slow cellular washout requiring at least a delay of approximately 2 hours after the injection to allow adequate clearance from normal background tissues.[104,110,111] Despite the limitations, useful clinical data have been generated (Fig. 7).[104,105,110–113] Cu-ATSM has been developed as an alternative hypoxia agent with faster pharmacokinetics leading to better sensitivity. The Cu-ATSM images show the best contrast early after injection but these images are confounded by blood flow and their mechanism of localization is 1 step removed from the intracellular O_2 concentration.[92,101] FMISO has been criticized because of its clearance characteristics, but its uptake after 2 hours is probably the most representative of regional P_{O2} at the time the radiopharmaceutical is used. ^{18}F]FAZA, the most recently studied of this class of agents, shows uptake similar to that of ^{18}F-FMISO but with faster blood clearance.[108]

Biodistribution

F-FMISO is metabolized by the liver and excreted by the kidney and bladder. Bowel uptake may be prominent, presumably secondary to intraluminal anaerobic bacteria. Biodistribution data in preclinical rat models have shown that the highest concentration of activity is in the urine, with uptake also evident in the intestine, liver, and kidney. The lowest activity is noted in the blood, spleen, heart, lung, muscle, bone, and brain.

MRI   **FDG**   **FMISO**

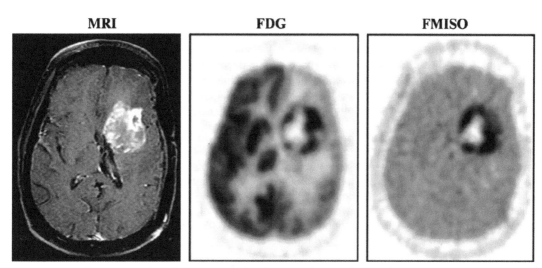

Fig. 7. Images of a recurrent left frontotemporal malignant pleomorphic xanthoastrocytoma in a 28-year-old woman. The top three images show similar tomographic planes imaged by (*left to right*): MRI, F[18]-FDG PET, and F[18]-fluoromisonidazole (FMISO) PET. Note the differences in distribution of tracer uptake between FDG and FMISO images reflecting different targeted mechanisms, glucose metabolism and tumor hypoxia, respectively. The quantitative showed that the tumor:blood ratio for FMISO was consistently below 1.2 (not shown) over a wide range of FDG SUVs in normal brain. The majority of tumor:blood ratios were greater than 1.2, indicative of hypoxia which emphasizes the objective identification of hypoxic regions of the tumor. (*From* Tatum JL, Kelloff GJ. Hypoxia: importance in tumor biology, noninvasive measurement by imaging, and value of its measurement in the management of cancer therapy. Int J Radiat Biol 2006;82(10):715; with permission.)

Timing

Selective retention of ^{18}F-FMISO is observed in hypoxic tissue by 1 hour after injection. The recommended time for FMISO PET imaging is between 90 and 120 minutes. The quantitation of ^{18}F-FMISO tumor/plasma ratio can be optimally performed at 2 hours after injection. The effective dose equivalent for ^{18}F-FMISO PET scan is 0.013 mSv/MBq in men and 0.014 mSv/MBq in women, with a standard dose of 3.7 MBq/kg (0.1 mCi/kg).[114]

Reproducibility

The intratumoral distribution of ^{18}F-FMISO is moderately reproducible with the definition of hypoxia as the tumor/muscle ratio of greater than 1.2. More work is required to identify the underlying causes of temporal variabilities in intratumoral distribution for ^{18}F-FMISO PET imaging at a single time point.

Sensitivity

Hypoxia is defined as the ratio of FMISO uptake in hypoxic cells compared with normoxic cells, which determines the uptake and specificity in vitro. The mean value for this ratio in all tissues is close to unity and almost all normoxic pixels have a value of less than 1.2.[115] Although this ratio reflects a low contrast between hypoxic tumor

tissue and normal tissues, previous studies have shown that tumor hypoxia can be assessed with ^{18}F-FMISO.[111,116]

Clinical Data and Applications in Radiotherapy

The aim of radiation treatment planning is to deliver the highest allowable radiation to the tumor with minimal radiation delivered to critical normal tissues to maintain a high therapeutic ratio. Molecular imaging methods provide the ability to better define tumor margins and help plan individualized treatments. Hypoxic cells require higher radiation doses for the same cytotoxic effect as normoxic cells.[117] Thus, a boost dose of radiation to hypoxic subvolumes may be beneficial to improve local tumor control.

The ability to incorporate the biologic imaging information provided by PET/CT technology with radiation treatment planning, particularly for intensity-modulated radiotherapy (IMRT), has facilitated dose-escalation schemes guided by hypoxic subvolumes. FMISO remains the most commonly used agent for PET-based hypoxia imaging (see **Fig. 7**).[105,113,116,118] Although most tumors are deprived of oxygen, the fractional hypoxic volumes can vary significantly.[105] More recent data revealed that high hypoxic volumes as determined by FMISO PET imaging were strongly associated with unfavorable time to progression and survival in patients with glioblastoma multiforme and head and neck cancers.[111,115] Rischin and colleagues[119] also showed that only those patients with significant FMISO uptake benefited from tirapazamine therapy to overcome radiotherapy resistance. In a multivariate analysis, pretherapy FMISO uptake and nodal status were both found to be independent prognostic measures in the prediction of survival in patients with HNSCC (n = 73).[115] However, further data are needed to establish the relationship between pretherapy tumor FMISO uptake and long-term clinical outcome. When FMISO was used to monitor tumor hypoxia after concomitant chemotherapy, normalization of FMISO activity was also associated with favorable response (Fig. 8).[119,120] Early resolution of FMISO uptake within 4 weeks of therapy was a harbinger of excellent locoregional control, with a 5-year

freedom-free relapse of 68% in patients with HNSCC receiving hypoxia-targeting agents.[121]

In advanced-stage HNSCC, only 5% of tirapazamine-treated patients experienced locoregional failure, as opposed to 61% of recurrences among those who were not given this hypoxia-targeting agent.[119] These data were important for subsequent FMISO PET/CT-guided IMRT trials with the goal of further improving locoregional control in HNSCC patients.[122] However, there are contradictory published data reporting excellent locoregional control in patients treated with concurrent chemotherapy and IMRT despite evidence of detectable hypoxia on the pretreatment FMISO PET studies.[123,124]

The heterogeneous distribution of FMISO reflects variable levels of hypoxia within the tumor volume. It is conceivable that hypoxia imaging may require delayed imaging to allow better accrual of

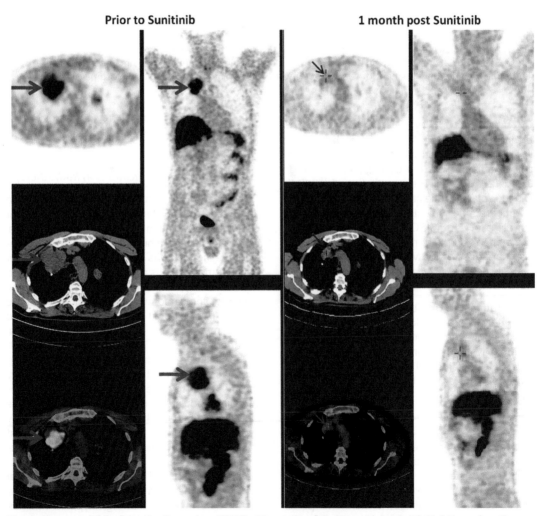

Fig. 8. Therapy response evaluation using FMISO. (*Courtesy of* Dr Marc Faraggi, Hôpital Européen Georges-Pompidou, France.)

radiotracer in hypoxic subvolumes; however, the ^{18}F label does not permit delayed imaging because of its short physical $T_{1/2}$ (110 minutes). Therefore, a longer-lived radiotracer such as [64]Cu-(II)-diacetyl-bis(N^4-methylthiosemicarbazone; ATSM) ($T_{1/2}$ 12.7 hours) is preferable.[125] Although labeled with a short-lived copper radioisotope, [62]Cu-ATSM ($T_{1/2}$, 9.7 minutes) guided IMRT by allowing for radiation dose escalation to the hypoxic gross tumor volume without compromising normal tissue protection in HNSCC.[126] To date, 38 patients with cancer of the uterine cervix have been imaged for hypoxia using another short-lived copper radiolabel [60]Cu-ATSM ($T_{1/2}$, 24 minutes).[127] [60]Cu-ATSM showed high contrast levels between hypoxic and normoxic tissues by as little as 10 to 15 minutes after injection,[128] a tumor/muscle ratio of 3.5 was a statistically significant cutoff for accurately differentiating relapsing patients from those who developed a recurrence after completing therapy. Progression-free survival and cause-specific survival were significantly better in patients with a tumor/muscle ratio of less than 3.5 ($P \leq .04$). In locally invasive primary or node-positive rectal cancer, [60]Cu-ATSM PET again showed promise as a predictor of the tumor response to neoadjuvant chemoradiotherapy and survival.[129] Thus far, there have been no data for determination of hypoxia in patients with lymphoma.

SUMMARY

Tissue hypoxic subvolume is an important factor that affects tumor microenvironment by conferring aggressive tumor behavior and promoting broad resistance to radiotherapy. The tumor hypoxic volume can be determined by using PET hypoxia imaging agents that may provide the ability to plan and deliver appropriate radiation doses to hypoxic subvolumes, mainly using IMRT. This advanced method can be beneficial in patients with lymphoma who are planned to undergo radiation therapy, particularly in those with bulky tumors and residual bulky masses. Potential clinical improvements include less toxicity with better tumor margin definition and the promise of delivering higher doses of radiation to these subvolumes without added morbidity.

IMAGING TUMOR ANGIOGENESIS

As one of the hallmarks of oncogenic transformation, the structurally and functionally deficient capillary endothelial cells of newly formed tumor blood vessels constitute an important target for cancer imaging and therapy (**Fig. 9**).[130–132] Tumor angiogenesis is often triggered under metabolic stress as an imbalance between proangiogenic and antiangiogenic signals, promoting tumor growth, invasion, and metastatic spread, usually when the tumor size exceeds 2 mm.[130,132,133] Essential to the process is the activation of vascular endothelial growth factor (VEGF), a crucial cytokine in the regulation of angiogenesis, through hypoxia-inducible factor α (HIFα). Following this step, proteolytic enzymes such as matrix metalloproteinases (MMPs) are produced to degrade the basement membrane and the extracellular matrix (ECM), providing sufficient space for the sprouting vessels.[133] One receptor class playing an important role during endothelial cell migration is the integrins.[134] It has been shown in murine tumor models that monoclonal antibodies as well as low-molecular-weight antagonists, recognizing the integrins $\alpha_v\beta_3$ and $\alpha_v\beta_5$, can counteract angiogenesis.[135,136] Another means to counteract tumor angiogenesis is the use of monoclonal antibodies targeting the VEGF signaling axis or by tyrosine kinases of VEGF receptors. However, not all patients are likely to respond to these therapies, so reliable biomarkers are of crucial importance and development of molecular imaging strategies to enable therapy monitoring could ensure therapeutic efficacy.

Noninvasive Detection of Angiogenesis

Contrary to expectations, tumor perfusion rate is lower than that of normal tissues even in the presence of extensive neoangiogenesis. As tumors grow, perfusion is further decreased because of a host of tumor environment and patient-related variables.[137] Hence, evaluation of tumor perfusion is not an accurate measure of angiogenesis. To predict the patient subpopulation who would benefit from antiangiogenic therapy and avoid unwarranted toxicity, various noninvasive imaging methods including magnetic resonance imaging, Doppler ultrasound, and PET techniques have been investigated.[138–140] The current PET strategies are concentrated on the development of radiolabeled small molecules and antibodies targeting VEGF and its receptor as well as $\alpha_v\beta_3$ integrin antagonists. Molecular imaging of radiolabeled $\alpha_v\beta_3$ expression is the only method that has entered clinical trials and [^{18}F]galacto-arginine-glycine-aspartate (RGD) sequence is the first molecule applied in patients. Prior experience with PET imaging with ^{64}Cu-labeled anti-VEGF receptor antibodies, the radiolabeled single-chain Fv antifibronectin antibody fragments, and the matrix metalloprotein (MMP) yielded limited success because of significant immunogenicity

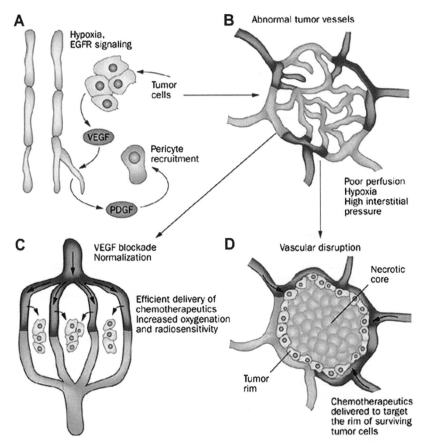

Fig. 9. The development of the tumor vasculature, and the effect of therapies that target it. (*A*) Hypoxia and EGFR signaling can lead to the production of VEGF by tumor cells. This induces the sprouting of endothelial cells and eventually the development of new vessels. PDGF produced by endothelial cells is involved in the recruitment of pericytes, which surround and stabilize new vessels. (*B*) The tumor vasculature is highly abnormal, tortuous, and lacks the normal architecture of arterioles, capillaries and venules. Consequently the tumor is poorly perfused and hypoxic. A lack of lymphatic drainage causes high interstitial pressure. (*C*) VEGF blockade causes vascular normalization, pruning and stabilization of the vasculature, resulting in good perfusion and the efficient delivery of chemotherapeutics. The increased oxygenation results in increased radiosensitivity of tumor cells. (*D*) Vascular-disrupting agents cause the collapse of tumor vessels, resulting in tumor-cell death and hemorrhagic necrosis. A surviving rim of tumor cells can be targeted by chemotherapeutics. EGFR, epidermal growth factor receptor; PDGF, platelet-derived growth factor; VEGF, vascular endothelial growth factor. (*From* Heath VL, Bicknell R. Anticancer strategies involving the vasculature. Nat Rev Clin Oncol 2009;6(7):397. DOI:10.1038/nrclinonc.2009.52; with permission.)

or unfavorable tumor/blood ratios.[141–144] In this article, only the strategies concentrated on the development of radiolabeled RGD peptides for imaging $\alpha_V\beta_3$ integrin expression are discussed.

Relevance in Lymphoma

The growth of lymphoma cells seems to be promoted by tumor microenvironment that takes part in modulating angiogenic response to proangiogenic growth factors via expression of VEGF.[11,145–153] There is evidence there is a correlation between the aggressiveness of NHLs and the magnitude of angiogenesis as reflected by

increase in VEGF expression and microvessel density and with proven upregulation of VEGF expression in peripheral T-cell lymphoma (PTCL), DLBCL, and MCL.[149–153] The level of expression of angiogenesis defines diverse prognostic groups in follicular lymphoma (FL) and DLBCL, based on gene expression profiling studies.[152,153] Although indolent lymphomas do not have consistently increased VEGF expression,[152] transformation to a high-grade histology is usually associated with high VEGF expression.[149,151,153] These data on the angiogenic properties of the lymphoma cells prepared the way for targeting tumor angiogenesis with antiangiogenic agents,[154] including receptor tyrosine kinase inhibitors as well as other compounds with antiangiogenic properties such asrapamycin (mTOR), and proteasome inhibitors.[150] Preliminary data support the feasibility and efficacy of antiangiogenic therapy using the therapeutic agents mentioned earlier in DLBCL, CLL, and MCL.[150] PET probes developed for imaging tumor angiogenesis may play a key role in selecting the proper patient population for an effective antiangiogenic treatment. It may also guide treatment by monitoring its efficacy using a real-time quantitative method. However, for a more meaningful clinical applicability, the first step should be the correlation between these PET imaging molecules and tissue angiogenic markers in an expanded clinical setting. Parallel to these efforts, the survival benefits of antiangiogenic therapy should be validated with or without combination chemotherapy.

Mechanism of Uptake

The $\alpha_v\beta_3$ integrin is a transmembrane cell adhesion receptor that is involved in tumor cell binding of extracellular matrix proteins. After activation of the endothelial cells, proteolytic enzymes, such as serine proteases and matrix metalloproteinases (MMPs), are excreted, allowing degradation of the basement membrane and the ECM surrounding the vessels.[155] At this stage, cell adhesion receptors, like the integrin $\alpha_v\beta_3$, play a crucial role by mediating migration of the endothelial cells in the basement membrane. The arginine-glycine-aspartic acid tripeptide recognizes the $\alpha_v\beta_3$ receptor. The radiotracer approach was one of the first to be used for molecular imaging of $\alpha_v\beta_3$ expression and is the most intensively studied strategy to date. The most investigated radiopharmaceutical for molecular imaging $\alpha_v\beta_3$ expression is [18F]Galacto-RGD.[156–159] In murine tumor models as well as in patients, this tracer showed receptor-specific tumor accumulation and favorable pharmocokinetics resulting in determination of $\alpha_v\beta_3$ expression with high contrast. Because of increasing availability in the last few years, metal-based PET isotopes such as ^{64}Cu and ^{68}Ga have also been introduced.[145] However, the high-activity concentration in the liver, intestine, and bladder indicate that further optimization of the radiolabeled product is needed.

Biodistribution

[18F]Galacto-RGD rapidly clears from the blood pool and is primarily eliminated through the kidneys, which may impair evaluation of lesions involving the urogenital tract. Intermediate to high tracer uptake is notable in the liver, spleen, and intestine, with SUVs ranging from 2.5 to 4.0. Background activity in lung and muscle tissue is low and the calculated effective dose was found to be similar to an [18F]FDG PET scan. Organ systems with low background tracer uptake, which are consequently well suited for PET imaging of $\alpha_v\beta_3$ expression, are the extremities, the skeletal system in general, the lungs, mediastinum, and thorax, including the breast and the head and neck area. For the brain, our results suggest that [18F]Galacto-RGD does not cross the blood-brain barrier, because tracer uptake in normal brain tissue is even lower than in muscle.[156] Distribution volumes, which reflect the tissue receptor concentration, are on average 4 times higher for tumor tissue than for muscle tissue, suggesting specific tracer binding. A high interindividual and intraindividual variance in tumor tracer accumulation was noted, suggesting substantial heterogeneity of $\alpha_v\beta_3$ expression.

Timing

Although still in an experimental phase, optimal imaging time is unknown. The previous studies were performed with an interval of 45 to 60 minutes between injection and start of image acquisition. Injection of a dose of radiotracer of 4 to 5 mCi (140–200 MBq) is recommended. No special patient preparation is necessary for imaging of $\alpha_v\beta_3$ expression with [18F]Galacto-RGD. The calculated effective dose found in our first studies was approximately 19 µSv/MBq, which is similar to an [18F]FDG scan.[156]

Clinical Data

Molecular imaging of angiogenesis with PET may be useful for the assessment of response to antiangiogenic or combined cytotoxic/antiangiogenic therapy as shown in preclinical studies suggesting a potential use for PET imaging of $\alpha_v\beta_3$ expression in response assessment. [18F]Galacto-RGD was the first PET radiopharmaceutical described for PET imaging of $\alpha_v\beta_3$ integrin expression with acceptable tumor/background ratios (Fig. 10).[140,156–159] [18F]Galacto-RGD uptake was correlated with tissue $\alpha_v\beta_3$ expression ($r = 0.92$) and the microvessel density ($r = 0.84$) in humans with solid tumors. The mean SUV was 3.8 ($\pm$ 2.3) with a tumor/background ratio of 3.4 ($\pm$ 2.2). Moreover, immunohistochemistry confirmed lack of $\alpha_v\beta_3$ expression in normal tissues and in the 2 tumors without tracer uptake.[157] In squamous cell carcinoma, [(18)F]Galacto-RGD PET allowed for specific imaging of $\alpha_v\beta_3$ expression in HNSCC with good tumor-to-background contrast. [18F]Galacto-RGD PET

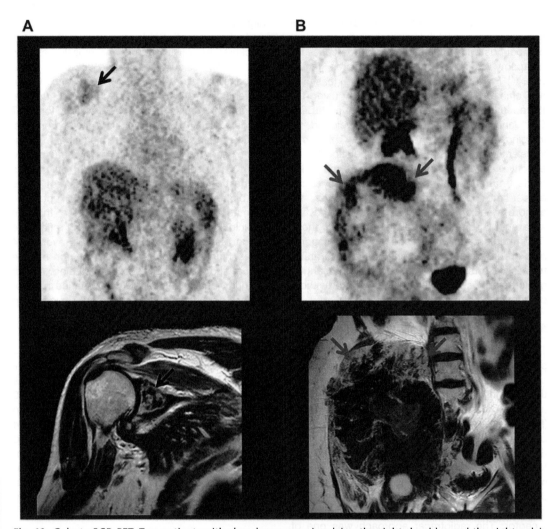

Fig. 10. Galacto-RGD PET. Two patients with chondrosarcoma involving the right shoulder and the right pelvis. Coronal images of RGD-PET (*upper panel*) and, Gd-DTPA MRI (*lower panel*). (*A*) The RGD images demonstrate mild uptake in a well-differentiated (grade 1) chondrosarcoma corresponding to the tumor showing contrast enhancement on the coronal MRI image. (*B*) Coronal RGD PET images demonstrate significantly higher uptake in a dedifferentiated (grade 3) chondrosarcoma in the right pelvis with contrast enhancement on MRI. The difference in differentiation between the tumors is reflected on the difference between the level of tracer uptake representing varing intensity of angiogenesis which is known to increase as the tumor grade increases. (*Courtesy of Dr Ambros J. Beer, Universität München, Germany.*)

identified 83% of tumors, with a mean SUV of 3.4. Immunohistochemistry showed predominantly microvessel $\alpha_v\beta_3$ expression, suggesting that, in HNSCC, [^{18}F]Galacto-RGD PET might be used as a surrogate marker of angiogenesis.[158] In patients with suspected or recurrent glioblastoma (GBM), although normal brain tissue did not show significant tracer accumulation, GBMs showed significant but heterogeneous tracer uptake, particularly in the highly proliferating and infiltrating areas of tumors (mean SUV, 1.6 ± 0.5), which correlated with immunohistochemical $\alpha_v\beta_3$ integrin expression of corresponding tumor samples. These data suggest that [^{18}F]Galacto-RGD PET successfully identifies $\alpha_v\beta_3$ expression in GBM and might be a promising tool for planning and monitoring individualized cancer therapies targeting this integrin.[160] However, [^{18}F]Galacto-RGD does not cross the intact blood-brain barrier, so this might be an important factor influencing tracer uptake in central nervous system (CNS) lesions. Therefore, data obtained in the CNS may not be compatible with those tumors that involve the body alone.

The $\alpha_v\beta_3$ integrin also plays a role in cancer metastasis, and is abundantly expressed on osteoclasts. There are data showing that ^{64}Cu-RGD localizes to areas in bone with increased osteoclast formation and that support the use of ^{64}Cu-RGD as an imaging biomarker for osteoclasts.[161,162] In a transgenic mouse model, ^{64}Cu-RGD successfully monitored physiologic changes in the bone metastatic microenvironment in osteolytic bone metastases after osteoclast-inhibiting bisphosphonate therapy.[161]

Another cyclic RGD-based radiotracer that has recently entered in clinical trials is ^{18}F-AH111585 (fluciclatide/GE 135)[163–165] and has shown safety as well as favorable biodistribution with predominantly renal excretion.[164,166] In a preliminary study of patients with solid tumors (melanoma, renal cell carcinoma, and renal oncocytoma), [^{18}F]fluciclatide-PET scan showed variable tumor uptake and retention.[163] In 7 patients with breast cancer, all 18 tumors were visualized on [^{18}F]-AH111585 PET images.[163] However, in the case of liver metastases, lesions were identified only as photopenic areas. In a patient with renal cell carcinoma, the images detect the mass of the primary as well as other sites within the liver and lymph nodes.[164] Thus far, no data have been published to elucidate whether PET imaging of $\alpha_v\beta_3$ expression is superior or complementary to functional imaging of angiogenesis with other imaging means including dynamic contrast-enhanced (DCE) MR imaging.

A recent study estimated the receptor-ligand binding of an RGD peptide in somatic tumors using dynamic PET data in patients with metastatic breast cancer, using [^{18}F]fluciclatide.[167] The volume of distribution was, on average, higher in lung metastases than in the healthy lung, but lower in liver metastases than in the healthy liver. In agreement with the expected higher $\alpha_v\beta_3$, this study indicated that the k(3)/k(4) ratio is a reasonable measure of specific binding, suggesting that this index can be used to estimate $\alpha_v\beta_3$ receptor expression in oncology, although further studies are necessary to validate this hypothesis.[167] Other promising compounds labeled with ^{64}Cu or ^{68}Ga that target $\alpha_v\beta_3$ receptors have been in the investigational phase and the results of these studies will show the optimal radiotracer with suitable characteristics to evaluate tumor angiogenesis.[168]

SUMMARY

PET with [^{18}F]Galacto-RGD might be used as a new marker of angiogenesis and for individualized planning of therapeutic strategies with $\alpha_v\beta_3$-targeted drugs; however, further validation of such biomarkers is required for a better understanding of antiangiogenic therapy. This field is rapidly evolving with development of different radiotracer techniques according to the structure of their $\alpha_v\beta_3$-specific ligands. Imaging characteristics may be substantially improved by multimeric ligands and with the use of radiolabeled nanoparticles, which can be functionalized for drug treatment or as multimodality imaging probes.

IMAGING APOPTOSIS

Evasion of apoptosis is an intrinsic cell death program, a hallmark of cancer that is widely applicable to hematological malignancies (Fig. 11). Targeting cellular death pathways, primarily apoptosis, has potential clinical implications for cancer imaging and therapy. Apoptosis is an organized, energy-dependent, complex process that is controlled by different B-cell lymphoma 2 (Bcl2) family members that are responsible for dysregulation of apoptosis and prevention of death in cancer cells.[169,170] When triggered by various signals, these cells undergo cytoplasmic shrinkage, membrane blebbing, and sequestration of intracellular contents followed by phagocytosis without provoking an inflammatory response. Initiation of apoptotic cell death leads to activation of caspases[171,172] and results in rapid externalization of phosphatidylserine (PS) from the inner leaflet of the plasma membrane to its outer surface. Annexin V and its derivatives, as members of the calcium and phospholipid binding family of annexin proteins, selectively binds to PS residues with a high affinity.[173–175] Annexin-mediated apoptosis imaging of externalized PS has, thus far, been extensively investigated using non–positron-emitting radionuclides such as ^{99m}Tc and ^{111}In, and data with positron-emitting radionuclides are currently scarce.[175] Current efforts are focused on development of low-molecular-weight, apoptosis-targeting probes that are potentially suitable to serve as PET tracers to improve rates of detectability.

Relevance in Lymphoma

Blocks in apoptotic pathways propagate the growth of cancer cells and potentiate progression by promoting genetic instability and gene mutations, conferring resistance to cytotoxic therapies, and by facilitating growth factor–independent survival.[169,170] Regulation of programmed cell death is relevant for lymphoma, because the hematopoietic system depends on a balance between newly formed cells and cell death, so the paucity of apoptosis may result in the development of lymphoma or leukemia.[176] In this regard, BCL2 proteins are important cell death regulators that interact in various ways to induce or prevent pore formation in the outer mitochondrial membrane. Bcl2 overexpression also promotes

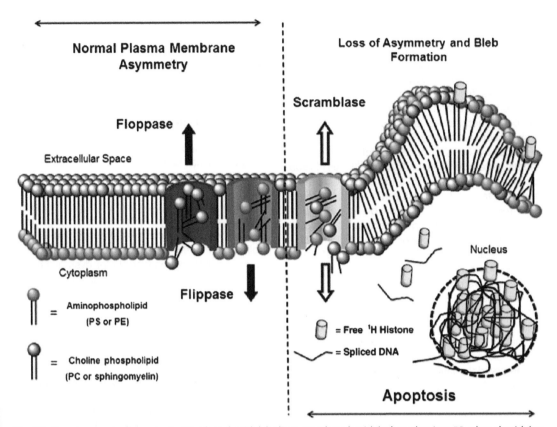

Fig. 11. Development of apoptosis. PC, phosphatidylcholine; PE, phosphatidylethanolamine; PS, phosphatidylserine. (*From* Blankenberg FG, Norfrau JF. Multimodality imaging of apoptosis in oncology. AJR Am J Roentgenol 2011;197:308–17; with permission.)

increased neoangiogenesis through upregulation of VEGF expression, and confers drug resistance.[177] From their close involvement in cancer propagation, the BCL2 family of proteins has been identified as an attractive target for diagnostic purposes and anticancer therapy.[178] An imaging agent that would monitor apoptotic activity induced by anticancer treatment may be of benefit to predict therapeutic efficacy and thereby prognosis. Some BCL2 family inhibitors have shown convincing evidence for efficacy in preclinical models and proceeded rapidly into phase I and II clinical trials.[179] As a proteasome inhibitor, bortezomib has been shown in preclinical studies to induce apoptosis and sensitize tumor cells to chemotherapy or radiation with potential activity in certain lymphoma subtypes. Bortezomib is approved for treatment of MCL[180] and, in relapsed or refractory patients with NHL, there are emerging data showing that bortezomib induces response in patients with DLBCL.[181] Similarly, other apoptotic biologic agents such as survivin, a member of the inhibitor of apoptosis gene family, might provide a useful therapeutic strategy for lymphomas.[182]

In summary, molecular imaging of programmed cell death, as one of the fundamental cellular processes, may be of clinical benefit by complementing biologic characterization of tumors, increasing the accuracy of staging algorithms, as well as monitoring disease course to assess therapy efficacy either early during or after completion of treatment. If successful results are obtained, the information from these molecular imaging techniques will probably help individualize treatment.

Mechanism of Uptake

In vivo imaging of apoptosis has focused on 2 main biologic targets: the externalized PS residues at the outer surface of the plasma membrane and the activated caspases.[183] The induction of apoptosis inactivates the enzymes, floppase and translocase, that maintain PS at the inner surface of the lipid bilayer, and simultaneously activates a third enzyme, scramblase, which externalizes PS. These cellular changes constitute the basis for annexin V, a 35-kDa human protein with high affinity for cell membrane–bound PS, as an apoptosis probe.[184] However, targeting PS can be misleading because the externalization occurs in reversible stress conditions and also in necrotic cell death.[184]

An alternative biologic target for imaging of apoptosis is the family of caspases, because the effector caspases function in the apoptosis signaling cascade. Caspase-3 in particular is a promising target for the development of apoptosis-specific molecular imaging probes.[185] Because caspases are intracellularly located, imaging probes should feature special properties for penetrating the membrane of the apoptotic cells.

Another class of apoptosis imaging radiotracers is the ApoSense family of biomarkers for apoptosis radiolabeled with PET radiotracers including ^{18}F-labeled 2-(5-fluoropentyl)-2-methylmalonic acid (^{18}F-ML-10).[186–188] These small molecules have an amphipathic structure, having both specific hydrophobic and charged moieties. Cellular uptake of the ApoSense compounds occurs in the early stages of apoptosis and runs parallel to the apoptotic features of PS externalization, caspase activation, and mitochondrial depolarization. On activation of apoptosis, the ^{18}F-ML-10 acquires enhanced affinity for selective binding, entrance, and accumulation within the apoptotic cell.

Biodistribution

Human studies are scarce in apoptosis imaging studies involving PET probes. Recent data in humans using ^{18}F-ML-10 reported a rapid excretion through the kidneys and rapid clearance from nontarget organs, with no significant uptake in any organ except in the testes; uptake was fivefold higher in the testes than in the muscle.[188] More data are necessary in humans.

Timing

There is no established timing for the various radiolabeled probes. However, an interval of 45 to 60 minutes between injection and imaging is acceptable, although longer time periods may allow better image contrast. Further data are required to establish an optimal time for apoptosis PET imaging. For ^{18}F-ML-10 PET imaging, the mean effective whole-body radiation dose related to ^{18}F-ML-10 administration was 15.4 ($\pm$ 3.7) μSv/MBq ($\sim$3.6 mSv per total injected dose; injected dose allowed up to 500 MBq).[188]

Clinical Data

An important aspect of noninvasive apoptosis imaging is to determine the efficacy of antiapoptotic treatment early during the course of therapy.

It was shown that imaging with technetium 99m (Tc-99m)-labeled annexin V early after therapy might help predict ultimate response.[189,190] ^{99m}Tc-labeled annexin V accumulation was documented with histologic evidence of apoptosis in response to transplanted murine B-cell lymphomas treated with cyclophosphamide.[184,191] In 15 patients with various malignancies, all patients with a subsequent objective tumor response had increased tumor uptake after initial treatment compared with baseline scans. Patients with no change in radiotracer uptake after the first dose of therapy had no subsequent objective clinical response.[189] However, because of unfavorable pharmacokinetic profile, low signal/noise ratio, and potential immunogenicity, the usefulness of annexin V was limited.[192]

The unmet need for an apoptosis-specific molecule yielding better resolution with favorable pharmacokinetic and safety profile has led to development of various PET probes. However, an optimal apoptosis marker labeled with a positron emitter has not been found. Annexin V and its derivatives have been radiolabeled with a wide variety of positron-emitting radionuclides including ^{18}F, ^{11}C, and ^{64}Cu.[173,175,193–195] The low uptake characteristics of ^{18}F-annexin A5 in liver, spleen, and kidney seem to be an advantage compared with the biodistribution behavior of the Tc-99m-annexin A5 analogue. Several other peptides and proteins have been proposed as PET probes recognizing membrane-bound phosphatidylserine,[196,197] but further preclinical studies are required to evaluate the potential of these radiolabeled molecules.

Radiolabeled caspase-3 substrates and inhibitors have been used as alternative approaches for apoptosis imaging.[198,199] For example, [^{18}F]ICMT-11 as a caspase-3 specific PET imaging radiotracer that has the potential for the assessment of tumor apoptosis was shown to bind to a range of drug-induced apoptotic cancer cells invitro and to 38C13 murine lymphoma xenografts in vivo. However, these studies are limited to several animal models without any published human data.[198] Results on in vivo tumor imaging with ^{18}F and other isotopes have yet to be published.

A fluorescent analogue of ApoSense was shown to be a specific marker of apoptosis.[200,201] The increased apoptosis was highly correlated with the increased uptake, and reflected evidence of a dose-response element. In a phase I trial on healthy volunteers, ^{18}F-ML-10 manifested high stability in vivo and favorable biodistribution and dosimetry profiles. In a phase IIa study, PET imaging of apoptosis of neurovascular cells has been achieved in patients with acute ischemic cerebral stroke. In patients with brain metastases treated with whole-brain radiation therapy, PET imaging with ^{18}F-ML-10 provided early detection of tumor response to treatment, which predicted an anatomic response evident on MR imaging 2 months later (Allen AM, unpublished data, 2010).[191] Phase II trials are ongoing with small-molecule apoptosis probes of the ApoSense family, ^{18}F-ML-10 [2-(5-fluoropentyl)-2-methylmalonic acid].

SUMMARY

Based on its crucial role in propagation of tumor progression, apoptosis provides an attractive framework for development of novel anticancer therapeutics, particularly for lymphoma. It has a good potential for radioisotope-based tumor detection, therapy planning, and assessment of treatment efficacy, or serving as a surrogate tool for drug development. A multitude of targets have been explored as potential probes for imaging apoptosis. Although PET emerges as the leading modality for molecular imaging, currently there are scant data for clinical use. Moreover, the definition and the understanding of the biochemical events in apoptosis are continuously evolving. Therefore, any proposed new specific imaging method that is potentially useful in monitoring apoptosis in vivo should take the definitions into consideration for a more clinically relevant approach. The results of ongoing clinical trials will further elucidate the potential role of molecular imaging of apoptosis.

IMAGING AMINO ACID METABOLISM

Malignant tumors may be characterized by alterations in amino acid transport and protein synthesis. ^{11}C-labeled methionine (C-MET), an essential amino acid for protein synthesis, is the most extensively investigated PET radiotracer as a marker of increased amino acid transport/metabolism in cancer imaging.[202] Artificial amino acids l-3-[^{18}F]fluoro-α-methyltyrosine (FMT)[203,204] have also been investigated. Although the original observations only included brain tumors, Jager and colleagues[205] showed similar kinetics in a variety of extracranial tumors including breast cancer, lung cancer, soft tissue sarcoma, and lymphoma.

Relevance in Lymphoma

Primary central nervous system lymphoma (PCNSL), mostly of diffuse large B-cell histology, accounts for 5% to 6% of all intracranial neoplasms and approximately 1% of all lymphomas, but its incidence has been steadily increasing in both immunocompromised and immunocompetent patients.[206] Even with the currently available advanced imaging technology, it may prove challenging to distinguish PCNSL from infectious causes and benign brain tumors. FDG PET imaging is useful in the differentiation of CNS lymphoma from infectious causes; however, C-MET has some advantages compared with FDG, primarily in its low uptake in the normal brain.[207,208] These prior reports have also shown its usefulness in evaluation of the histologic grade of malignancy as well as response to therapy. However, the role of MET PET is yet to be established in patients with PCNSL.

The amino acids that enter protein synthesis (eg, THY and MET) are deemed to reflect malignant transformation and increased proliferation rate more than other amino acids that are only transported into the cell without incorporation into proteins. In this context, the tissue distribution of large neutral amino acid transporter (LAT1) suggests that it is involved mainly in transporting amino acids into growing cells and across some endothelial/epithelial secretory barriers. Hence, the cellular transportation of l-methionine, l-tyrosine, and other neutral amino acids is suggested to be increased in lymphoma cells through upregulated LAT1.[209] In light of this evidence, it can be hypothesized that radiolabeled MET or THY can be used to determine proliferation rates in lymphoma. However, this hypothesis is yet to be proved. Moreover, this may not produce faithfully accurate results because increased protein synthesis is, at best, an indirect measurement of proliferation.

Mechanism of Uptake

The mechanism of malignant tumor uptake is based on the increase in membrane amino acid transport as a result of changes in cell-surface structure and function that occur in association with oncogenic transformation as well as increased protein synthesis.[205,210] Thus, increase in radiolabeled amino acid uptake reflects both the increased rate of amino acid transport and protein synthesis. However, amino acids are also precursors for many other biomolecules, and are involved in other metabolic cycles, including transamination and transmethylation. Hence, the measurement of amino acid transport may not accurately represent protein synthesis alone but rather they may represent a measure of the cellular amino acid turnover.[211] Non–protein-synthesis processes can contribute to increased transport rather than to increased protein synthesis. It is also conceivable that protein synthesis may also reflect repair mechanisms.[212,213] The importance of blood flow in tumor methionine uptake was also shown, suggesting that at least part of MET uptake may result from passive diffusion,[214] particularly, with the loss of integrity of the blood-brain barrier for neuro-oncologic imaging.

Biodistribution

Virtually all amino acids have been radiolabeled with ^{11}C to maintain the authenticity of the molecule because the replacement of a carbon atom by ^{11}C maintains the chemical composition. High methionine uptake is observed in the pituitary gland and pancreas; moderate uptake in liver, bowel, salivary glands, lacrimal glands, and bone marrow; and low uptake in the normal brain.[205] MET and TYR show only moderate uptake in the renal cortex.

Timing

Patients are instructed to fast for at least 4 to 6 hours before PET imaging. Image acquisition starts between 15 and 20 minutes after an intravenous injection of C-MET (6 MBq/kg or 12–15 mCi). The total body effective dose is 5.2×10^{-3} mSv/MBq (2.3 mSv for a dose of 444 MBq [12 mCi]).[215]

Specificity

Because inflammatory cells have a low protein metabolism in comparison with glucose metabolism, amino acid imaging is deemed more tumor specific than FDG. However, active inflammatory cells and the increased tissue perfusion in infectious processes may still contribute to nonspecific uptake. Therefore, the tumor-specific quotient for radiolabeled amino acids is probably higher than that of FDG but is not 100%. However, in a mouse model, accumulation of (Fluoroethyl)-L-Tyrosine (L-FET) showed no overlap between inflammation and tumor-infiltrated lymph nodes.[216] However, there needs to be further validation of specificity of imaging using radiolabeled amino acids based on various conflicting reports and the belief that at least a fraction of the tracer uptake is the result of passive diffusion.

Clinical Data

Based on the overexpression of amino acid transporters in brain tumors and with no accumulation in the normal brain tissue, C-MET is considered to be a suitable candidate for applications in neuro-oncologic imaging.[217] The role of C-MET has been investigated in detection and grading of primary or recurrent tumor,[202,207,208,212,214,218] as a prognostic marker,[219–221] in radiotherapy planning,[222–224] and for assessment of treatment response.[225–227] For high-grade gliomas, C-MET PET was found to be highly sensitive (84%–97%) but, in low-grade tumors including low-grade astrocytomas, oligodendrogliomas, and astrocytomas, the detection rate was low at 61%.[207,208,228] In addition, nontumor accumulation of C-MET raised questions about its specificity. Herholz and colleagues[227] attained high accuracy (79%) in a large patient population in distinguishing glioma from nonneoplastic lesions. C-MET PET imaging can also contribute to the planning of surgical margins and may guide stereotactic biopsies and radiotherapy planning by delineating necrotic from anaplastic components in large tumors.

Evaluation of response

Preclinical studies validating the use of C-MET in the evaluation of response to chemotherapy or radiotherapy showed that MET and TYR uptake is reduced rapidly following chemotherapy or radiotherapy, suggesting immediate inactivation of protein synthesis and/or damage to the membrane transport system.[213,229,230] Terakawa and colleagues[231] showed that the values for each measured index of C-MET PET tended to be higher for tumor recurrence than for radiation necrosis and that C-MET PET could provide quantitative values to help differentiate tumor recurrence from radiation. A decline in C-MET after 3 cycles of temozolomide chemotherapy yielded a more favorable time to progression than in those with an increased tracer uptake (23 vs 3.5 months; $P = .01$).[225] In patients with newly diagnosed glioblastoma multiforme, pretreatment C-MET PET seemed to identify areas of highest risk for recurrence. Thus, it is reasonable to test a strategy of incorporating C-MET PET into radiation treatment planning, particularly for identifying areas suitable for radiation boost.[232]

Limited data exist in extracranial tumors, but the general feasibility of amino acid imaging has been shown as a proof of principle for detection of primary tumors of greater than 1.0 cm.[222,233] In lung cancer and gliomas, tumor C-MET uptake correlated well with the proliferation indices (S phase fraction, Ki-67).[228,234] However, because of the small sample sizes, the predictive value of C-MET-PET remains to be established.

In lymphoma, C-MET avidly accumulated in lymphomas of both low-grade and of high-grade histologies, thus its uptake did not seem to correlate with tumor grade.[222] However, kinetic analysis of C-MET data allowed separation of high-grade lymphomas from lymphomas of lower grades (n = 32),[235] but final outcome was independent of MET uptake. In detection of PCNSLC-MET PET showed equal sensitivity to FDG PET (100%) (n = 13). However, the uptake of MET in PCNSL was significantly lower than that of FDG (4.27 ± 1.91 vs 13.94 ± 5.65; $P<.002$).[202] Although preliminary, these results could not prove the hypothesized superiority of MET PET compared with FDG PET in PCNSL. More recently, Kawai and colleagues[236] reported that visual analysis of both FDG and C-MET uptake in atypical PCNSLs was not useful for delineation of the lesions in the brain. FDG and MET uptake values (SUVmax) and quantitative FDG influx rate constant (Ki) are significantly lower in atypical PCNSL compared with those in typical PCNSL. These corresponding MR findings were also not useful for differentiating PCNSL from other tumors. However, the kinetic analysis (k3) in atypical PCNSL provided valuable information in the diagnosis of PCNSL.

Despite the convenient radiotracer synthesis of C-MET, the generation of considerable nonprotein metabolites rendered quantification of protein synthesis difficult.[203–205] In addition, the limitations associated with short $T_{1/2}$ of ^{11}C have stimulated efforts to develop ^{18}F-labeled amino acids. An nonmetabolizable analogue of tyrosine, O-(2-^{18}F-fluoroethyl)-L-tyrosine (^{18}F-FET),[204] and, ^{18}F-labeled another amino acid 1-amino-3-fluoro-cyclobutane carboxylic acid (^{18}F-FACBC), were synthesized.[237] Based on the preliminary data, ^{18}F-FET may complement FDG PET by providing an additional tool in selected patients to differentiate tumor from inflammatory process.[238,239] Recently, a novel PET tracer targeting intermediary tumor metabolism, 4-[^{18}F]fluoroglutamic acid (TIM-1), has been introduced with favorable preclinical data.[240] In patients with breast cancer and melanoma, tumors can be visualized with TIM-1. A rapid renal clearance and little background from healthy tissues were observed. TIM-1 uptake was observed in 71% of the lesions identified by FDG. However, these data are not complete and require further elucidation to establish the role of imaging amino acid transport/metabolism in cancer.

SUMMARY

Amino acids may have a potential role in the characterization of the biologic properties of lymphomas by determining increased amino acid transport and/or protein synthesis. In brain tumors, the use of radiolabeled amino acids is established but the scarcity of clinical data in extracranial tumors does not allow a definitive description of the role of PET imaging of amino acid metabolism. It may be beneficial that amino acid imaging is less influenced by inflammation than is FDG PET; however, tumor specificity of C-MET is not highly promising. Its potential for evaluation of response and patient outcome remain to be established. Prognostic information cannot be deduced from the existing MET PET data. Although the advantages compared with FDG imaging are suggested in the management of PCNSLs, its superiority compared with FDG PET could not be proved despite better contrast ratios. The role of amino acids for monitoring the treatment response of tumors as well as the differentiation between inflammation and tumor tissue has to be established with further studies.

RADIOLABELED THERAPEUTIC DRUGS

The preclinical and clinical studies using radiolabeled therapeutic drugs with PET tracers are in the early stages of development but have been gradually gaining importance to prove a clinical role for patient management. These small molecules will allow direct determination of drug concentration at its target to predict efficacy and also monitoring of the effectiveness of these agents, particularly for phase II studies. These developments, if proved successful, will lead to a true individualization of anticancer treatment.

SUMMARY

This article discusses possible roles for emerging novel PET radiotracers for diagnosis and during the follow-up period in patients with lymphomas. In a more clinically oriented approach, evaluation of tumor response at the level of biomolecular therapeutic targets would be a priority to select the proper therapy option for therapeutically relevant phenotypes. Building on the foundation of FDG PET, novel imaging probes are being developed to fulfill the need of a more specific radiopharmaceutical to target subcomponents of tumor microenvironment to individualize management approaches. Noninvasive molecular imaging probes other than FDG are being developed to revolutionize characterization of tumor biology and response to therapy in more specific ways for the host, tumor microenvironment, and therapeutic regimens. Although further refinement of preclinical and clinical data is warranted, the new clinical PET probes seem promising in fostering clinical gains that would lead to better survival outcomes.

REFERENCES

1. Yamada S, Kubota K, Kubota R, et al. High accumulation in fluorine-18-fluordeoxyglucose in turpentine-induced inflammatory tissue. J Nucl Med 1995;36:1301–6.

2. Strauss LG. Fluorine-18 deoxyglucose and false-positive results: a major problem in the diagnostics of oncological patients. Eur J Nucl Med 1996;23:1409–15.

3. Stumpe KD, Dazzi H, Schaffner A, et al. Infection imaging using whole-body FDG-PET. Eur J Nucl Med 2000;27:822–32.

4. Familiari D, Glaudemans AW, Vitale V, et al. Can sequential 18F-FDG PET/CT replace WBC imaging in the diabetic foot? J Nucl Med 2011;52:1012–9.

5. Hanahan D, Weinberg RA. Hallmarks of cancer: the next generation. Cell 2011;144:646–74.

6. Lemmon MA, Schlessinger J. Cell signaling by receptor tyrosine kinases. Cell 2010;25(141):1117–34.

7. Hynes NE, MacDonald G. ErbB receptors and signaling pathways in cancer. Curr Opin Cell Biol 2009;21:177–84.

8. Shields AF, Grierson JR, Dohmen BM, et al. Imaging proliferation in vivo with F-18-FLT and positron emission tomography. Nat Med 1998;4:1334–6.

9. Bading JR, Shields AF. Imaging of cell proliferation: status and prospects. J Nucl Med 2008;49(Suppl 2):64S–80S.

10. Shields AF. PET imaging with 18F-FLT and thymidine analogs: promise and pitfalls. J Nucl Med 2003;44:1432–4.

11. Alshenawy HA. Prognostic significance of vascular endothelial growth factor, basic fibroblastic growth factor, and microvessel density and their relation to cell proliferation in B-cell non-Hodgkin's lymphoma. Ann Diagn Pathol 2010;14:321–7.

12. Salles G, de Jong D, Xie W, et al. Prognostic significance of immunohistochemical biomarkers in diffuse large B-cell lymphoma: a study from the Lunenburg Lymphoma Biomarker Consortium. Blood 2011;117:7070–8.

13. Gaudio F, Giordano A, Perrone T, et al. High Ki67 index and bulky disease remain significant adverse prognostic factors in patients with diffuse large B cell lymphoma before and after the introduction of rituximab. Acta Haematol 2011;126:44–51.

14. Galbán CJ, Bhojani MS, Lee KC, et al. Evaluation of treatment-associated inflammatory response on diffusion-weighted magnetic resonance imaging and 2-[18F]-fluoro-2-deoxy-D-glucose-positron emission tomography imaging biomarkers. Clin Cancer Res 2010;16:1542–52.

15. Spaepen K, Stroobants S, Dupont P, et al. [(18)F]FDG PET monitoring of tumour response to chemotherapy: does [(18)F]FDG uptake correlate with the viable tumour cell fraction? Eur J Nucl Med Mol Imaging 2003;30:682–8.

16. Hoffmann M, Kletter K, Becherer A, et al. 18F-fluorodeoxyglucose positron emission tomography (18F-FDG–PET) for staging and follow-up of marginal zone B-cell lymphoma. Oncology 2003;64:336–40.

17. Elstrom R, Guan L, Baker G, et al. Utility of FDG–PET scanning in lymphoma by WHO classification. Blood 2003;101:3875–6.

18. Gill S, Wolf M, Prince HM, et al. [18F]fluorodeoxyglucose positron emission tomography scanning for staging, response assessment, and disease surveillance in patients with mantle cell lymphoma. Clin Lymphoma Myeloma 2008;8:159–65.

19. Rasey JS, Grierson JR, Wiens LW, et al. Validation of FLT uptake as a measure of thymidine kinase-1 activity in A549 carcinoma cells. J Nucl Med 2002;43:1210–7.

20. Sherley JL, Kelly TJ. Regulation of human thymidine kinase during the cell cycle. J Biol Chem 1988;263:8350–8.

21. Grierson JR, Schwartz JL, Muzi M, et al. Metabolism of 3'-deoxy-3'-[F-18]fluorothymidine in proliferating A549 cells: validations for positron emission tomography. Nucl Med Biol 2004;31:829–37.

22. Salskov A, Tammisetti VS, Grierson J, et al. FLT: measuring tumor cell proliferation in vivo with positron emission tomography and 3-deoxy-3-[18F]fluorothymidine. Semin Nucl Med 2007;37:429–39.

23. Sun H, Sloan A, Mangner T, et al. Imaging DNA synthesis in vivo with [F-18]FMAU and positron emission tomography in patients with cancer. Eur J Nucl Med Mol Imaging 2005;32:15–22.

24. Collins JM, Klecker RW, Katki AG. Suicide prodrugs activated by thymidylate synthase: rationale for treatment and noninvasive imaging of tumors with deoxyuridine analogues. Clin Cancer Res 1999;5:1976–81.

25. Buchmann I, Neumaier B, Schreckenberger M, et al. [18F]3'-deoxy-3'-fluorothymidine-PET in NHL patients: whole-body biodistribution and imaging of lymphoma manifestations–a pilot study. Cancer Biother Radiopharm 2004;19:436–42.

26. Shields AF, Lawhorn-Crews JM, Briston DA, et al. Analysis and reproducibility of 3'-deoxy-3'-[18F]fluorothymidine positron emission tomography imaging in patients with non-small cell lung cancer. Clin Cancer Res 2008;14:4463–8.

27. de Langen AJ, Klabbers B, Lubberink M, et al. Reproducibility of quantitative 18F-3'-deoxy-3'-fluorothymidine measurements using positron emission tomography. Eur J Nucl Med Mol Imaging 2009;36:389–95.

28. Hatt M, Cheze-Le Rest C, Aboagye EO, et al. Reproducibility of 18F-FDG and 3'-deoxy-3'-18F-

fluorothymidine PET tumor volume measurements. J Nucl Med 2010;51:1368–76.

29. Moroz MA, Kochetkov T, Cai S, et al. Imaging colon cancer response following treatment with AZD1152: a preclinical analysis of [18F]fluoro-2-deoxyglucose and 3'-deoxy-3'-[18F]fluorothymidine imaging. Clin Cancer Res 2011;17:1099–110.

30. Dittmann H, Dohmen BM, Kehlbach R, et al. Early changes in [18F]FLT uptake after chemotherapy: an experimental study. Eur J Nucl Med Mol Imaging 2002;29:1462–9.

31. Viertl D, Bischof Delaloye A, Lanz B, et al. Increase of FLT tumor uptake in vivo mediated by FdUrd: toward improving cell proliferation positron emission tomography. Mol Imaging Biol 2011; 13:321–31.

32. Kenny LM, Contractor KB, Stebbing J, et al. Altered tissue 3'-deoxy-3'-[18F]fluorothymidine pharmacokinetics in human breast cancer following capecitabine treatment detected by positron emission tomography. Clin Cancer Res 2009;15:6649–57.

33. Menda Y, Boles Ponto LL, Dornfeld KJ, et al. Kinetic analysis of 3'-deoxy-3'-(18)F-fluorothymidine ((18)F-FLT) in head and neck cancer patients before and early after initiation of chemoradiation therapy. J Nucl Med 2009;50:1028–35.

34. Francis DL, Visvikis D, Costa DC, et al. Potential impact of [18F]-3-fluoro-3-deoxy-thymidine versus [18F]-fluoro-2-deoxy-D-glucose in positron emission tomography for colorectal cancer. Eur J Nucl Med Mol Imaging 2003;30:988–94.

35. Yamamoto Y, Nishiyama Y, Ishikawa S, et al. Correlation of 18F-FLT and 18F-FDG uptake on PET with Ki-67 immunohistochemistry in non-small cell lung cancer. Eur J Nucl Med Mol Imaging 2007;34: 1610–6.

36. Yap CS, Czernin J, Fishbein MC, et al. Evaluation of thoracic tumors with 18F-fluorothymidine and 18F-fluorodeoxyglucose-positron emission tomography. Chest 2006;129:393–401.

37. Cobben DC, van der Laan BF, Maas B. 18F-FLT PET for visualization of laryngeal cancer: comparison with 18F-FDG PET. J Nucl Med 2004;45:226–31.

38. Yang W, Zhang Y, Fu Z, et al. Imaging of proliferation with 18F-FLT PET/CT versus 18F-FDG PET/CT in non-small-cell lung cancer. Eur J Nucl Med Mol Imaging 2010;37:1291–9.

39. Buck AK, Hetzel M, Schirrmeister H, et al. Clinical relevance of imaging proliferative activity in lung nodules. Eur J Nucl Med Mol Imaging 2005;32: 525–33.

40. Herrmann K, Eckel F, Schmidt S, et al. In vivo characterization of proliferation for discriminating cancer from pancreatic pseudotumors. J Nucl Med 2008;49:1437–44.

41. Yamamoto Y, Kameyama R, Izuishi K, et al. Detection of colorectal cancer using 18F-FLT PET: comparison with 18F-FDG PET. Nucl Med Commun 2009;30:841–5.

42. Hoshikawa H, Nishiyama Y, Kishino T, et al. Comparison of FLT-PET and FDG-PET for visualization of head and neck squamous cell cancers. Mol Imaging Biol 2011;13:172–7.

43. Troost EG, Bussink J, Slootweg PJ, et al. Histopathologic validation of 3'-deoxy-3'-18F-fluorothymidine PET in squamous cell carcinoma of the oral cavity. J Nucl Med 2010;51:713–9.

44. Linecker A, Kermer C, Sulzbacher I, et al. Uptake of (18)F-FLT and (18)F-FDG in primary head and neck cancer correlates with survival. Nuklearmedizin 2008;47:80–5.

45. Been LB, Hoekstra HJ, Suurmeijer AJ, et al. [18F]FLT-PET and [18F]FDG-PET in the evaluation of radiotherapy for laryngeal cancer. Oral Oncol 2009;45:211–5.

46. Smyczek-Gargya B, Fersis N, Dittmann H, et al. PET with [18F]fluorothymidine for imaging of primary breast cancer: a pilot study. Eur J Nucl Med Mol Imaging 2004;31:720–4.

47. Been LB, Elsinga PH, de Vries J, et al. Positron emission tomography in patients with breast cancer using 18F-3'-deoxy-3'-fluoro-L-thymidine (18F-FLT): a pilot study. Eur J Surg Oncol 2006; 32:39–43.

48. Buck AK, Bommer M, Stilgenbauer S, et al. Molecular imaging of proliferation in malignant lymphoma. Cancer Res 2006;66:11055–61.

49. Lee TS, Ahn SH, Moon BS, et al. Comparison of 18F-FDG, 18F-FET and FLT for differentiation between tumor and inflammation in rats. Nucl Med Biol 2009;36:681–6.

50. van Waarde A, Cobben DC, Suurmeijer AJ, et al. Selectivity of 18F-FLT and FDG for differentiating tumor from inflammation in a rodent model. J Nucl Med 2004;45:695–700.

51. Yue J, Chen L, Cabrera AR, et al. Measuring tumor cell proliferation with 18F-FLT PET during radiotherapy of esophageal squamous cell carcinoma: a pilot clinical study. J Nucl Med 2010;514:528–34.

52. Nakagawa Y, Yamada M, Suzuki Y. 18F-FDG uptake in reactive neck lymph nodes of oral cancer: relationship to lymphoid follicles. J Nucl Med 2008; 49:1053–9.

53. Troost EG, Vogel WV, Merkx MA, et al. 18F-FLT PET does not discriminate between reactive and metastatic lymph nodes in primary head and neck cancer patients. J Nucl Med 2007;48:726–35.

54. Vesselle H, Grierson J, Muzi M, et al. In vivo validation of 3'deoxy-3'-[(18)F] fluorothymidine ([(18)F]FLT) as a proliferation imaging tracer in humans: correlation of [(18)F]FLT uptake by positron emission tomography with Ki-67 immunohistochemistry and flow cytometry in human lung tumours. Clin Cancer Res 2002;8:3315–23.

55. Kenny L, Coombes RC, Vigushin DM, et al. Imaging early changes in proliferation at 1 week post chemotherapy: a pilot study in breast cancer patients with 3′-deoxy-3′-[(18)F]fluorothymidine positron emission tomography. Eur J Nucl Med Mol Imaging 2007;34:1339–47.

56. Wagner M, Seitz U, Buck A, et al. 3′-[18F]fluoro-3′-deoxythymidine ([18F]-FLT) as positron emission tomography tracer for imaging proliferation in a murine B-cell lymphoma model and in the human disease. Cancer Res 2003;63:2681–7.

57. Kenny LM, Vigushin DM, Al-Nahhas A, et al. Quantification of cellular proliferation in tumor and normal tissues of patients with breast cancer by [18F] fluorothymidine-positron emission tomography imaging: evaluation of analytical methods. Cancer Res 2005;65:10104–12.

58. Lee WC, Chang CH, Ho CL, et al. Early detection of tumor response by FLT/microPET imaging in a C26 murine colon carcinoma solid tumor animal model. J Biomed Biotechnol 2011;2011: 535902.

59. Cullinane C, Dorow DS, Jackson S, et al. Differential 18F-FDG and 3′-deoxy-3′-18F-fluorothymidine PET responses to pharmacologic inhibition of the c-MET receptor in preclinical tumor models. J Nucl Med 2011;52:1261–7.

60. Barthel H, Cleij MC, Collingridge DR, et al. 3-Deoxy-3-18F-fluorothymidine as a new marker for monitoring tumour response to antiproliferative therapy in vivo with positron emission tomography. Cancer Res 2003;63:3791–8.

61. Oyama N, Hasegawa Y, Kiyono Y, et al. Early response assessment in prostate carcinoma by 18F-fluorothymidine following anticancer therapy with docetaxel using preclinical tumour models. Eur J Nucl Med Mol Imaging 2011;38:81–9.

62. Aide N, Kinross K, Cullinane C, et al. 18F-FLT PET as a surrogate marker of drug efficacy during mTOR inhibition by everolimus in a preclinical cisplatin-resistant ovarian tumor model. J Nucl Med 2010;51:1559–64.

63. Shah C, Miller TW, Wyatt SK, et al. Imaging biomarkers predict response to anti-HER2 (ErbB2) therapy in preclinical models of breast cancer. Clin Cancer Res 2009;15:4712–21.

64. Ott K, Herrmann K, Schuster T, et al. Molecular imaging of proliferation and glucose utilization: utility for monitoring response and prognosis after neoadjuvant therapy in locally advanced gastric cancer. Ann Surg Oncol 2011;18(12):3316–23.

65. Pfannenberg C, Aschoff P, Dittmann H, et al. PET/CT with 18F-FLT: does it improve the therapeutic management of metastatic germ cell tumors? J Nucl Med 2010;51:845–53.

66. Nygren P, Glimelius B. The Swedish Council on Technology Assessment in Health Care (SBU) report on cancer chemotherapy–project objectives, the working process, key definitions and general aspects on cancer trial methodology and interpretation. Acta Oncol 2001;40:155–65.

67. Waldherr C, Mellinghoff IK, Tran C, et al. Monitoring antiproliferative responses to kinase inhibitor therapy in mice with 3′-deoxy-3′-18F-fluorothymidine PET. J Nucl Med 2005;46:114–20.

68. Fuereder T, Wanek T, Pflegerl P, et al. Gastric cancer growth control by BEZ235 in vivo does not correlate with PI3K/mTOR target inhibition but with [18F]FLT uptake. Clin Cancer Res 2011;17: 5322–32.

69. Chen W, Delaloye S, Silverman DH, et al. Predicting treatment response of malignant gliomas to bevacizumab and irinotecan by imaging proliferation with [18F] fluorothymidine positron emission tomography: a pilot study. J Clin Oncol 2007;25:4714–21.

70. Yang M, Gao H, Yan Y, et al. PET imaging of early response to the tyrosine kinase inhibitor ZD4190. Eur J Nucl Med Mol Imaging 2011;38:1237–47.

71. Takeuchi S, Zhao S, Kuge Y, et al. 18F-Fluorothymidine PET/CT as an early predictor of tumor response to treatment with cetuximab in human lung cancer xenografts. Oncol Rep 2011;26: 725–30.

72. Atkinson DM, Clarke MJ, Mladek AC, et al. Using fluorodeoxythymidine to monitor anti-EGFR inhibitor therapy in squamous cell carcinoma xenografts. Head Neck 2008;30:790–9.

73. Ullrich RT, Zander T, Neumaier B, et al. Early detection of erlotinib treatment response in NSCLC by 3′-deoxy-3′-[F]-fluoro-L-thymidine ([F]FLT) positron emission tomography (PET). PLoS One 2008; 3:e3908.

74. Zander T, Scheffler M, Nogova L, et al. Early prediction of nonprogression in advanced non-small-cell lung cancer treated with erlotinib by using [(18)F]fluorodeoxyglucose and [(18)F] fluorothymidine positron emission tomography. J Clin Oncol 2011;29:1701–8.

75. Mileshkin L, Hicks RJ, Hughes BG, et al. Changes in 18F-fluorodeoxyglucose and 18F-fluorodeoxythymidine positron emission tomography imaging in patients with non-small cell lung cancer treated with erlotinib. Clin Cancer Res 2011;17:3304–15.

76. Sohn HJ, Yang YJ, Ryu JS, et al. [18F]Fluorothymidine positron emission tomography before and 7 days after gefitinib treatment predicts response in patients with advanced adenocarcinoma of the lung. Clin Cancer Res 2008;14:7423–9.

77. Witzig TE, Reeder CB, LaPlant BR, et al. A phase II trial of the oral mTOR inhibitor everolimus in relapsed aggressive lymphoma. Leukemia 2011; 25:341–7.

78. Johnston PB, Inwards DJ, Colgan JP, et al. A phase II trial of the oral mTOR inhibitor everolimus in

relapsed Hodgkin lymphoma. Am J Hematol 2010; 85(5):320–4.

79. Sugiyama M, Sakahara H, Sato K, et al. Evaluation of 3-deoxy-3-^{18}F-fluorothymidine for monitoring of tumour response to radiotherapy and photodynamic therapy in mice. J Nucl Med 2004;45: 1754–8.

80. Yang YJ, Ryu JS, Kim SY, et al. Use of 3'-deoxy-3'-[^{18}F]fluorothymidine PET to monitor early responses to radiation therapy in murine SCCVII tumors. Eur J Nucl Med Mol Imaging 2006;33:412–9.

81. Everitt S, Hicks RJ, Ball D, et al. Imaging cellular proliferation during chemo-radiotherapy: a pilot study of serial 18F-FLT positron emission tomography/computed tomography imaging for non-small-cell lung cancer. Int J Radiat Oncol Biol Phys 2009;75:1098–104.

82. Menda Y, Ponto LL, Dornfeld KJ, et al. Investigation of the pharmacokinetics of 3'-deoxy-3'-[^{18}F]fluorothymidine uptake in the bone marrow before and early after initiation of chemoradiation therapy in head and neck cancer. Nucl Med Biol 2010;37(4): 433–8.

83. Wieder HA, Geinitz H, Rosenberg R, et al. PET imaging with [18F]3'-deoxy-3'-fluorothymidine for prediction of response to neoadjuvant treatment in patients with rectal cancer. Eur J Nucl Med Mol Imaging 2007;34:878–83.

84. Herrmann K, Wieder HA, Buck AK, et al. Early response assessment using 3'-deoxy-3'-[18F]fluorothymidine-positron emission tomography in high-grade non-Hodgkin's lymphoma. Clin Cancer Res 2007;13:3552–8.

85. Herrmann K, Buck AK, Schuster T, et al. Predictive value of initial 18F-FLT uptake in patients with aggressive non-Hodgkin lymphoma receiving R-CHOP treatment. J Nucl Med 2011;52:690–6.

86. Buck AK, Kratochwil C, Glatting G, et al. Early assessment of therapy response in malignant lymphoma with the thymidine analogue [18F]FLT. Eur J Nucl Med Mol Imaging 2007;34:1775–82.

87. Brepoels L, Stroobants S, Verhoef G, et al. (18)F-FDG and (18)F-FLT uptake early after cyclophosphamide and mTOR inhibition in an experimental lymphoma model. J Nucl Med 2009;50: 1102–9.

88. Graf N, Herrmann K, den Hollander J, et al. Imaging proliferation to monitor early response of lymphoma to cytotoxic treatment. Mol Imaging Biol 2008;10:349–55.

89. Chao KS. 3'-Deoxy-3'-(18)F-fluorothymidine (FLT) positron emission tomography for early prediction of response to chemoradiotherapy–a clinical application model of esophageal cancer. Semin Oncol 2007;34(2 Suppl 1):S31–6.

90. Kasper B, Egerer G, Gronkowski M, et al. Functional diagnosis of residual lymphomas after radiochemotherapy with positron emission tomography comparing FDG- and FLT-PET. Leuk Lymphoma 2007;48:746–53.

91. Vanderhoek M, Juckett MB, Perlman SB, et al. Early assessment of treatment response in patients with AML using [(18)F]FLT PET imaging. Leuk Res 2011;35:310–6.

92. Rajendran JG, Krohn KA. Imaging hypoxia and angiogenesis in tumors. Radiol Clin North Am 2005;43:169–87.

93. Graeber TG, Osmanian C, Jacks T, et al. Hypoxia-mediated selection of cells with diminished apoptotic potential in solid tumours. Nature 1996; 379:88–91.

94. Hockel M, Schlenger K, Aral B, et al. Association between tumor hypoxia and malignant progression in advanced cancer of the uterine cervix. Cancer Res 1996;56:4509–15.

95. Wang R, Zhou S, Li S. Cancer therapeutic agents targeting hypoxia-inducible factor-1. Curr Med Chem 2011;18:3168–89.

96. Ford EC, Kinahan PE, Hanlon L, et al. Tumor delineation using PET in head and neck cancers: threshold contouring and lesion volumes. Med Phys 2006;33(11):4280–8.

97. Hoppe R. Radiotherapy planning for the lymphomas: expanding roles for biologic imaging. Front Radiat Ther Oncol 2011;43:331–43.

98. Evens AM, Schumacker PT, Helenowski IB, et al. Hypoxia inducible factor-alpha activation in lymphoma and relationship to the thioredoxin family. Br J Haematol 2008;141:676–80.

99. Hasenclever D, Diehl V, for the International Prognostic Factors Project on Advanced Hodgkin's Disease. A prognostic score for advanced Hodgkin's disease. N Engl J Med 1998;339:1506–14.

100. Shipp MA. Prognostic factors in aggressive non-Hodgkin's lymphoma: who has "high-risk" disease? Blood 1994;83:1165–73.

101. Padhani AR, Krohn KA, Lewis JS, et al. Imaging oxygenation of human tumors. Eur Radiol 2007; 17:861–72.

102. Jones DP. Radical-free biology of oxidative stress. Am J Physiol Cell Physiol 2008;295:C849–68.

103. Varghese AJ, Whitmore GF. Binding to cellular macromolecules as a possible mechanism for the cytotoxicity of misonidazole. Cancer Res 1980;40: 2165–9.

104. Koh WJ, Rasey JS, Evans ML, et al. Imaging of hypoxia in human tumors with [F-18]fluoromisonidazole. Int J Radiat Oncol Biol Phys 1992;22: 199–212.

105. Rajendran JG, Wilson DC, Conrad EU, et al. [18F]FMISO and [18F]FDG PET imaging in soft tissue sarcomas: correlation of hypoxia, metabolism and VEGF expression. Eur J Nucl Med Mol Imaging 2003;30:695–704.

106. Rasey JS, Koh WJ, Evans ML, et al. Quantifying regional hypoxia in human tumors with positron emission tomography of [18F] fluoromisonidazole: a pretherapy study of 37 patients. Int J Radiat Oncol Biol Phys 1996;36:417–28.

107. Lewis JS, McCarthy DW, McCarthy TJ, et al. Evaluation of Cu-64-ATSM in vitro and in vivo in a hypoxic model. J Nucl Med 1999;40:177–83.

108. Piert M, Machulla HJ, Picchio M, et al. Hypoxia-specific tumor imaging with 18F-fluoroazomycin arabinoside. J Nucl Med 2005;46:106–13.

109. Postema EJ, McEwan AJ, Riauka TA, et al. Initial results of hypoxia imaging using 1-alpha-D: -(5-deoxy-5-[18F]-fluoroarabinofuranosyl)-2-nitroimidazole (18FFAZA). Eur J Nucl Med Mol Imaging 2009;36:1565–73.

110. Cherk MH, Foo SS, Poon AM, et al. Lack of correlation of hypoxic cell fraction and angiogenesis with glucose metabolic rate in non–small cell lung cancer assessed by 18F-fluoromisonidazole and 18F-FDG PET. J Nucl Med 2006;47: 1921–6.

111. Spence AM, Muzi M, Swanson KR, et al. Regional hypoxia in glioblastoma multiforme quantified with [18F]fluoromisonidazole positron emission tomography before radiotherapy: correlation with time to progression and survival. Clin Cancer Res 2008; 14:2623–30.

112. Hoogsteen J, Marres HA, van der Kogel AJ, et al. The hypoxic tumour microenvironment, patient selection and hypoxia-modifying treatments. Clin Oncol 2007;19:385–96.

113. Hendrickson K, Phillips M, Smith W, et al. Hypoxia imaging with [F-18] FMISO-PET in head and neck cancer: potential for guiding intensity modulated radiation therapy in overcoming hypoxia-induced treatment resistance. Radiother Oncol 2011; 101(3):369–75.

114. Graham MM, Peterson LM, Link JM, et al. Fluorine-18-fluoromisonidazole radiation dosimetry in imaging studies. J Nucl Med 1997;38:1631–6.

115. Rajendran JG, Schwartz DL, O'Sullivan J, et al. Tumor hypoxia imaging with [F-18]fluoromisonidazole positron emission tomography in head and neck cancer. Clin Cancer Res 2006;12:5435–41.

116. Rajendran JG, Mankoff DA, O'Sullivan F, et al. Hypoxia and glucose metabolism in malignant tumors: evaluation by [18F]fluoromisonidazole and [18F]fluorodeoxyglucose positron emission tomography imaging. Clin Cancer Res 2004;10: 2245–52.

117. Hall EJ, Giaccia AJ. Radiobiology for the radiologist. 6th edition. Philadelphia: Lippincott Williams & Wilkins; 2006.

118. Liu RS, Chu LS, Yen SH, et al. Detection of anaerobic odontogenic infections by fluorine-18 fluoromisonidazole. Eur J Nucl Med 1996;23:1384–7.

119. Rischin D, Hicks RJ, Fisher R, et al. Prognostic significance of [18F]misonidazole positron emission tomography-detected tumor hypoxia in patients with advanced head and neck cancer randomly assigned to chemoradiation with or without tirapazamine: a substudy of Trans-Tasman Radiation Oncology Group Study 98.02. J Clin Oncol 2006;24:2098–104.

120. Eschmann SM, Paulsen F, Bedeshem C, et al. Hypoxia-imaging with (18)F-misonidazole and PET: changes of kinetics during radiotherapy of head-and-neck cancer. Radiother Oncol 2007;83: 406–10.

121. Hicks RJ, Rischin D, Fisher R, et al. Utility of FMISO PET in advanced head and neck cancer treated with chemoradiation incorporating a hypoxia-targeting chemotherapy agent. Eur J Nucl Med Mol Imaging 2005;32:1384–91.

122. Lee NY, Mechalakos JG, Nehmeh S, et al. Fluorine-18-labeled fluoromisonidazole positron emission and computed tomography-guided intensity-modulated radiotherapy for head and neck cancer: a feasibility study. Int J Radiat Oncol Biol Phys 2008;70:2–13.

123. Lee N, Nehmeh S, Schöder H, et al. Prospective trial incorporating pre-/mid-treatment [(18)F]-misonidazole positron emission tomography for head-and-neck cancer patients undergoing concurrent chemoradiotherapy. Int J Radiat Oncol Biol Phys 2009;75:101.

124. Rajendran JG, Hendrickson KR, Spence AM, et al. Hypoxia imaging-directed radiation treatment planning. Eur J Nucl Med Mol Imaging 2006;33(Suppl 1): 44–53.

125. Yuan H, Schroeder T, Bowsher JE, et al. Intertumoral differences in hypoxia selectivity of the PET imaging agent 64Cu(II)-diacetyl-bis(N4-methylthio-semicarbazone). J Nucl Med 2006;47:989–98.

126. Ling CC, Humm J, Larson S, et al. Towards multidimensional radiotherapy (MD-CRT): biological imaging and biological conformality. Int J Radiat Oncol Biol Phys 2000;47:551–60.

127. Chao KS, Bosch WR, Mutic S, et al. A novel approach to overcome hypoxic tumor resistance: Cu-ATSM-guided intensity-modulated radiation therapy. Int J Radiat Oncol Biol Phys 2001;49: 1171–82.

128. Dehdashti F, Grigsby PW, Lewis JS, et al. Assessing tumor hypoxia in cervical cancer by positron emission tomography with 60Cu-ATSM. J Nucl Med 2008;49:201–5.

129. Dietz DW, Dehdashti FD, Grigsby PW, et al. Tumor hypoxia detected by positron emission tomography with 60Cu-ATSM as a predictor of response and survival in patients undergoing neoadjuvant chemoradiotherapy for rectal carcinoma: a pilot study. Dis Colon Rectum 2008;51:1641–8.

130. Gullino PM. Angiogenesis and neoplasia. N Engl J Med 1981;305:884–5.

131. Koukourakis MI, Giatromanolaki A, Sivridis E, et al. Cancer vascularization: implications in radiotherapy? Int J Radiat Oncol Biol Phys 2000;48: 545–53.

132. Folkman J. Tumor angiogenesis: therapeutic implications. N Engl J Med 1971;285:1182–6.

133. Zhao Y, Bao Q, Renner A, et al. Cancer stem cells and angiogenesis. Int J Dev Biol 2011;55:477–82.

134. Hynes RO. Integrins: bidirectional, allosteric signaling machines. Cell 2002;110:673–87.

135. McDonald DM, Teicher BA, Stetler-Stevenson W, et al. Report from the Society for Biological Therapy and Vascular Biology Faculty of the NCI Workshop on Angiogenesis Monitoring. J Immunother 2004; 27:161–75.

136. Costouros NG, Diehn FE, Libutti SK, et al. Molecular imaging of tumor angiogenesis. J Cell Biochem Suppl 2002;39:72–8.

137. Jain RK, Safabakhsh N, Sckell A, et al. Endothelial cell death, angiogenesis, and microvascular function after castration in an androgen-dependent tumor: role of vascular endothelial growth factor. Proc Natl Acad Sci U S A 1998;95:10820–5.

138. Sipkins DA, Cheresh DA, Kazemi MR, et al. Detection of tumor angiogenesis in vivo by alphaVbeta3-targeted magnetic resonance imaging. Nat Med 1998;4:623–6.

139. Leong-Poi H, Christiansen JP, Klibanov AL, et al. Noninvasive assessment of angiogenesis by contrast ultrasound imaging with microbubbles targeted to alpha-V integrins. J Am Coll Cardiol 2003; 41:430–1.

140. Haubner R, Wester HJ, Weber WA, et al. Noninvasive imaging of alpha(v)beta3 integrin expression using 18F-labeled RGD-containing glycopeptide and positron emission tomography. Cancer Res 2001;61:1781–5.

141. Haubner R, Beer AJ, Wang H, et al. Positron emission tomography tracers for imaging angiogenesis. Eur J Nucl Med Mol Imaging 2010;37(Suppl 1): S86–103.

142. Levashova Z, Backer M, Backer JM, et al. Direct site-specific labeling of the Cys-tag moiety in scVEGF with technetium 99m. Bioconjug Chem 2008;19:1049–54.

143. Rossin R, Berndorff D, Friebe M, et al. Small-animal PET of tumor angiogenesis using a (76)Br-labeled human recombinant antibody fragment to the ED-B domain of fibronectin. J Nucl Med 2007;48: 1172–9.

144. Zheng QH, Fei X, Liu X, et al. Comparative studies of potential cancer biomarkers carbon-11 labeled MMP inhibitors (S)-2-(4'-[11C]methoxybiphenyl-4-sulfonylamino)-3-methylbutyric acid and N-hydroxy-(R)-2-[[(4'-[11C]methoxyphenyl)sulfonyl] benzylamino]-3-methylbutanamide. Nucl Med Biol 2004;31:77–85.

145. Chen X, Park R, Tohme M, et al. MicroPET and autoradiographic imaging of breast cancer alpha v-integrin expression using 18F- and 64Cu-labeled RGD peptide. Bioconjug Chem 2004;15:41–9.

146. Ruan J, Hyjek E, Kermani P, et al. The magnitude of stromal hemangiogenesis correlates with histologic subtype of non-Hodgkin's lymphoma. Clin Cancer Res 2006;12:5622–31.

147. Ganjoo KN, An CS, Robertson MJ, et al. Rituximab, bevacizumab and CHOP (RA-CHOP) in untreated diffuse large B-cell lymphoma: safety, biomarker and pharmacokinetic analysis. Leuk Lymphoma 2006;47:998–1005.

148. Wang ES, Teruya-Feldstein J, Wu Y, et al. Targeting autocrine and paracrine VEGF receptor pathways inhibits human lymphoma xenografts in vivo. Blood 2004;104:2893–902.

149. Jorgensen JM, Sorensen FB, Bendix K, et al. Angiogenesis in non-Hodgkin's lymphoma: clinico-pathological correlations and prognostic significance in specific subtypes. Leuk Lymphoma 2007;48:584–95.

150. Ruan J, Hajjar K, Rafii S, et al. Angiogenesis and antiangiogenic therapy in non-Hodgkin's lymphoma. Ann Oncol 2009;20:413–24.

151. Dave SS, Wright G, Tan B, et al. Prediction of survival in follicular lymphoma based on molecular features of tumor-infiltrating immune cells. N Engl J Med 2004;351:2159–69.

152. Koster A, Van Krieken JH, Mackenzie MA, et al. Increased vascularization predicts favorable outcome in follicular lymphoma. Clin Cancer Res 2005;11:154–61.

153. Shipp MA, Ross KN, Tamayo P, et al. Diffuse large B-cell lymphoma outcome prediction by gene-expression profiling and supervised machine learning. Nat Med 2002;8:68–74.

154. Stopeck AT, Unger J, Rimsza LM, et al. A phase II trial of single agent bevacizumab in patients with relapsed, aggressive non-Hodgkin lymphoma: Southwest Oncology Group study S0108. Leuk Lymphoma 2009;50(5):728–35.

155. Rundhaug JE. Matrix metalloproteinases and angiogenesis. J Cell Mol Med 2005;9:267–85.

156. Beer AJ, Haubner R, Wolf I, et al. PET-based human dosimetry of 18F-galacto-RGD, a new radiotracer for imaging alpha v beta3 expression. J Nucl Med 2006;47:763–9.

157. Beer AJ, Haubner R, Sarbia M, et al. Positron emission tomography using [18F]galacto-RGD identifies the level of integrin alpha(v)beta3 expression in man. Clin Cancer Res 2006;12:3942–9.

158. Beer AJ, Grosu AL, Carlsen J, et al. [18F]Galacto-RGD positron emission tomography for imaging of {alpha}v{beta}3 expression on the neovasculature

in patients with squamous cell carcinoma of the head and neck. Clin Cancer Res 2007;13:6610–6.

159. Haubner R, Wester HJ, Burkhart F, et al. Glycosy-lated RGD-containing peptides: tracer for tumor targeting and angiogenesis imaging with improved biokinetics. J Nucl Med 2001;42:326–36.

160. Schnell O, Krebs B, Carlsen J, et al. Imaging of integrin {alpha}v{beta}3 expression in patients with malignant glioma by [18F] galacto-RGD posi-tron emission tomography. Neuro Oncol 2009;11: 861–70.

161. Wadas TJ, Deng H, Sprague JE, et al. Targeting the alphavbeta3 integrin for small-animal PET/CT of os-teolytic bone metastases. J Nucl Med 2009;50: 1873–80.

162. Zheleznyak A, Wadas TJ, Sherman CD, et al. Integ-rin α (v)β (3) as a PET imaging biomarker for oste-oclast number in mouse models of negative and positive osteoclast regulation. Mol Imaging Biol 2011. [Epub ahead of print].

163. Kenny LM, Coombes RC, Oulie I, et al. Phase I trial of the positron emitting ArgGlyAsp (RGD) peptide radioligand 18 F-AH111585 in breast cancer patients. J Nucl Med 2008;49:879–86.

164. Indrevoll B, Kindberg GM, Solbakken M, et al. NC-100717: a versatile RGD peptide scaffold for angiogenesis imaging. Bioorg Med Chem Lett 2006;16:6190–3.

165. Mena E, Turkbey I, McKinney Y, et al. A novel PET imaging approach for detection of tumor angiogen-esis via the expression of v_3 integrin using an RGD peptide, [18F]fluciclatide (AH111585). J Nucl Med 2010;51(Suppl 2):505.

166. McParland BJ, Miller MP, Spinks TJ, et al. The bio-distribution and radiation dosimetry of the Arg-Gly-Asp peptide ^{18}F-AH111585 in healthy volunteers. J Nucl Med 2008;49:1664–7.

167. Tomasi G, Kenny L, Mauri F, et al. Quantification of receptor-ligand binding with [(18)F]fluciclatide in metastatic breast cancer patients. Eur J Nucl Med Mol Imaging 2011;38(12):2186–97.

168. Dumont RA, Deininger F, Haubner R, et al. Novel (64)Cu- and (68)Ga-labeled RGD conjugates show improved PET imaging of α($ν$)β(3) integrin expression and facile radiosynthesis. J Nucl Med 2011;52:1276–84.

169. Reed J. Dysregulation of apoptosis in cancer. J Clin Oncol 1999;17:2941–53.

170. Nagata S. Apoptosis by death factor. Cell 1997;88: 355–65.

171. Blankenberg FG. In vivo imaging of apoptosis. Cancer Biol Ther 2008;7:1525–32.

172. Hengartner MO. The biochemistry of apoptosis. Nature 2000;407:770–6.

173. Blankenberg FG, Norfray JF. Multimodality molec-ular imaging of apoptosis in oncology. AJR Am J Roentgenol 2011;197:308–17.

174. Lahorte CM, Vanderheyden JL, Steinmetz N, et al. Apoptosis-detecting radioligands: current state of the art and future perspectives. Eur J Nucl Med Mol Imaging 2004;31:887–919.

175. Boersma HH, Kietselaer BL, Stolk LM, et al. Past, present, and future of annexin A5: from protein discovery to clinical applications. J Nucl Med 2005;46:2035–50.

176. Fulda S. Cell death in hematological tumors. Apoptosis 2009;14:409–23.

177. Biroccio A, Candiloro A, Mottolese M, et al. Bcl-2 overexpression and hypoxia synergistically act to modulate vascular endothelial growth factor expression and in vivo angiogenesis in a breast carcinoma cell line. FASEB J 2000;14:652–60.

178. Kang MH, Reynolds CP. Bcl-2 inhibitors: targeting mitochondrial apoptotic pathways in cancer therapy. Clin Cancer Res 2009;15:1126–32.

179. Pro B, Leber B, Smith M, et al. Phase II multicenter study of oblimersen sodium, a Bcl-2antisense oligo-nucleotide, in combination with rituximab in patients with recurrent B-cell non-Hodgkin lymphoma. Br J Haematol 2008;143:355–60.

180. Wang M, Zhou Y, Zhang L, et al. Use of bortezomib in B-cell non-Hodgkin's lymphoma. Expert Rev Anticancer Ther 2006;6:983–91.

181. Goy A, Younes A, McLaughlin P, et al. Phase II study of proteasome inhibitor bortezomib in relapsed or refractory B-cell non-Hodgkin's lymphoma. J Clin Oncol 2005;23:667–75.

182. Ansell SM, Arendt BK, Grote DM, et al. Inhibition of sur-vivin expression suppresses the growth of aggressive non-Hodgkin's lymphoma. Leukemia 2004;18:616–23.

183. Martin SJ, Reutelingsperger CP, McGahon AJ. Early redistribution of plasma membrane phosphatidyl-serine is a general feature of apoptosis regardless of the initiating stimulus: inhibition by overexpres-sion of Bcl-2 and Abl. J Exp Med 1995;182:1545–56.

184. Blankenberg FG, Katsikis PD, Tait JF, et al. Imaging of apoptosis (programmed cell death) with 99mTc annexin V. J Nucl Med 1999;40:184–91.

185. Huerta S, Goulet EJ, Huerta-Yepez S, et al. Screening and detection of apoptosis. J Surg Res 2007;139:143–56.

186. Cohen A, Shirvan A, Levin G, et al. From the Gla domain to a novel small-molecule detector of apoptosis [Erratum appears in Cell Res 2011;21: 1642]. Cell Res 2009;19:625–37.

187. Reshef A, Shirvan A, Akselrod-Ballin A, et al. Small-molecule biomarkers for clinical PET imaging of apoptosis. J Nucl Med 2010;51(6):837–40.

188. Höglund J, Shirvan A, Antoni G, et al. 18F-ML-10, a PET tracer for apoptosis: first human study. J Nucl Med 2011;52:720–5.

189. Belhocine T, Steinmetz N, Hustinx R, et al. Increased uptake of the apoptosis-imaging agent 99mTc recombinant human annexin V in human

tumours after one course of chemotherapy as a predictor of tumour response and patient prognosis. Clin Cancer Res 2002;8:2766–74.

190. Kartachova MS, Valdés Olmos RA, Haas RL, et al. 99mTc-HYNIC-rh-annexin-V scintigraphy: visual and quantitative evaluation of early treatment-induced apoptosis to predict treatment outcome. Nucl Med Commun 2008;29:39–44.

191. Haberkorn U, Kinscherf R, Krammer PH, et al. Investigation of a potential scintigraphic marker of apoptosis: radioiodinated Z-Val-Ala-DL-Asp(O-methyl)-fluoromethyl ketone. Nucl Med Biol 2001; 28:793–8.

192. Collingridge DR, Glaser M, Osman S, et al. In vitro selectivity, in vivo biodistribution and tumour uptake of annexin V radiolabelled with a positron emitting radioisotope. Br J Cancer 2003;89:1327–33.

193. Li X, Link JM, Stekhova S, et al. Site-specific labeling of annexin V with F-18 for apoptosis imaging. Bioconjug Chem 2008;19:1684–8.

194. Bauwens M, De Saint-Hubert M, Devos E, et al. Site-specific 68Ga-labeled annexin A5 as a PET imaging agent for apoptosis. Nucl Med Biol 2011; 38:381–92.

195. Oltmanns D, Zitzmann-Kolbe S, Mueller A, et al. Zn(II)-bis(cyclen) complexes and the imaging of apoptosis/necrosis. Bioconjug Chem 2011;22: 2611–24.

196. Thapa N, Kim S, So IS, et al. Discovery of a phosphatidylserine recognizing peptide and its utility in molecular imaging of tumour apoptosis. J Cell Mol Med 2008;12(5A):1649–60.

197. Wang K, Purushotham S, Lee JY, et al. In vivo imaging of tumor apoptosis using histone H1-targeting peptide. J Control Release 2010;148:283–91.

198. Nguyen QD, Smith G, Glaser M, et al. Positron emission tomography imaging of drug-induced tumor apoptosis with a caspase-3/7 specific [18F]-labeled isatin sulfonamide. Proc Natl Acad Sci U S A 2009;106:16375–80.

199. Smith G, Glaser M, Perumal M, et al. Design, synthesis, and biological characterization of a caspase 3/7 selective isatin labeled with 2-[18F]fluoroethylazide. J Med Chem 2008;51:8057–67.

200. Damianovich M, Ziv I, Heyman SN, et al. ApoSense: a novel technology for functional molecular imaging of cell death in models of acute renal tubular necrosis. Eur J Nucl Med Mol Imaging 2006;33:281–91.

201. Cohen A, Ziv I, Aloya T, et al. Monitoring of chemotherapy-induced cell death in melanoma tumors by N,N'-didansyl-L-cystine. Technol Cancer Res Treat 2007;6:221–33.

202. Kawase Y, Yamamoto Y, Kameyama R, et al. Comparison of (11)C-methionine PET and (18)F-FDG PET in patients with primary central nervous system lymphoma. Mol Imaging Biol 2011;13:1284–9.

203. Inoue T, Tomiyoshi K, Higuichi T, et al. Biodistribution studies on L-3-[fluorine-18]fluoro-alpha-methyl tyrosine: a potential tumor-detecting agent. J Nucl Med 1998;39:663–6.

204. Wester HJ, Herz M, Weber W, et al. Synthesis and radiopharmacology of O-(2- [18F]fluoroethyl)-L-tyrosine for tumor imaging. J Nucl Med 1999;40:205–12.

205. Jager PL, Plaat BE, Vries de EG, et al. Imaging of soft-tissue tumors using L-3-[iodine-123]iodo-alpha-methyl-tyrosine SPECT: comparison with proliferative and mitotic activity, cellularity and vascularity. Clin Cancer Res 2000;6:2252–9.

206. Behin A, Hoang-Xuan K, Caroentier AF, et al. Primary brain tumours in adults. Lancet 2003;361:323–31.

207. Yamamoto Y, Nishiyama Y, Kimura N, et al. 11C-Acetate PET in the evaluation of brain glioma: comparison with 11C-methionine and 18F-FDG-PET. Mol Imaging Biol 2008;10:281–7.

208. Sasaki M, Kuwabara Y, Yoshida T, et al. A comparative study of thallium-201 SPET. Carbon-11 methionine PET and fluorine-18 fluoro-deoxyglucose PET for the differentiation of astrocytic tumours. Eur J Nucl Med 1998;25:1261–9.

209. Kühne A, Kaiser R, Schirmer M, et al. Genetic polymorphisms in the amino acid transporters LAT1 and LAT2 in relation to the pharmacokinetics and side effects of melphalan. Pharmacogenet Genomics 2007;17:505–17.

210. Isselbacher KJ. Sugar and amino acid transport by cells in culture: differences between normal and malignant cells. N Engl J Med 1972;286:929–33.

211. Souba WW. Glutamine and cancer. Ann Surg 1993; 218:715–28.

212. Ishiwata K, Kubota K, Murakami M, et al. Re-evaluation of amino acid PET studies: can the protein synthesis rates in brain and tumor tissues be measured in vivo? J Nucl Med 1993;34:1936–43.

213. Daemen BJ, Elsinga PH, Ishiwata K, et al. A comparative PET study using different 11C-labelled amino acids in Walker 256 carcinosarcoma-bearing rats. Int J Rad Appl Instrum B 1991;18:197–204.

214. Roelcke U, Radu E, Ametamey S, et al. Association of rubidium and C-methionine uptake in brain tumors measured by positron emission tomography. J Neurooncol 1996;27:163–71.

215. Deloar HM, Fujiwara T, Nakamura T, et al. Estimation of internal absorbed dose of L-[methyl-11C] methionine using whole-body positron emission tomography. Eur J Nucl Med 1998;25:629–33.

216. Rau FC, Weber WA, Wester HJ, et al. O-(2-[(18)F] Fluoroethyl)-L-tyrosine (FET): a tracer for differentiation of tumour from inflammation in murine lymph nodes. Eur J Nucl Med Mol Imaging 2002; 29:1039–46.

217. Singhal T, Narayan TK, Jain V, et al. 11C-L-methionine positron emission tomography in the clinical

management of cerebral gliomas. Mol Imaging Biol 2008;10:1–18.

218. Ogawa T, Kanno I, Shishido F, et al. Clinical value of PET with 18F-fluorodoxyglucose and L-methyl-11C-methionine for diagnosis of recurrent brain tumour and radiation injury. Acta Radiol 1991;32:197–202.

219. Kaschten B, Stevenaert A, Sadzot B, et al. Preoperative evaluation of 54 gliomas by PET with fluorine-18-fluorodeoxyglucose and/or carbon-11-methionine. J Nucl Med 1998;39:778–85.

220. De Witte O, Goldberg I, Wikler D, et al. Positron emission tomography with injection of methionine as a prognostic factor in glioma. J Neurosurg 2001;95:746–50.

221. Potzi C, Becherer A, Marosi C, et al. 11C Methionine and 18F fluorodeoxyglucose PET in the follow-up of glioblastoma multiforme. J Neurooncol 2007;84: 305–14.

222. Nuutinen J, Sonninen P, Lehikoinen P, et al. Radiotherapy treatment planning and long-term follow-up with [(11)C]methionine PET in patients with low-grade astrocytoma. Int J Radiat Oncol Biol Phys 2000;48:43–52.

223. Wurker M, Herholz K, Voges J, et al. Glucose consumption and methionine uptake in low grade gliomas after iodine-125 brachytherapy. Eur J Nucl Med 1996;23:583–6.

224. Grosu AL, Weber WA, Astner ST, et al. 11C-methionine PET improves the target volume delineation of meningiomas treated with stereotactic fractionated radiotherapy. Int J Radiat Oncol Biol Phys 2006;66:339–44.

225. Galldiks N, Kracht LW, Burghaus L, et al. Use of 11C-methionine PET to monitor the effects of temozolomide chemotherapy in malignant gliomas. Eur J Nucl Med Mol Imaging 2006;33:516–24.

226. Tang BN, Sadeghi N, Branle F, et al. Semi-quantification of methionine uptake and flair signal for the evaluation of chemotherapy in low-grade oligodendroglioma. J Neurooncol 2005;71:161–8.

227. Herholz K, Kracht LW, Heiss WD. Monitoring the effect of chemotherapy in a mixed glioma by C-11-methionine PET. J Neuroimaging 2003;13: 268–71.

228. Torii K, Tsuyuguchi N, Kawabe J, et al. Correlation of amino-acid uptake using methionine PET and histological classifications in various gliomas. Ann Nucl Med 2005;19:677–83.

229. Jansson T, Westlin JE, Ahlström H, et al. Positron emission tomography studies in patients with locally advanced and/or metastatic breast cancer: a method for early therapy evaluation? J Clin Oncol 1995;13:1470–7.

230. Daemen BJ, Elsinga PH, Paans AM, et al. Radiation-induced inhibition of tumor growth as monitored by PET using L-[1-11C]tyrosine and fluorine-18-fluorodeoxyglucose. J Nucl Med 1992;33:373–9.

231. Terakawa Y, Tsuyuguchi N, Iwai Y, et al. Diagnostic accuracy of 11C-methionine PET for differentiation of recurrent brain tumors from radiation necrosis after radiotherapy. J Nucl Med 2008;49: 694–9.

232. Lee IH, Piert M, Gomez-Hassan D, et al. Association of 11C-methionine PET uptake with site of failure after concurrent temozolomide and radiation for primary glioblastoma multiforme. Int J Radiat Oncol Biol Phys 2009;73:479–85.

233. Lindholm P, Lapela M, Någren K. Preliminary study of carbon-11 methionine PET in the evaluation of early response to therapy in advanced breast cancer. Nucl Med Commun 2009;30:30–6.

234. Miyazawa H, Arai T, Iio M, et al. PET imaging of non-small-cell lung carcinoma with carbon-11-methionine: relationship between radioactivity uptake and flow-cytometric parameters. J Nucl Med 1993;34:1886–91.

235. Nishiyama Y, Yamamoto Y, Monden T, et al. Diagnostic value of kinetic analysis using dynamic FDG PET in immunocompetent patients with primary CNS lymphoma. Eur J Nucl Med Mol Imaging 2007;34:78–86.

236. Kawai N, Okubo S, Miyake K, et al. Use of PET in the diagnosis of primary CNS lymphoma in patients with atypical MR findings. Ann Nucl Med 2010; 24(5):335–43.

237. McConathy J, Voll RJ, Yu W, et al. Improved synthesis of anti-[18F]FACBC: improved preparation of labeling precursor and automated radiosynthesis. Appl Radiat Isot 2003;58:657–66.

238. Pauleit D, Zimmermann A, Stoffels G, et al. 18F-FET PET compared with 18FFDG PET and CT in patients with head and neck cancer. J Nucl Med 2006;47: 256–61.

239. Nye JA, Schuster DM, Yu W, et al. Biodistribution and radiation dosimetry of the synthetic nonmetabolized amino acid analogue anti-18F-FACBC in humans. J Nucl Med 2007;48:1017–20.

240. Krasikova RN, Kuznetsova OF, Fedorova OS, et al. 4-[18F]Fluoroglutamic acid (BAY 85-8050), a new amino acid radiotracer for PET imaging of tumors: synthesis and in vitro characterization. J Med Chem 2011;54:406–10.

241. Cobben DC, Elsinga PH, Suurmeijer AJ, et al. Detection and grading of soft tissue sarcomas of the extremities with (18)F-3'-fluoro-3'-deoxy-L-thymidine. Clin Cancer Res 2004;10:1685–90.

242. Buck AK, Herrmann K, Büschenfelde CM, et al. Imaging bone and soft tissue tumors with the proliferation marker [18F]fluorodeoxythymidine. Clin Cancer Res 2008;14:2970–7.

Prediction and Early Detection of Response by NMR Spectroscopy and Imaging

Seung-Cheol Lee, PhD[a],
Fernando Arias-Mendoza, MD, PhD[b], Harish Poptani, PhD[a],
E. James Delikatny, PhD[a], Mariusz Wasik, MD[c],
Michal Marzec, MD, PhD[d], Stephen J. Schuster, MD[e,f],
Sunita D. Nasta, MD[g], Jakub Svoboda, MD[h,i],
Owen A. O'Connor, MD, PhD[j], Mitchell R. Smith, MD, PhD[k],
Jerry D. Glickson, PhD[a,*]

KEYWORDS

- Phosphorus-31 magnetic resonances spectroscopy
- Hydrogen-1 magnetic resonance spectroscopy
- Lactate • Choline

The authors' laboratory was the first to demonstrate that ^{31}P NMR spectroscopy was able to detect early metabolic changes in subcutaneous tumors in mice in response to chemotherapy, radiation therapy, and hyperthermia.[1] In addition, the authors and others[2,3] showed that nuclear magnetic resonance (NMR) detectable changes during untreated growth reflected changes in tumor perfusion, energetics, and pH, which could serve as sensitive predictors of therapeutic

This work has been supported by National Institute of Health grants CA101700, CA41078 and CA118559. Animal studies were performed at the Small Animal Imaging Facility of the University of Pennsylvania, which is operated with partial support from an National Cancer Institute Small Animal Resource grant. Much of this research has been conducted by members of the Cooperative Group on 5U24CA08315-07 and as a core facility of the Abramson Comprehensive Cancer Center, which is supported by 5P30CA016520-34.

[a] Laboratory of Molecular Imaging, Department of Radiology, The University of Pennsylvania School of Medicine, B6 Blockley Hall, 423, Guardian Drive, Philadelphia, PA 19104-6069, USA
[b] Department of Radiology and Hatch Imaging Center, Columbia University College of Physicians & Surgeons, 710 West 168th Street, New York, NY 10032, USA
[c] Department of Pathology & Laboratory Medicine, The University of Pennsylvania School of Medicine, Philadelphia, 6 Founders, 3400 Spruce Street, Philadelphia, PA 19104, USA
[d] The Children's Hospital of Philadelphia, Abramson Research Building, 3516 Civic Center Boulevard, Philadelphia, PA 19104, USA
[e] Division of Hematology-Oncology, Department of Medicine, Hospital of the University of Pennsylvania, Philadelphia, PA 19104, USA
[f] Abramson Cancer Center of the University of Pennsylvania, 3400 Civic Center Boulevard, Philadelphia, PA 19104, USA
[g] Hospital of the University of Pennsylvania, 3400 Civic Center Boulevard, Philadelphia, PA 19104, USA
[h] Hospital of the University of Pennsylvania, Philadelphia, PA 19104, USA
[i] Department of Medicine, University of Pennsylvania School of Medicine, 3400 Civic Center Boulevard, Philadelphia, PA 19104
[j] Department of Hematology/Oncology, Columbia University Medical Center, 1130 Street Nicholas Avenue, ICRC 2216, New York, NY 10032, USA
[k] Lymphoma Service, Fox Chase Cancer Center, 333 Cottman Avenue, Philadelphia, Pennsylvania, 19111-2497, USA
* Corresponding author.
E-mail address: glickson@mail.med.upenn.edu

PET Clin 7 (2012) 119–126
doi:10.1016/j.cpet.2011.12.007

response. These seminal observations were subsequently translated into the clinic and led to the initiation of a National Institutes of Health supported multi-institutional program to evaluate the potential utility of ^{31}P magnetic resonance spectroscopy (MRS) for the prediction and early detection of therapeutic response. This program was initially headed by Dr Truman Brown at the Fox Chase Cancer Center and included Memorial Sloan-Kettering, Wayne State University, Duke, University of California in San Francisco (UCSF), Johns Hopkins, and The Royal Marsden and St George's Hospitals in London. Initially the study included 4 malignancies rgR exhibited approximately a 50:50 response rate—non-Hodgkin lymphoma (NHL), squamous cell carcinoma of the head and neck (HNSCC), soft tissue sarcomas (STS), and locally advanced breast cancer (LABC). Because of limited accrual, HNSCC, STS, and LABC were dropped from the study, and Wayne State, Duke, and UCSF left the study. However, the Radboud University Nijmegen Medical Center in the Netherlands joined the study. The participants call themselves Cooperative Group for NMR Spectroscopy of Cancer. While the participants in this program have continued to work together for over a decade, some have changed institutions. Dr Brown moved from Fox Chase to Columbia Presbyterian Medical Center and more recently to the Medical College of South Carolina, but a new principal investigator (PI), Dr Fernando Arias-Mendoza, has remained at Columbia. The Johns Hopkins Group under Dr Glickson moved to the University of University of Pennsylvania in 1996, and St George's group under Dr Griffiths recently transferred to Cambridge University in the United Kingdom. Despite changes of institutions among some of the participants, and the use of different commercial imaging systems (General Electric, Siemens, and Philips), a uniform protocol has been developed for acquisition and analysis of MRS data,[4] with statistical evaluation being performed at the PI institution (Columbia). Both the Columbia and University of Pennsylvania programs are participating in this report. Until now, all the ^{31}P studies were performed on 1.5 T instruments, although future plans are to continue the studies at 3 T. Because of the limited sensitivity of ^{31}P MRS, studies have been limited to large ($\geq 3 \times 3 \times 3$ cm^3) mostly superficial lesions in the axial, inginal, or head and neck lymph nodes. Data were generally analyzed from a single voxel, although data acquisition was performed by 2-dimensional chemical shift imaging followed by voxel shifting to optimally localize the tumor in one voxel (**Fig. 1**). Visualization of the tumor was achieved by T$_2$-weighted ^{1}H magnetic resonance

imaging (MRI). Recently, a number of institutions have initiated ^{1}H MRS (lactate [Lac]) or (total choline [tCho]) and MRI (diffusion-weighted imaging [DWI]), which can accommodate substantially smaller lesions (approximately 1 cm^3 for Lac and tCho and smaller for DWI).

The scope and operational procedure has evolved over about 15 years of the study. Overall, more than 200 NHL patients have participated in the 31P MRS study. The initial plan was to perform MRS measurements before and after treatment, but it soon became apparent that because the examination required that the patient be confined in the magnet for about an hour, few patients returned for the follow-up examination. Therefore, the study focused on evaluating the utility of pretreatment metabolic data for predicting complete response (CR) defined according to WHO criteria as complete disappearance of all detectable lesions and on time to treatment failure (TTF). **Fig. 1** shows the 31P NMR spectrum of a typical NHL tumor in a human patient.

Based on animal data and anecdotal clinical reports, the ratio of phosphocholine (PCh) plus phosphoethanolamine (PEth), 2 phospholipid precursors, to total nucleoside triphosphate (NTP) (ie, [PCho + PEth])/NTP also called the phosphatemonoester/NTP or PME/NTP ratio) was chosen as the biomarker for predicting therapeutic response. Initially patients with all forms of NHL treated with any therapeutic modality or combination of modalities were accepted into the study. Remarkably, despite this diversity of tumor histology and treatment method, the pretreatment PME/NTP ratio proved to be a robust predictor of response failure. When patients were stratified with respect to risk of tumor progression in accordance with the International Prognostic Index as low- (L), low-to-Intermediate (LI), high-to-intermediate (IH) and high- (H) risk and the PME/NTP values were plotted for each risk category, it was noted that simply drawing a line between the median of the L and IL PME/NTP ratios and extending this line to the HI and H risk categories segregated the PME/NTP ratios into 2 groups (**Fig. 2**).[5] With few exceptions, all the ratios above this line originated from tumors that were not destined to exhibit a CR, whereas those tumors whose PME/NTP ratios fell below this line were approximately equally distributed between patients with CRs and non-CRs (NCR). Thus with a sensitivity of 0.92 and specificity of 0.79, it was possible to predict CR or non-CR in these patients. An even better prediction has recently been achieved by defining an optimum cut-off value of PME/NTP for each tumor grade (Cooperative Group in NMR Spectroscopy of Cancer, unpublished data, 2011).

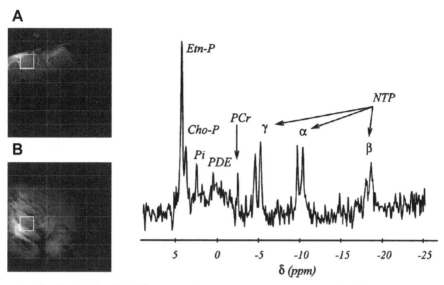

Fig. 1. Example of an in vivo localized ^{31}P magnetic resonance spectroscopy study of a non-Hodgkin lymphoma. Insets (*A*) and (*B*) show two orthogonal magnetic resonance images (axial and coronal, respectively), illustrating tumor localization, in this case the right inguinal area. The images were overlaid with the ^{31}P 3-dimensional localization chemical shift imaging (CSI) grid, a cubic matrix with 8 steps per spatial dimension with a nominal cubic voxel of 30 mm^3. The ^{31}P spectrum was sampled from the single tumor voxel projected on the images shown by a thick-lined square. The assignments are phosphoethanolamine **(Etn-P)** and phosphocholine **(Cho-P)** in the phosphomonoester region; inorganic phosphate **(Pi)**; phosphodiester region **(PDE)**; phosphocreatine **(PCr)**; and phosphates α, β, and γ of nucleotide triphosphates **(NTP)**. The chemical shift (δ) is expressed in parts per million **(ppm)** using the phosphoric acid as reference at 0 ppm (internal reference Pα of NTP at −10.01 ppm). The leftover glitch of PCr in the spectrum is minimal contamination from neighboring voxels caused by the CSI point spread function. The (Etn-P Cho-P)/NTP ratios reported throughout the article were obtained by summing the integrals of the Etn-P and Cho-P signals in the tumor spectra and dividing the result by the integral of the β−phosphate of NTP (assignments in bold). (*From* Arias-Mendoza F, Smith MR, Brown TR. Predicting treatment response in non-Hodgkin's lymphoma from the pretreatment tumor content of phosphoethanolamine plus phosphocholine. Acad Radiol 2004;11(4):370; with permission.)

However, in a more recent study of 27 patients with the most common form of NHL, diffuse large B-cell lymphoma all of whom were treated wtih RCHOP or "RCHOP-like" therapy, a similar analysis was able to predict CR or non-CR with a sensitivity of 1.0 and specificity of 0.90.

The key limitation of the ^{31}P MRS technique is its low sensitivity. To overcome this limitation, the University of Pennsylvania component of the Cooperative Group undertook preclinical ^{1}H MRS and MRI as well as ^{31}P MRS studies of human diffuse large B-cell lymphoma (DLBCL) xenografts in nude mice using the DLCL2 tumor model introduced by Mohammed and colleagues[6,7] Treatment of these xenografts with cyclophosphamide, hydroxydaunorubicin, oncovin (vincristine), prednisone or prednisolone (CHOP), rituximab (R), RCHOP, CHOP plus bryostatin (CHOPB) or radiation therapy (RTX) were evaluated using protocols similar to the clinical protocols except that the drug doses were slightly modified; the time per cycle of drug therapy was decreased from 3 weeks to 1 week because of the shorter

doubling time of the tumor in the mouse, and the RTX was administered as a single 15 Gy bolus instead of multiple 2 Gy fractions.[8–11] Tumor volume, measured with calipers, was the response end-point. Relative response followed the order RTX>CHOPB> CHOP = RCHOP>R, with R producing only a slight growth delay. The ^{1}H MRS studies indicated that decreases in steady state lactic acid (Lac) were statistically significant following 1 cycle of therapy with CHOP, CHOPB, or within 24 hours following RTX, whereas treatment with R alone had no effect on Lac but decreased total choline (tCho), which was also decreased by RCHOP, CHOPB, or RTX. CHOPB and RTX also decreased the PME/NTP ratio of the tumor, but none of the other treatments had a significant effect on metabolites detected by ^{31}P MRS. Of potentially greatest clinical significance was the observation that with respect to treatment of the DLCL2 xenograft model with CHOP or RCHOP, which are the 2 most common therapies for DLBCL patients, Lac was selectively responsive to CHOP, whereas tCho

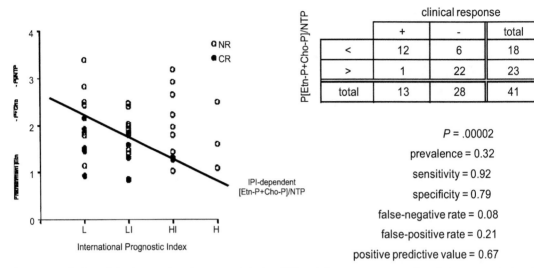

IPI-dependent [Etn-P+Cho-P]/NTP

clinical response			
P[Etn-P+Cho-P]/NTP	+	-	total
<	12	6	18
>	1	22	23
total	13	28	41

P = .00002

prevalence = 0.32

sensitivity = 0.92

specificity = 0.79

false-negative rate = 0.08

false-positive rate = 0.21

positive predictive value = 0.67

Fig. 2. Correlation of the international prognostic index (IPI) and the pretreatment phosphatemonoester/ nucleoside triphosphate per patient in the whole non-Hodgkin lymphoma cohort. The long-term response to treatment outcome of each patient was also plotted as CR, complete response (*filled circles*) and noncomplete responders (*open circles*). Tumors were stratified on the basis of the IPI as low grade (L), low-to-intermediate (LI), high-to-intermediate (HI) and high-grade (H) tumors. A line was drawn between the medians of the L and LI points and extended through the HI and H columns. This line was a useful threshold for predicting failure to exhibit a CR.

was selectively responsive to R; hence, a decrease of Lac but an increase in tCho following RCHOP therapy could indicate rituximab resistance, which could be treated in the clinic with lenalidomide or other agents that restores immunologic response of NHL tumors. This principle is demonstrated in **Fig. 3**, which shows data from a DLBCL patient who was examined on a Monday, started RCHOP therapy on Wednesday and was re-examined on Friday. His tumor exhibited a 70% decrease in Lac and a 15% increase in tCho, suggesting that this patient may have been rituximab refractive, but no confirmatory data of this were obtained. The patient went on to exhibit a CR and is still in remission several months after treatment.

Recent ^{13}C MRS studies of the DLCL2 model using the 2-compartment analysis technique of Artemov and colleagues[12] demonstrate that the decrease in steady-state lactate levels following CHOP chemotherapy resulted from a 16% decrease in glycolytic flux and a 55% increase in lactate washout rate (S.C. Lee and J.D. Glickson, unpublished data, 2011); hence, the changes in lactate levels appear to be perfusion driven and probably could be detected by dynamic contrast enhanced (DCE) MRI. Such studies are now in progress.

The University of Pennsylvania group has recently performed a pilot study of 1 chronic lymphocytic leukemia/small lymphocytic lymphoma (CLL/SLL)

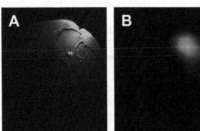

	48h before treatment	48h after treatment	Relative changes
Tumor volume	351 cm3	261 cm3	25 % ↓
Lac:H$_2$O	2.7e-4	0.8e-4	70 % ↓
tCho:H$_2$O	9.5e-4	10.9e-4	15 % ↑

Fig. 3. 63-year-old man with inguinal node diffuse large B-cell lymphoma. (*A*) T2-weighted image, echo time = 15 milliseconds, repetition time = 3000 milliseconds (*B*) Lactate image measured with Had-SelMQC- chemical shift imaging sequence.

patient who had developed resistance to R. This patient was examined by ^{1}H MRS/MRI at 5 time points in the UPCC-02408 protocol for restoring R-sensitivity with lenalidomide (**Fig. 4**A). **Fig. 4**B summarizes the NMR results. After 4 weeks of R following lenalidomide, tCho was decreasing throughout the R treatment portion of the protocol, and the tumor began to shrink after 4 cycles of R. These results are consistent with the authors' animal studies, but obviously data on more patients are required to draw definitive conclusions. The decrease in tumor volume is small, comes only late in the treatment schedule, and is preceded by decreases in tCho. The authors have also performed DWI measurements of the apparent diffusion constant (ADC) of this patient's tumor. The gradual increase in ADC after treatment with lenolidamide is consistent with restoration of R response (see **Fig. 4**B). In these preliminary studies, the authors only recorded the average ADC of the entire tumor; a detailed image multivoxel analysis of ADC values of coregistered data over the entire course of therapy is planned for the future.

It is important to note that the authors are dealing with an indolent lymphoma for which complete regression may not be anticipated. The key point is that the disease is not progressing. The authors are intrigued by the increase in tCho during the initial lenalidomide treatment. Lenalidomide may produce an inflammatory response that caused this increase. Increases in Lac might have confirmed this, but unfortunately technical problems interfered with obtaining these data. The authors plan to pursue this in future experiments.

The utility of 2 forms of MRI (DWI and T$_2$-weighted [T2WI]) was evaluated on DLCL2 xenografts treated with CHOPB.[13] These imaging methods produce tumor images showing submillimeter in-plane resolution at acquisition times on the order of 10 minutes. Bryostatin produces a more robust response of this tumor model to CHOP chemotherapy by inhibiting multidrug resistance or Bcl-2 expression.[7] A significant increase in the ADC was detected by DWI following only 1 cycle of CHOPB, whereas T2WI required 2 therapy cycles to detect a statistically significant but anomalous decrease in the average T$_2$.[13] However, the most interesting observation was that in 3of the 5 tumors examined, the changes in ADC or T$_2$ were not uniform over the entire tumor but were limited to distinct regions of the tumor. This regional response pattern could be due to various causes including heterogeneity in tumor perfusion, oxygenation, or apoptotic ability or drug resistance (which are energy- and hence perfusion-dependent). The exact mechanism producing this heterogeneity is under examination, but it is

apparent that if, for example, it proves to be related to perfusion, then there are various interventions that could be used to produce a more homogeneous and, therefore, extensive response of the tumor. Thus, image-guided therapy is a distinct possibility if not a probability for the future.

About 30% of all the new cancer drugs under development by pharmaceutical companies target signal transduction pathways. These drugs usually act by inhibiting key kinases that modify critical cell properties such as proliferation, apoptosis, angiogenesis, bioenergetics, gene expression, protein expression, and others. However, there are no noninvasive imaging method for monitoring the actual kinase inhibition in the malignant cells in patients. There is, however, a great need to monitor these processes within the individual patient. To develop such a method, the authors proceeded on the assumption that to modify vital cellular functions, signal transduction pathways had to modify cellular metabolism; cellular metabolism can be monitored by NMR and positron emission tomography (PET) methods. The goal was, therefore, to identify specific metabolic pathways that were modified when specific signaling pathways were inhibited. As proof of principle, the authors chose the mTORC1 pathway, which is selectively inhibited by rapamycin and its analogs. Treatment with 7 doses of rapamycin (10 mg/kg × 2 doses/d) of mice transplanted with the human DLCL2 lymphoma cell line produced a 90% decrease in tumor Lac detected by ^{1}H MRS (Lee S-C, Marzec M, Liu X, et al. submitted for publication). There was no significant change in tCho. Gene chip and Western blot analysis indicated an approximate 35% decrease in the expression of hexokinase-2, the key enzyme involved in regulating tumor glycolysis. A number of other glycolytic enzymes exhibited smaller decreases in expression following rapamycin treatment including phosphofructokinase (15% to 20%), enolase 1 (18%) and pyruvate kinase (5%). There was a small decrease in choline kinase and a small increase in phospholipase A$_2$. Therefore, the glycolytic pathway appears to be selectively inhibited. Similar findings were made with another human lymphoma cell line Ramos. Thus, it appears that inhibition of mTOR can be monitored selectively by ^{1}H MRS using lactate imaging methods[14–16] and probably also by fluorodeoxyglucose (18F) or 2-deoxy-2-(18F)fluoro-D-glucose (FDG) PET.

In summary, the authors have shown that pretreatment ^{31}P MRS can predict about two-thirds of the response failures among human NHL patients. These patients could be directed to more vigorous therapeutic regimens followed

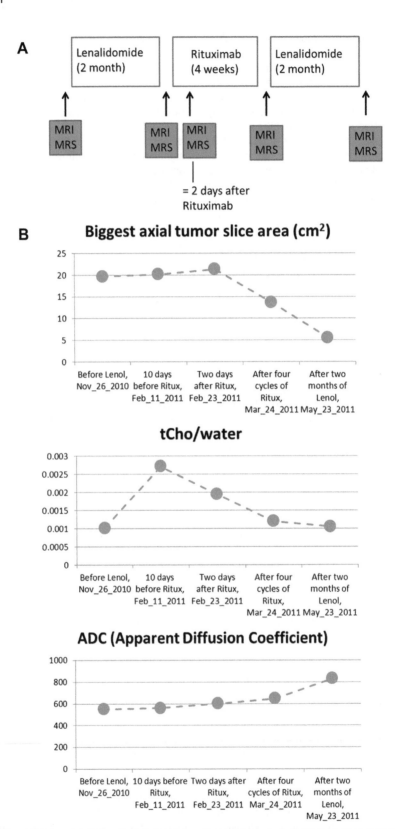

Fig. 4. (*A*) Treatment protocol and time points for magnetic resonance imaging/magnetic resonance spectroscopy studies of CLL/SLL patient. Results shown in **Fig. 3**B. (*B*) Summary of tumor size, total choline (tCho) and apparent diffusion constant (ADC) of a patient on 5 examinations.

by bone marrow transplantation or to experimental new therapeutic agents. Phosphorus-31 NMR is limited to large superficial tumors and only provides a predictor of response failure rather than successful response unless the method is applied to populations of patients with DLBCL tumors treated with RCHOP or equivalent therapy. Proton NMR data can be used to monitor much smaller tumors in any site in the human body. Proton spectroscopy has 2 response markers, lactate and choline, which can selectively detect response to CHOP chemotherapy and rituximab immunotherapy, respectively. This may provide a noninvasive method for detecting patients refractory to rituximab therapy who can be treated with thalidomide-related agents that restore rituximab response. Finally, the authors have demonstrated a general strategy for noninvasively monitoring response to inhibitors of specific signal transduction pathways by monitoring the corresponding metabolic pathway that is modified by signal transduction inhibition. The authors have demonstrated that in the case of mTOR, inhibition of this signaling pathway can be detected by inhibition of glycolysis, which can be detected by ^{1}H MRS lactate imaging or FDG PET.

ACKNOWLEDGMENTS

This work has been supported by NIH grants CA101700, CA41078CA041078 and CA118559, CA89194, CA96856. Animal studies were performed at the Small Animal Imaging Facility of the University of Pennsylvania that is operated with partial support from an NCI Small Animal Resource grant. Much of this research has been conducted by members of the Cooperative Group on 5U24CA08315-0708 and as a core facility of the Abramson Comprehensive Cancer Center that is supported by 5P30CA016520-34. Clinical studies have been performed by the NMR Spectroscopy in Cancer Cooperative Group that includes the following participants: Columbia University (Fernando Arias-Mendoza), Memorial Sloan-Kettering Cancer Center (Jason A. Koutcher, Kirsten Zakian, Amita Shukla-Dave), The Royal Marsden Hospital, London, UK (Martin O. Leach, Geoffrey S. Payne, Adam J. Schwarz, David Cunningham), CR UK Cambridge Research Institute, Cambridge, United Kingdom (John R. Griffiths, Marion Stubbs), Radboud University Nijmegen Medical Center, The Netherlands (Arend Heerschap), Medical Univesity of Charleston, SC (Truman R. Brown), The University of Pennsylvania (Harish Poptani, Seung-Cheol Lee and Jerry D. Glickson).

REFERENCES

1. Ng TC, Evanochko WT, Hiramoto RN, et al. P-31 NMR-spectroscopy of in vivo tumors. J Magn Reson 1982;49(2):271–86.
2. Evelhoch JL, Sapareto SA, Nussbaum GH, et al. Correlation between 31P NMR spectroscopy and 15O perfusion measurements in the RIF1 murine tumor in-vivo. Radiat. Res 1986;106(1):122–31.
3. Glickson JD, Wehrle JP, Rajan SS, et al. NMR spectroscopy of tumors. In: Pettegrew JW, editor. NMR in Biomedical Research. New York: Springer-Verlag; 1989. p. 253–307.
4. Arias-Mendoza F, Zakian K, Schwartz A, et al. Methodological standardization for a multi-institutional in vivo trial of localized P-31 MR spectroscopy in human cancer research. In vitro and normal volunteer studies. NMR Biomed 2004;17(6):382–91.
5. Arias-Mendoza F, Smith MR, Brown TR. Predicting treatment response in non-Hodgkin's lymphoma from the pretreatment tumor content of phosphoethanolamine plus phosphocholine. Acad Radiol 2004; 11(4):368–76.
6. Al-Katib AM, Smith MR, Kamanda WS, et al. Bryostatin 1 down-regulates mdr1 and potentiates vincristine cytotoxicity in diffuse large cell lymphoma xenografts. Clin Cancer Res 1998;4(5):1305–14.
7. Mohammad RM, Wall NR, Dutcher JA, et al. The addition of bryostatin 1 to cyclophosphamide, doxorubicin, vincristine, and prednisone (CHOP) chemotherapy improves response in a CHOP-resistant human diffuse large cell lymphoma xenograft model. Clin Cancer Res 2000;6(12):4950–6.
8. Huang MQ, Nelson DS, Pickup S, et al. In vivo monitoring response to chemotherapy of human diffuse large B-Cell lymphoma xenografts in SCID mice by H-1 and P-31 MRS. Acad Radiol 2007;14(12): 1531–9.
9. Lee SC, Huang MQ, Nelson DS, et al. In vivo MRS markers of response to CHOP chemotherapy in the WSU-DLCL2 human diffuse large B-cell lymphoma xenograft. NMR Biomed 2008;21(7): 723–33.
10. Lee SC, Delikatny EJ, Poptani H, et al. In vivo H-1 MRS of WSU-DLCL2 human non-Hodgkin's lymphoma xenografts: response to rituximab and rituximab plus CHOP. NMR Biomed 2009;22(3): 259–65.
11. Lee SC, Poptani H, Jenkins WT, et al. Early detection of radiation therapy response in non-Hodgkin's lymphoma xenografts by in vivo 1H magnetic resonance spectroscopy and imaging. NMR Biomed 2010;23(6):624–32.
12. Artemov D, Bhujwalla ZM, Pilatus U, et al. Two-compartment model for determination of glycolytic rates of solid tumors by in vivo C-13 NMR spectroscopy. NMR Biomed 1998;11(8):395–404.

13. Huang MQ, Pickup S, Nelson DS, et al. Monitoring response to chemotherapy of non-Hodgkin's lymphoma xenografts by T-2-weighted and diffusion-weighted MRI. NMR Biomed 2008;21(10): 1021–9.

14. Serrai H, Nadal-Desbarats L, Poptani H, et al. Lactate editing and lipid suppression by continuous wavelet transform analysis: application to simulated and H-1 MRS brain tumor time–domain data. Magn Reson Med 2000;43(5):649–56.

15. Pickup S, Lee SC, Mancuso A, et al. Lactate imaging with Hadamard-encoded slice-selective multiple quantum coherence chemical-shift imaging. Magn Reson Med 2008;60(2):299–305.

16. Mellon EA, Lee SC, Pickup S, et al. Detection of lactate with a hadamard slice selected, selective multiple quantum coherence, chemical shift imaging sequence (HDMD-SelMQC-CSI) on a clinical MRI scanner: application to tumors and muscle ischemia. Magn Reson Med 2009;62(6):1404–13.

Diffuse Optical Technology: A Portable and Simple Method for Noninvasive Tissue Pathophysiology

So Hyun Chung, PhD

KEYWORDS

- Diffuse optical technology • Noninvasive
- Treatment monitoring • Tissue pathophysiology
- Bed-side • Portable

In this article, noninvasive diffuse optical technologies are briefly introduced for the future application for lymphoma diagnosis/treatment monitoring. Diffuse optical technologies measure tumor physiology in deep tissues in vivo, and demonstrate efficacy for tumor detection and chemotherapy response monitoring in breast cancer.[1–8] In fact, light has been used to see tumors in thick human tissues for more than 80 years.[9] Based on the same fundamental idea that the interaction between the light and tumor provides its pathology related information, biomedical optics technology has advanced to be more quantitative and more accurate so that it can be used for tumor diagnosis and treatment monitoring.

One of the most commonly used optical imaging technologies is bright-field microscopy, which is generally employed to see histologically stained cells in a small piece of excised tissue. Although its role is invaluable in tumor diagnosis, the excised tissues lose significant amount of information that can be only preserved in embedded tissues. Diffuse optics, a relatively new technology to clinicians, provides pathophysiological changes in thick in vivo tissues noninvasively.[3–5,10–12]

Diffuse optics uses near-infrared (NIR) light and a mathematical model that describes transport of photons in a diffusion regime; photons are modeled to behave as stochastic particles that travel in proportion to a gradient, similar to diffusion of molecules (**Fig. 1**).[13] In the NIR, there is a therapeutic window (approximately from 600–1000 nm) where absorption of water and hemoglobin is lower than visual and infrared wavelength range (**Fig. 2**).[14,15] As a result, more photons survive to be detected after interacting with the tissues, making the diffuse optics suitable for deep tissue measurement.

When photons travel in thick tissues (1–2 mm), they scatter against the tissue components and dominate over absorption. The photons are scattered more often (typically after traveling approximately 20 μm) than absorbed (after approximately 10 cm) in tissues. The scattering reflects size and density of intracellular structures such as nuclei[16] and mitochondria,[17] and extracelluar matrix, such as collagen.[18] Dynamic motion of scatters, such as red blood cells, are also measured as a blood flow index using diffuse correlation spectroscopy (DCS).[14]

This work was supported by NIH R01-CA75124, R01-EB002109 and Susan G. Komen for the Cure Postdoctoral Fellowship.
Department of Physics and Astronomy, University of Pennsylvania, 209 South 33rd Street, Philadelphia, PA, USA
E-mail address: sochung@sas.upenn.edu

PET Clin 7 (2012) 127–131
doi:10.1016/j.cpet.2011.12.008

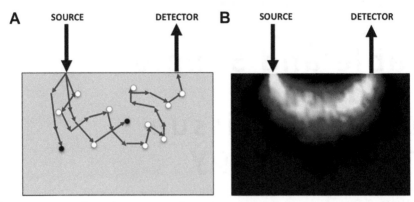

Fig. 1. (*A*) Photons come out from the source on the surface of the skin then undergo scattering and absorption while interacting with the tissues. (*B*) A simulated photon sensitivity map. The photons survived after going through multiple absorption, and scattering steps in a banana-shaped region are detected, also on the surface of the skin a few centimeters away from the source.

Most tissue components have their unique absorption profile in the NIR, and their concentration or molecular binding state can be quantified when the effect of multiscattering is cancelled using the mathematical diffusion model and modulated light either in time, frequency, or spatial domain.[19–21] The scattering in thick tissues is measured first using a photon migration model, a diffusion approximation to the radiative transfer equation, and the Mie theory (**Fig. 3**).[22,23] Then, the power–law fit scattering spectrum is subtracted from the overall light measurement, which leaves only an absorption spectrum.[6,19] Most frequently obtained physiologic information from the tissue absorption spectrum are tissue oxygenation and concentrations of oxy-, deoxy- and total hemoglobin, lipid, and water. Also, the molecular binding state of water and deep tissue temperature are measured using quantitative water absorption spectra.[5,6,19] In breast cancer clinical studies, the tumor tissues have been detected with high sensitivity (98%) and specificity (90%) by measuring total hemoglobin concentration ratio of tumor to normal tissues.[10] Optically measured tissue bound water index (BWI) showed a high correlation (R = −0.96, $P = .002$) with histopathologically assessed tumor grades.[5] Diffuse optical spectroscopy (DOS) can also predict pathologic response to neoadjuvant chemotherapy (NAC) in a few days, even on day 1 into the therapy by measuring tissue physiologic changes noninvasively.[24,25] A recent publication also suggested that the combination of DOS measured deep tissue temperature and tissue oxygenation may provide apoptotic status of cells during neoadjuvant chemotherapy.[11] The DOS measured spectra can be mapped into a 2-dimensional spectroscopic image as shown in **Fig. 4**, and this method was called diffuse optical spectroscopic imaging (DOSI) by the Tromberg group at the Univeristy of California, Irvine.[13]

For lymphoma measurement, a hand-held probe with optical fibers coupled to a source and detector can be placed on the lesion area directly. With a hand-held probe, DOS/DCS can detect photons reflected back after traveling a tissue volume at depths up to several centimeters. Thus, with this set-up, DOS/DCS can only measure palpable lymphoma. However, the instrument can be brought into the examination room and does not require special shielding. Furthermore, it is capable of providing tumor pathophysiology in real time so that the physician can use the information during the patient's visit. DOS/DCS is also harmless (no risk of ionizing radiation) and does not need injection of any contrast agents or radioactive material. Instead, it can quantify endogenous biochemical composition, which can consequently provide the pathologic state of the

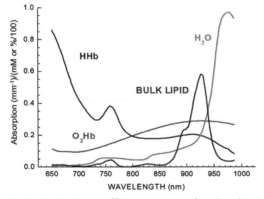

Fig. 2. Extinction coefficient spectra of major tissue chromophores measured in the near infrared.

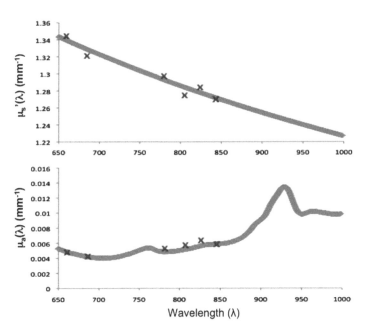

Fig. 3. Reduced scattering $\mu_s'(\lambda)$ (*top*) and absorption $\mu_a(\lambda)$ (*bottom*) coefficients spectra from in vivo human tissues. The reduced scattering spectra is fit to a power law according to the Mie theory then subtracted from a reflectance spectrum to obtain the absorption spectrum shown below.

tumor. For example, the diffuse optics measured hemoglobin concentration and blood flow can communicate vascular structure changes that occur in response to chemotherapy or molecularly targeted therapy.[24,26,27] Alteration of tissue structural composition during the therapy can be monitored by measuring lipid concentration variations using DOS.[1] Water concentration variation may reflect edema, inflammation, or interstitial fluid pressure changes.[5,28] Tissue water binding state measurement can communicate the invasiveness of the tumor that may appear as an overall extracellular composition change that also alters the association of macromolecules with water.[5,29] Noninvasive tissue temperature measurement provides enthalpy variation in the tumor due to mitochondrial changes, such as uncoupling of their membranes as a part of apoptotic process.[11]

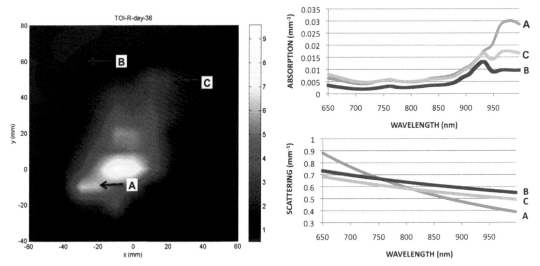

Fig. 4. An example of a diffuse optical spectroscopic imaging (DOSI) image (*left*). TOI stands for tissue optical index, which is a combined optical index of multiplication of deoxy-hemoglobin and water divided by lipid concentrations. The shown image is a spectroscopic map of 50 × 55 mm diameter infiltrating ducal carcinoma tumor in a 43-year-old subject. (*Right*) Near infrared absorption and reduced scattering spectra obtained by DOSI shown for specific regions of the image.

Additionally, tissue oxygen measurement communicates if the tumor is under hypoxia, which may predict bad prognosis.[30] Lastly, antibodies, drugs, or biologic agents tagged with a US Food and Drug Administration (FDA)-approved NIR dye (such as indocyanine green) could be injected into the body to be measured with diffuse optical technologies to study certain signal pathways in tissues in vivo.

Ongoing clinical studies using diffuse optical technologies include differentiating various types of non-Hodgkin lymphoma (diffuse large B-cell lymphoma, mantle cell lymphoma, follicular lymphoma, and chronic lymphocytic leukemia/small lymphocytic lymphoma) and monitoring tumor response during chemotherapy/molecularly targeted therapy. During the author's clinical studies using diffuse optical technologies, patients volunteered cheerfully due to its noninvasiveness and simplicity. Although the diffuse optical technologies have just begun to be used for lymphoma measurement, they hold a great potential for providing tumor pathophysiological information conveniently in the examination room, which might help physicians to optimize the therapy for each patient during the visit.

REFERENCES

1. Cerussi AE, Shah N, Hsiang D, et al. In vivo absorption, scattering, and physiologic properties of 58 malignant breast tumors determined by broadband diffuse optical spectroscopy. J Biomed Opt 2006; 11(4):044005.
2. Chance B, Nioka S, Zhang J, et al. Breast cancer detection based on incremental biochemical and physiological properties of breast cancers: a six-year, two-site study. Acad Radiol 2005;12:925–33.
3. Chung SH, Cerussi A, Mehta R, et al. Noninvasive detection and monitoring of tumor pathological grade during neoadjuvant chemotherapy by measuring tissue water state using diffuse optical spectroscopic imaging. Cancer Res 2009;69(2):101S.
4. Chung SH, Cerussi AE, Hsiang D, et al. Non-invasive measurement of pathological heterogeneity of cancer tissues using water state information from diffuse optical spectroscopic imaging. Cancer Res 2009;69(24):767S.
5. Chung SH, Cerussi AE, Klifa C, et al. In vivo water state measurements in breast cancer using broadband diffuse optical spectroscopy. Phys Med Biol 2008;53(23):6713–27.
6. Chung SH, Cerussi AE, Merritt SI, et al. Noninvasive tissue temperature measurements based on quantitative diffuse optical spectroscopy (DOS) of water. Phys Med Biol 2010;55(13):3753–65.
7. Pogue BW, Jiang S, Dehghani H, et al. Characterization of hemoglobin, water, and NIR scattering in breast tissue: analysis of intersubject variability and menstrual cycle changes. J Biomed Opt 2004;9: 541–52.
8. Spinelli L, Torricelli A, Pifferi A, et al. Bulk optical properties and tissue components in the female breast from multiwavelength time-resolved optical mammography. J Biomed Opt 2004;9:1137–42.
9. Cutler M. Transillumination of the breast. Surg Gynecol Obstet 1929;48:721–7.
10. Choe R, Konecky SD, Corlu A, et al. Differentiation of benign and malignant breast tumors by in-vivo three-dimensional parallel-plate diffuse optical tomography. J Biomed Opt 2009;14(2):024020.
11. Chung SH, Mehta R, Tromberg BJ, et al. Noninvasive measurement of deep tissue temperature changes caused by apoptosis during breast cancer neoadjuvant therapy: a case study. J Innov Opt Health Sci 2011;4(4):361–72.
12. Tromberg BJ, Pogue BW, Paulsen KD, et al. Assessing the future of diffuse optical imaging technologies for breast cancer management. Med Phys 2008; 35(6):2443–51.
13. Tromberg BJ, Cerussi AE, Chung SH, et al. Broadband diffuse optical spectroscopic imaging. In: Boas DA, Pitris C, Ramanujam N, editors. Handbook of biomedical optics. CRC Press; 2011.
14. Durduran T, Choe R, Baker WB, et al. Diffuse optics for tissue monitoring and tomography. Rep Progr Phys 2010;73(7):1–43.
15. Jöbis-vander VF. Discovery of the near-infrared window into the body andthe early development of near-infrared spectroscopy. J Biomed Opt 1999;4: 392–6.
16. Mourant JR, Canpolat M, Brocker C, et al. Light scattering from cells: the contribution of the nucleus and the effects of proliferative status. J Biomed Opt 2000;5:131–7.
17. Beauvoit B, Chance B. Time-resolved spectroscopy of mitochondria, cells and tissues under normal and pathological conditions. Mol Cell Biochem 1998; 184:445–55.
18. Weingarten MS, Papazoglou ES, Zubkov L, et al. Correlation of near infrared absorption and diffuse reflectance spectroscopy scattering with tissue neovascularization and collagen concentration in a diabetic rat wound healing model. Wound Repair Regen 2008;16:234–42.
19. Bevilacqua F, Berger AJ, Cerussi AE, et al. Broadband absorption spectroscopy in turbid media by combined frequency-domain and steady-state methods. Appl Opt 2000;39(34):6498–507.
20. Cuccia DJ, Bevilacqua F, Durkin AJ, et al. Quantitation and mapping of tissue optical properties using modulated imaging. J Biomed Opt 2009;14(2): 024012.

21. Sevick EM, Change B, Leigh J, et al. Quantitation of time-resolved and frequency-resolved optical spectra for the determination of tissue oxygenation. Anal Biochem 1991;195:330–51.

22. Haskell RC, Svaasand LO, Tsay TT, et al. Boundary conditions for the diffusion equation in radiative transfer. J Opt Soc Am A Opt Image Sci Vis 1994; 11:2727–41.

23. Nilsson AM, Sturesson KC, Liu DL, et al. Changes in spectral shape of tissue optical properties in conjunction with laser-induced thermotherapy. Appl Opt 1998;37:1256–67.

24. Cerussi A, Hsiang D, Shah N, et al. Predicting response to breast cancer neoadjuvant chemotherapy using diffuse optical spectroscopy. Proc Natl Acad Sci U S A 2007;104(10):4014–9.

25. Roblyer D, Ueda S, Cerussi A, et al. Optical imaging of breast cancer oxyhemoglobin flare correlates with neoadjuvant chemotherapy response one day after starting treatment. Proc Natl Acad Sci U S A 2011; 108(35):14626–31.

26. Tromberg BJ, Cerussi A, Shah N, et al. Imaging in breast cancer: diffuse optics in breast cancer: detecting tumors in pre-menopausal women and monitoring neoadjuvant chemotherapy. Breast Cancer Res 2005;7:279–85.

27. Zhou C, Choe R, Shah N, et al. Diffuse optical monitoring of blood flow and oxygenation in human breast cancer during early stages of neoadjuvant chemotherapy. J Biomed Opt 2007;12(5):051903.

28. Tromberg BJ, Cerussi AE. Imaging Breast Cancer Chemotherapy Responses with Light, Commentary on Soliman et al., p. 2605. Clin Cancer Res 2010; 16:2486–8.

29. Toole BP. Hyaluronan: from extracellular glue to pericellular cue. Nat Rev Cancer 2004;4(7):528–39.

30. Schindl M, Schoppmann SF, Samonigg H, et al; Austrian Breast and Colorectal Cancer Study Group. Overexpression of hypoxia-induced factor 1α is associated with an unfavorable prognosis in lymph node-positive breast cancer. Clin Cancer Res 2002;8:1831–7.

Index

Note: Page numbers of article titles are in **boldface** type.

A

Abdomen, structural imaging for, 10–11
Aggressive lymphoma, 36–37, 92–93
[^{18}F]AH111585 (fluciclatide/GE 135), 103
Amino acid metabolism, radiotracers for, 106–108
Angiogenesis, radiotracers for, 99–103
Ann Arbor staging system, 1, 22, 35–36
Annexins, in apoptosis, 103–106
Apoptosis, radiotracers for, 103–106
ApoSense, 105–106
Autologous hematopoietic stem cell transplantation, 28–29, 61–62

B

BCL2 proteins, in apoptosis, 103–106
BEACOPP (bleomycin, etoposide, adriamycin, cyclophosphamide, vincristine, procarbazine, prednisone) regimen, 60–61
Biologic therapy, 42
Bone marrow
    biopsy of, 40
        for staging, 22–24
        in pediatric patients, 52–53
    PET and PET/CT evaluation of, 40, 52–53
    structural imaging for, 11–12
Bortezomib, 104
Brain, structural imaging for, 7–8

C

Cancer, hallmarks of, 83
Cancer and Leukemia Group B study, 60–61
Caspases, in apoptosis, 105–106
Central nervous system, structural imaging for, 7–8
Chemotherapy, for lymphoma
    diffuse large B-cell, 57–60
    mantle cell, 63
    radiation therapy after, **67–72**
    radiotracers as, 108
    response to
        assessment of, 40–41, 78–80
        for radiation therapy planning, 67–71
        MR imaging for, 15
        NMR spectroscopy for, 121–123
        PET and PET/CT for, 25–26, 49–51
    salvage, 28–29, 37, 87
Chest, structural imaging for, 8–9
Chest radiography, 38

Colon

    lesions of, in pediatric patients, 54
    structural imaging for, 10–11
Color Doppler evaluation, for lymphoma, 7
Compound ultrasonography, for lymphoma, 15–16
Contrast-enhanced ultrasonography, for lymphoma, 15–16
Copper(II) complex (Cu-ATSM), 96–98
CORAL study group, 59–60
Costs, PET and, 26–27
CT, for lymphoma, 4–5. *See also* PET and PET/CT.
    advanced techniques for, 12–14
    for staging, 22–23, 38
    in various body systems, 7–12
Cu-ATSM (^{64}Cu-labeled acetyl derivative of pyruvaldehyde bis [N-ethylthiosemicarbazonato] copper(II) complex), 96–98

D

dBiopsy, lymph node, 37
3'-Deoxy-3'- [^{18}F]-fluorothymidine (FLT). *See* Proliferation, radiotracers for (FLT).
1-(2'-Deoxy-2'-fluoro-β-D-arabinofuranosyl)thymine (FMAU), 85–86
Diagnosis, PET and PET/CT for, 37
Diffuse large B-cell lymphoma, treatment of, 57–60
Diffuse optical technology, for lymphoma, **127–131**
Diffuse-weighted MR imaging, for lymphoma, 14–15
Doppler evaluation, for lymphoma, 7
Dual-energy CT, for lymphoma, 12–14
Dynamic contrast-enhanced MR imaging, for lymphoma, 14–15

E

Economic issues, PET and, 26–27
European Organisation for the Research and Treatment of Cancer, 61
European Society of Medical Oncology guidelines, for follow-up, 42
Event-free survival, prediction of, 25

F

FAZA ([^{18}F]Fluoroazomycinarabinoside), 96–98
FDG- PET and FDG-PET/CT, for lymphoma, **21–33**
    clinical applications of, **47–56**
    disadvantages of, 40

PET Clin 7 (2012) 133–137
doi:10.1016/S1556-8598(12)00014-4
1556-8598/12/$ – see front matter © 2012 Elsevier Inc. All rights reserved.

FDC- PET (*continued*)
    for follow-up, 28, 41–42
    for staging, 22–24, 38–42
    for treatment response assessment, 24–27
    for treatment response prediction, 28–29
    in pediatric patients, **47–56**
    versus MR imaging, 73–74
    with personalized therapy, **57–65**
    with radiation therapy, **67–72**
FET (*O*-(2- [^{18}F]-Fluoroethyl)-L-tyrosine), 106
Flare phenomenon, 87
FLT (3'-Deoxy-3'- [^{18}F]-fluorothymidine (FLT)).
    See Proliferation, radiotracers for (FLT).
Fluciclatide/GE 135 ([^{18}F]AH111585), 103
[^{18}F]Fluoro-α-methyltyrosine (FMT), 105–106
[^{18}F]Fluoroazomycinarabinoside (FMISO), 96–98
[^{18}F]-Fluorodeoxyglucose. *See* FDG- PET and
    FDG-PET/CT.
O-(2- [^{18}F]-Fluoroethyl)-L-tyrosine), 106
[^{18}F]Fluoromisonidazole (FMISO), 96–98
2-(5-Fluoropentyl)-2-methylmalonic acid
    ([^{18}F]-ML-10), 105–106
FMAU (1-(2'-Deoxy-2'-fluoro-β-D-arabinofuranosyl)
    thymine), 85–86
FMISO ([^{18}F]Fluoromisonidazole), 96–98
[^{18}F]-ML-10 (2-(5-fluoropentyl)-2-methylmalonic
    acid), 105–106
FMT ([^{18}F]fluoro-α-methyltyrosine), 105–106
Follicular lymphoma, treatment of, 62–63
Follicular Lymphoma International Prognostic
    Index, 36

G

[^{18}F]Galacto-arginine-glycine-aspartate sequence,
    99–103
Gallamini Criteria, 62
Gallium-67 scans, for lymphoma
    in pediatric patients, 49
    in staging, 38
Gastrointestinal lesions
    in pediatric patients, 54
    structural imaging for, 10–11
German Hodgkin Study Group, 60

H

Head and neck, structural imaging for, 8
Highly aggressive lymphoma, 36–37
HIV/AIDS, PET results in, 40
Hodgkin lymphoma
    CT for, 4–5, 7–12
    diffuse optical technology for, **127–131**
    distribution patterns of, 1
    growth of, 1
    hallmarks of, 83
    MR imaging for, 5–7

    advanced techniques for, 14–15
    in various body systems, 7–12
    whole-body diffusion-weighted, **73–82**
    NMR spectroscopy for, **119–126**
    PET and PET/CT for, **21–33**
        for management, **35–46**
        for personalized therapy, 60–62
        in pediatric patients, **47–56**
        radiotracers for, **83–117**
        with radiation therapy, **67–72**
    response assessment in, 1
    staging of, systems for, 1, 3
    structural imaging for, **1–19**
    ultrasonography for. *See* Ultrasonography.
Hypoxia, radiotracers for, 95–99
Hypoxia-inducible factor α, in angiogenesis, 99–103

I

Immunotherapy, for diffuse large B-cell lymphoma,
    57–60
Indolent lymphoma, 36–37, 92–93
Infections, with lymphoma, 54
Inflammation, 54, 88
Intergruppo Italiano Linfomi, 61
International Harmonization Project, 39–40, 58, 62
International Prognostic Index, 36
International Prognostic Score, 36
International Working Group
    follow-up guidelines of, 42
    Revised response criteria of, 1, 4
Iron oxide-enhanced MR imaging, for lymphoma,
    14–15

K

Ki-67, in lymphoma, 84, 89
Kidney, structural imaging for, 11

L

Liver, structural imaging for, 10
London Criteria, 62
Lung lesions, in pediatric patients, 54
Lymph nodes
    biopsy of, 37
    PET/CT evaluation of, in pediatric patients, 51–52
Lymphography, 38
Lymphoid hyperplasia, reactive, FLT uptake in, 88–89
Lymphoma
    classification of, 35, 92–93
    CT for, 4–5
        advanced techniques for, 12–14
        in various body systems, 7–12
    diffuse optical technology for, **127–131**
    hallmarks of, 83
    incidence of, 35

infections and inflammation with, 54
MR imaging for, 5–7, **73–82**
   advanced techniques for, 14–15
   in various body systems, 7–12
NMR spectroscopy for, **119–126**
overview of, 35–37
PET and PET/CT for, **21–33**
   for management, **35–46**
   for personalized therapy, **57–65**
   in pediatric patients, 2, **47–56**
   radiotracers for, **83–117.** See also specific
      tracers, eg FDG-PET and FDG-PET/CT.
   with radiation therapy, **67–72**
staging of. See Staging.
structural imaging for, **1–19**
ultrasonography for. See Ultrasonography.

M

Magnetic resonance imaging. See MR imaging.
Magnetic resonance spectroscopy, nuclear, **119–126**
Mantle cell lymphoma, treatment of, 63
Matrix metalloproteinases, in angiogenesis, 99–103
Mediastinum, structural imaging for, 8–9
[^{11}C]-Methionine, 106–108
MR imaging, for lymphoma, 5–7, 42, **73–82**
   challenges with, 76–77
   development of, 75–76
   for staging, 38, 77–78
   for treatment response assessment, 78–80
   in various body systems, 7–12
   principles of, 74–75
   versus FDG-PET/CT, 73–74
   whole-body diffusion-weighted, **73–82**
MR imaging spectroscopy, for lymphoma, 14–15
Murphy description of St Jude staging system, 1
Musculoskeletal system, structural imaging for,
   11–12

N

National Cancer Center Network guidelines, for
   follow-up, 41–42
Natural history, 36–37
Neck, structural imaging for, 8
NMR spectroscopy, for lymphoma, **119–126**
Non-Hodgkin lymphoma
   CT for, 4–5, 7–12
   diffuse optical technology for, **127–131**
   distribution patterns of, 1
   growth of, 1
   hallmarks of, 83
   MR imaging for, 5–7
      advanced techniques for, 14–15
      in various body systems, 7–12
      whole-body diffusion-weighted, **73–82**

NMR spectroscopy for, **119–126**
PET and PET/CT for, **21–33**
   for management, **35–46**
   for personalized therapy, **57–65**
   in pediatric patients, 2, **47–56**
   radiotracers for, **83–117**
   with radiation therapy, **67–72**
response assessment in, 1
staging of, systems for, 1, 3
structural imaging for, **1–19**
ultrasonography for. See Ultrasonography.
Nuclear magnetic resonance spectroscopy,
   119–126

O

Observational treatment, 37
Optical technology, diffuse, for lymphoma, **127–131**

P

Pediatric patients, lymphoma in, **47–56**
   extranodal lesion evaluation in, 51–54
   nodal evaluation in, 51–52
   staging of, 2, 47–49
   treatment assessment for, 49–51
Pelvis, structural imaging for, 10–11
Peripheral nervous system, structural imaging for,
   7–8
PET and PET/CT, for lymphoma, **35–46**
   diagnostic, 37
   for personalized therapy, **57–65**
   for response assessment, **21–33**
   for staging, **21–33,** 37–40
   history of, 21–22
   in bone marrow, 40
   in pediatric patients, 2, **47–56**
   novel radiotracers for, **83–117**
   radiotracers for, **83–117.** See also specific tracers,
      eg FDG-PET and FDG-PET/CT.
   with radiation therapy. See Radiation therapy.
Primary Rituximab and Maintenance (PRIMA) study
   group, 62–63
Prognosis, for lymphoma, 36, 58–59
Proliferation, radiotracers for (FLT), 83–94
   applications of, 92–94
   biodistribution of, 86
   factors influencing uptake of, 86–88
   histology and, 89–90
   in reactive lymphoid hyperplasia, 88–89
   in treatment response assessment, 90–92
   mechanism of uptake of, 85–86
   relevance of, 84–85
   reproducibility of, 86
   sensitivity of, 88
   specificity of, 88

Proliferation (*continued*)
    timing of, 86
    versus inflammation, 88
Proliferative index, FLT and, 89–90

R

Radiation therapy, PET and PET/CT with, 59–60,
    67–72
    after chemotherapy, 61
    interference with, 71
    omitting consolidative radiation and, 67–68
    planning for, 68–71
    radiotracers for, 92
Radioimmunotherapy, 37
Radiotracers, **83–117**. *See also specific tracers,*
    eg FDG-PET and FDG-PET/CT.
    for amino acid metabolism, 106–108
    for angiogenesis, 99–103
    for apoptosis, 103–106
    for hypoxia, 95–99
    for proliferation, 83–94
    therapeutic drugs as, 108
RAPID trial, 61
R-CHOP regimen, 58–59
Reactive lymphoid hyperplasia, FLT uptake in, 88–89
Relapsed disease
    criteria for, 3
    monitoring for, 41–42
    treatment of
        monitoring of, 41, 59–60
        options for, 37
Remission, criteria for, 3
Residual disease, PET and PET/CT for, 25–27, 41, 68
Retroperitoneal disease, structural imaging for, 10–11
Revised International Working Group response
    criteria, 1.4
Revised Response Criteria for Malignant Melanoma,
    23–24
Rituximab, 62–63

S

St Jude staging system, 1
Salvage pathway, in proliferation, 87
Salvage therapy, 28–29, 37
Skeletal system, structural imaging for, 11–12
Small intestinal lesions
    in pediatric patients, 54
    structural imaging for, 10–11
Spectroscopy, NMR, **119–126**
Spinal cord, structural imaging for, 7–8
Splenic lesions
    in pediatric patients, 53
    structural imaging for, 10

Staging
    MR imaging for, 77–78
    PET and PET/CT for, 37–40
        in pediatric patients, 47–49
        initial, 22–24
        radiotracers for, 92
    systems for, 1, 35–37
Stem cell transplantation, 28–29, 61–62
Structural imaging, for lymphoma, **1–19**
Superparamagnetic iron oxide-enhanced MR
    imaging, for lymphoma, 14–15

T

Testis, structural imaging for, 11
Thoracic disease, structural imaging for, 8–9
Thymidine, in FLT uptake, 87–88
[^{11}C]-Thymidine, 106–108
Thymus, lesions of, in pediatric patients, 53
Tissue harmonic ultrasonography, for lymphoma,
    15–16
TK-1, in lymphoma, 89–90
Tracers. *See* Radiotracers.
Treatment. *See also* Chemotherapy; Radiation
    therapy.
    diffuse large B-cell lymphoma, 57–60
    future directions in, 42
    omitting radiation in, 67–68
    personalized, **57–65**
    salvage, 28–29, 37
    versus classification, 37
Treatment response
    assessment of
        MR imaging for, 15, 78–80
        NMR spectroscopy for, **119–126**
        PET and PET/CT for, 1, 24–27
            after relapse, 40–41
            end of therapy, 49–51
            FLT for, 90–92
            follow-up for, 28, 41–42
            for radiation therapy planning, 67–71
            in diffuse large B-cell lymphoma, 57–60
            in pediatric patients, 49–51
            interim, 49
            radiotracers for, 93–94
            surveillance, 51
    prediction of, 28–29

U

Ultrasmall superparamagnetic iron oxide-enhanced
    MR imaging, for lymphoma, 14–15
Ultrasonography, for lymphoma, 7
    advanced techniques for, 15–16
    in staging, 38
    in various body systems, 7–12

V

Vascular endothelial growth factor, in angiogenesis, 99–103

W

Whole-body diffusion-weighted MR imaging, **73–82**
  challenges with, 76–77

description of, 74
development of, 75–76
for staging, 77–78
for treatment response assessment, 78–80
principles of, 74–75
versus FDG-PET/CT, 73–74
"Will Rogers phenomenon," in staging, 23

Moving?

Make sure your subscription moves with you!

To notify us of your new address, find your **Clinics Account Number** (located on your mailing label above your name), and contact customer service at:

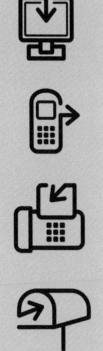

Email: journalscustomerservice-usa@elsevier.com

800-654-2452 (subscribers in the U.S. & Canada)
314-447-8871 (subscribers outside of the U.S. & Canada)

Fax number: 314-447-8029

Elsevier Health Sciences Division
Subscription Customer Service
3251 Riverport Lane
Maryland Heights, MO 63043

*To ensure uninterrupted delivery of your subscription, please notify us at least 4 weeks in advance of move.

ELSEVIER

Printed and bound by CPI Group (UK) Ltd, Croydon, CR0 4YY

03/10/2024

01040356-0004